Positron Emission Tomography

Edited by

Malik E. Juweid

Department of Radiology, University of Iowa, Iowa City, IA, USA

Otto S. Hoekstra

*Department of Nuclear Medicine & PET Research, VU University Medical Centre,
Amsterdam, The Netherlands*

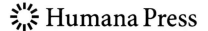

Humana Press

Editors
Malik E. Juweid, MD
Department of Radiology
and the Holden Comprehensive
Cancer Center, University of Iowa
Iowa City, IA, USA
malik-juweid@uiowa.edu

Otto S. Hoekstra, MD
Department of Nuclear Medicine & PET
Research, VU University Medical Centre
Amsterdam, The Netherlands
os.hoekstra@vumc.nl

ISSN 1064-3745   e-ISSN 1940-6029
ISBN 978-1-61779-061-4   e-ISBN 978-1-61779-062-1
DOI 10.1007/978-1-61779-062-1
Springer New York Dordrecht Heidelberg London

Library of Congress Control Number: 2011921313

Printed on acid-free paper

Humana Press is part of Springer Science+Business Media (www.springer.com)

Preface

Oncological imaging has thoroughly changed in the past decade, especially due to the introduction of PET and ^{18}FDG. For the first time, technology was challenged to provide evidence of (cost-) effectiveness, and this demand has resulted in many excellent trials. Meanwhile, PET-CT was introduced, and this made the PET technology even more appealing for those who were still getting used to the anatomy-deprived PET images. At the same time, oncological patient care evolved toward a truly multidisciplinary effort, combining the expertise of oncologists, surgeons, radiotherapists, radiologists, nuclear medicine physicians, and pathologists.

The current challenge is to use common language and develop skills at the boundaries of each other's area of expertise. There is more to that than providing accurate scan reports accurately describing the findings of the technology at hand. The communicative competences need to be improved: to communicate scan findings so that the referring specialist receives proper advice from the imager, and that, alternatively, the referring one provides the imager with appropriate clinical details to allow for a proper interpretation, and that the referring specialist is aware of possibilities and limitations of the requested technology. With PET-CT, the first challenge is to properly combine the expertises of nuclear medicine and radiology.

This book aims to help and bridge some of the knowledge gaps in several oncological domains. Chapters are typically written by a referring specialist and an imager so that either discipline can benefit. The focus is clearly on applications with FDG PET, but, where appropriate, other radiopharmaceuticals are covered as well.

Iowa City, IA
Amsterdam, The Netherlands

Malik E. Juweid
Otto S. Hoekstra

Contents

Contributors

ABASS ALAVI • *Division of Nuclear Medicine, Hospital of the University of Pennsylvania, University of Pennsylvania School of Medicine, Philadelphia, PA, USA*

MARTIN S. ALLEN-AUERBACH • *Ahmanson Biological Imaging Division, Department of Molecular and Medical Pharmacology, David Geffen School of Medicine at the University of California Los Angeles, Los Angeles, CA, USA*

NORBERT AVRIL • *Department of Nuclear Medicine, Barts and The London School of Medicine, Queen Mary, University of London, London, UK*

ESTHER BASTIAANNET • *Department of Surgical Oncology, University Medical Centre, Groningen, The Netherlands*

SANDIP BASU • *Division of Nuclear Medicine, Hospital of the University of Pennsylvania, University of Pennsylvania School of Medicine, Philadelphia, PA, USA; Radiation Medicine Centre (BARC), Tata Memorial Hospital Annexe, Parel, Mumbai, India*

ALEXANDER BECHERER • *LKH Feldkirch, Abteilung für Nuklearmedizin, Feldkirch, Austria*

AMBROS J. BEER • *Nuklearmedizinische Klinik und Poliklinik, Technische Universität München, München, Germany*

MATTHIAS R. BENZ • *Ahmanson Biological Imaging Division, Department of Molecular and Medical Pharmacology, David Geffen School of Medicine at the University of California Los Angeles, Los Angeles, CA, USA*

RONALD BOELLAARD • *Department of Nuclear Medicine & PET Research, VU University Medical Centre, Amsterdam, The Netherlands*

ANDREAS K. BUCK • *Nuklearmedizinische Klinik und Poliklinik, Technische Universität München, München, Germany*

SARAH CEYSSENS • *Department of Nuclear Medicine, Antwerp University Hospital, Edegem, Belgium*

JOHANNES CZERNIN • *Ahmanson Biological Imaging Division, Department of Molecular and Medical Pharmacology, David Geffen School of Medicine at the University of California Los Angeles, Los Angeles, CA, USA*

DIRK DE RUYSSCHER • *Department of Radiotherapy (Maastro Clinic), GROW Research Institute, Maastricht University Medical Center, Maastricht, The Netherlands*

DOMINIQUE DELBEKE • *Department of Radiology and Radiological Sciences, Vanderbilt University Medical Center, Nashville, TN, USA*

FLORIAN ECKEL • *Nuklearmedizinische Klinik und Poliklinik, Technische Universität München, München, Germany*

SERGE GOLDMAN • *PET-Biomedical Cyclotron Unit, ERASME Hospital, Université Libre de Bruxelles, Brussels, Belgium*

SOFIA GOURTSOYIANNI • *Centre for Cancer Imaging, University Hospital of Heraklion, Medical School of Crete, Crete, Greece*

MICHAEL M. GRAHAM • *Division of Nuclear Medicine, Department of Radiology, Carver College of Medicine, University of Iowa, Iowa City, IA, USA*

KEN HERRMANN • *Department of Nuclear Medicine, Klinikum rechts der Isar, Technische Universität München, München, Germany*

HARALD J. HOEKSTRA • *Department of Surgical Oncology, University Medical Centre, Groningen, The Netherlands*

OTTO S. HOEKSTRA • *Department of Nuclear Medicine & PET Research, VU University Medical Centre, Amsterdam, The Netherlands*

HOSSEIN JADVAR • *Department of Radiology, Keck School of Medicine, University of Southern California, Los Angeles, CA, USA*

MALIK E. JUWEID • *Department of Radiology and the Holden Comprehensive Cancer Center, University of Iowa, Iowa City, IA, USA*

WOLFRAM KARGES • *Department of Endocrinology, University Hospital Aachen, Aachen, Germany*

BERND J. KRAUSE • *Department of Nuclear Medicine, Klinikum rechts der Isar, Technische Universität München, München, Germany*

THOMAS C. KWEE • *Department of Radiology, University Medical Center Utrecht, Utrecht, The Netherlands*

WILLIAM H. MARTIN • *Vanderbilt University Medical Center, Nashville, TN, USA*

YUSUF MENDA • *Division of Nuclear Medicine, Department of Radiology, Carver College of Medicine, University of Iowa, Iowa City, IA, USA*

FELIX M. MOTTAGHY • *Department of Nuclear Medicine, University Hospital Leuven, Leuven, Belgium*

BENOIT J.M. PIROTTE • *Department of Neurosurgery, ERASME Hospital, Université Libre de Bruxelles, Brussels, Belgium*

RODNEY REZNEK • *Centre for Cancer Imaging, Chelsea and Westminster Hospital, London, UK*

JOSHUA ROSENBAUM • *Division of Nuclear Medicine, Hospital of the University of Pennsylvania, University of Pennsylvania School of Medicine, Philadelphia, PA, USA*

HANS C. STEINERT • *Division of Nuclear Medicine, University Hospital of Zürich, Zürich, Switzerland*

SIGRID STROOBANTS • *Department of Nuclear Medicine, Antwerp University Hospital, Edegem, Belgium*

MUAMMER URHAN • *Department of Nuclear Medicine, GATA Haydarpasa Training Hospital, Istanbul, Turkey*

SOFIE VAN BINNEBEEK • *Department of Nuclear Medicine, University Hospital Leuven, Leuven, Belgium*

HINRICH A. WIEDER • *Department of Radiology, Klinikum rechts der Isar, Technische Universität München, München, Germany*

Chapter 1

FDG-PET/CT in Lymphoma

Malik E. Juweid

Abstract

Molecular Imaging has played a prominent role in the assessment of lymphoma for now almost three decades since the introduction of ^{67}Ga-citrate imaging for staging and restaging of both Hodgkin's and non-Hodgkin's lymphoma (HL and NHL). Since then other molecular probes have been investigated for more accurate pre- and posttreatment assessment of lymphomas but none of these probes was widely accepted and utilized until the emergence of ^{18}F-fluorodeoxyglucose positron emission tomography (FDG-PET). FDG-PET or FDG-PET/CT, which combines FDG-PET with CT scanning, is now widely utilized for response assessment of lymphoma after completion of therapy, for pretreatment staging, and, increasingly, also for assessment of response during therapy (therapy monitoring). Particularly for response assessment at therapy conclusion, FDG-PET has been shown to be considerably more accurate than CT or conventional MRI because of its ability to distinguish between viable tumor and necrosis or fibrosis in posttherapy residual mass (es) that are frequently present in patients with lymphoma without any other clinical or biochemical evidence of disease. FDG-PET/CT is therefore the noninvasive modality of choice for response classifications of HL and aggressive NHLs consistent with the recently revised, primarily FDG-PET/CT-based, response criteria for lymphoma. This review will highlight the most important applications of FDG-PET (FDG-PET/CT) in lymphoma emphasizing the strengths and pitfalls of this imaging approach, past and ongoing efforts to standardize the use of FDG-PET, particularly in response assessment and therapy monitoring. Other promising molecular probes for lymphoma imaging will also be briefly discussed.

Key words: Hodgkin's lymphoma, Non-Hodgkin's lymphoma, Response assessment of lymphoma, FDG-PET/CT in lymphoma, Pretreatment staging of lymphoma, Therapy monitoring of lymphoma

1. Introduction

Conventional imaging, primarily using CT, was clearly the dominant radiologic tool for lymphoma assessment for the last three decades or so, although it was long recognized that its use for response assessment of lymphoma following treatment is highly problematic (1–7). This is primarily due to the inability of CT to differentiate between viable tumor and necrosis or fibrosis in patients presenting

Malik E. Juweid and Otto S. Hoekstra (eds.), *Positron Emission Tomography*, Methods in Molecular Biology, vol. 727,
DOI 10.1007/978-1-61779-062-1_1, © Springer Science+Business Media, LLC 2011

with persistent masses posttherapy, who make about one-third of patients with aggressive non-Hodgkin's lymphoma (NHL) and two-thirds of those with Hodgkin's lymphoma (HL) (1, 3, 8). In fact, several studies have shown that, overall, the progression-free-survival (PFS) of aggressive NHL or HL patients with a positive posttherapy CT is not significantly different from that in patients with a negative CT (4–7). The addition of the first molecular imaging agent for lymphoma assessment, namely ^{67}Ga-citrate, significantly improved the accuracy of response assessment of patients with lymphoma (4–7). Unlike with CT, several studies showed that there is a significant difference in PFS between lymphoma patients with a positive or negative ^{67}Ga scan posttherapy (4–7). Nevertheless, both the positive and negative predictive values of ^{67}Ga scanning remained suboptimal. Importantly, ^{67}Ga imaging has not found widespread use and acceptability because of its low spatial resolution, lack of specificity, low sensitivity for low grade lymphomas and for abdominal disease due to physiologic bowel uptake and the time involved in performing the required scans, which may extend to 7–14 days post-^{67}Ga injection. Use of ^{67}Ga scanning was further complicated by the lack of a universally uniform approach for imaging with ^{67}Ga which should include the consistent use of single-photon-emission computer tomography (SPECT) and appropriately high doses of radioactivity. Because of these shortcomings and recent problems with the availability of ^{67}Ga citrate, ^{67}Ga scanning has been largely replaced by positron emission tomography (PET) scanning, particularly using ^{18}F-fluorodeoxyglucose (FDG), a marker of glucose metabolism.

Currently, FDG-PET, and more recently, FDG-PET/CT which combines an FDG-PET and a CT scan in a single study, has become an integral part of assessment of lymphoma, particularly in the posttherapy setting (8–15). FDG-PET or FDG-PET/CT is now widely utilized in North America, Europe, and Australia and, increasingly, also in developing countries with several studies clearly demonstrating its superiority to the now "outdated" [67]Ga scanning in both staging and restaging of lymphoma (16). Interestingly, FDG-PET is currently the only clinical PET study approved by the US Food and Drug Administration (FDA) and the Center of Medicare and Medicaid Services (CMS) for assessment of lymphoma.

2. Applications of FDG-PET in Lymphoma

Major applications of FDG-PET or FDG-PET/CT in lymphoma may reasonably be divided into pretreatment staging, restaging, therapy monitoring, assessment of transformation, and posttherapy surveillance and will be reviewed separately below.

3. FDG-PET for Pretreatment Staging

FDG-PET has been clearly shown to be quite sensitive for detection of nodal and extranodal lymphoma prior to treatment as well as the time of established or suspected relapse (Fig. 1) (17–27).

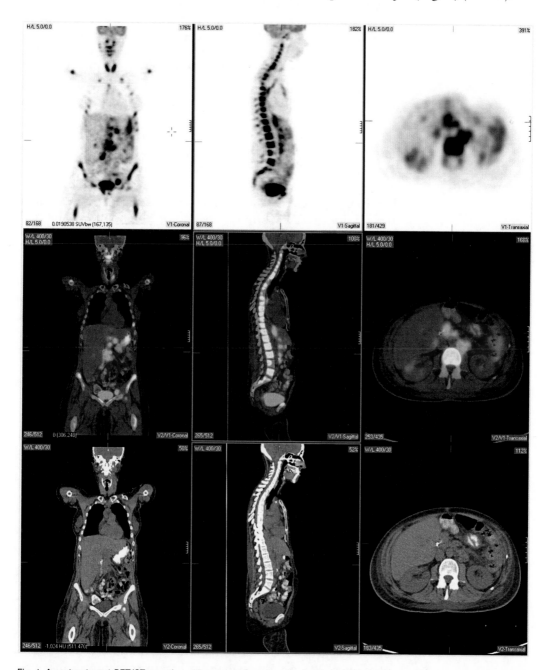

Fig. 1. A pretreatment PET/CT scan in a 48-year-old female patient with Burkitt's lymphoma showing widespread nodal and extranodal disease including periaortic, iliac, and mediastinal lymphadenopathy in addition to extensive involvement of the bone/bone marrow, both thyroid lobes, and focal liver involvement.

Compared with CT, FDG-PET clearly detects an additional number of presumed lymphoma manifestations, particularly at extranodal sites such as the liver, spleen, bone marrow, and muscle, in patients with diffuse large B cell (DLBCL), follicular lymphomas (FL), and HL (17–27). Overall, compared with conventional staging methods, including CT and iliac crest bone marrow biopsy (BMB), FDG-PET results in a modification of disease stage (usually upstaging) in about 15–20% of patients with an impact on management in about 5–15% (17–27). Pretreatment FDG-PET also facilitates the interpretation of posttherapy FDG-PET studies in patients with DLBCL and HL that should be routinely performed after the conclusion of therapy according to the recommendations of the International Harmonization Project (IHP) in lymphoma (8, 9).

FDG-PET has been shown to detect focal or multifocal bone marrow involvement in patients with negative iliac crest BMB (17, 18, 27–29). However, it is important to note that FDG-PET alone is unreliable in detecting a limited degree of bone marrow involvement (i.e., ≤10–20% of marrow space) and, hence, cannot replace iliac crest BMB in the staging of lymphomas of any type in the sense that a negative PET scan cannot rule out lymphomatous involvement of the marrow (30, 31). On the other hand, widespread multifocal bone marrow involvement seen on FDG-PET probably obviates the need for iliac crest BMB.

Pretreatment staging with FDG-PET is not without pitfalls. Diffuse bone marrow uptake in pretherapy FDG-PET scans should not automatically be interpreted as evidence of bone marrow involvement since this uptake may be due to reactive myeloid hyperplasia at least in patients with HL (12). Even focal bone marrow hyperplasia can occasionally occur. Degenerative changes can also result in discrete uptake in the skeleton that may be mistaken for bone or marrow involvement (Fig. 2). Uptake in braun fat represents yet another pitfall but the recognition of braun fat is now relatively straightforward with the advent of PET/CT. It is essential to recognize these and other pitfalls to avoid over-interpreting the FDG-PET findings. Planned treatment for a particular patient should not change based on "FDG-PET-only" findings; every effort should be made to confirm these findings by biopsy and/or other imaging methods before a treatment change is contemplated (12, 15).

While FDG-PET generally detects a larger number of lesions compared with CT in patients with DLBCL and FL with only a very small fraction of disease sites detected by CT by not FDG-PET in these histologic subtypes, several reports indicate that in HL, CT may demonstrate abnormalities consistent with lymphoma that are undetectable by FDG-PET with impact on disease stage in 10–20% of patients (20–26). Although the reverse also occurs with an impact of a similar magnitude, it is clear that FDG-PET alone cannot

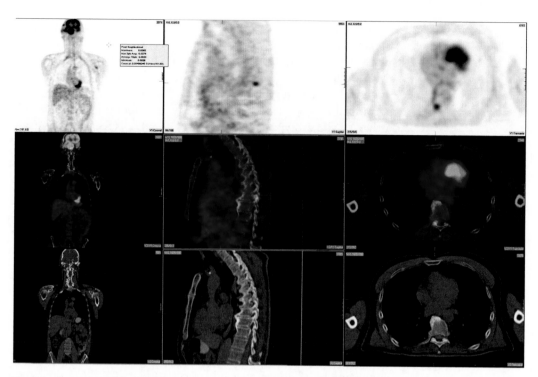

Fig. 2. Pretherapy fused PET/CT images in a patient with cavernous sinus diffuse large B-cell lymphoma (DLBCL) showing a mild focus of increased uptake in the spine, clearly representing facet joint degenerative disease and not lymphomatous bone/bone marrow involvement.

replace CT for pretreatment staging of HL (20, 21, 23, 25). However, this shortcoming of FDG-PET in HL may have been addressed to a large extent by the current widespread utilization of modern PET/CT scanners where information from both FDG-PET and diagnostic CT is available. On the other hand, FDG-PET has been reported to have low sensitivity compared with CT in patients with small-lymphocytic lymphoma (SLL) and extranodal marginal-zone lymphoma (MZL) of the mucosa-associated lymphoid tissue (MALT) (32, 33). In these subtypes, a diagnostic CT scan alone is probably sufficient for radiologic staging and FDG-PET is clearly not indicated.

Only limited data is available regarding the sensitivity of FDG-PET in peripheral T-cell lymphoma (PTCL), which includes multiple subtypes such as systemic PTCL unclassified (PTCL-U), systemic anaplastic large cell lymphoma (ALCL), angioimmuno-plastc T-cell lymphoma (AITL), natural killer T-cell-nasal type (NK/T), coetaneous T-cell lymphoma (CTCL)-PTCL-U and CTCL-ALCL. Available reports invariably show high sensitivity for FDG-PET in patients with systemic ALCL (30, 34–36). There are conflicting reports with respect to patients with systemic PTCL-U where two reports including a total of 17 patients showed high sensitivity for lesion detection (i.e., >90%) while one report on five patients with systemic PTCL-U showed a sensitivity of only 40% (30, 34–36). Several studies demonstrated that the sensitivity of FDG-PET is very poor at cutaneous sites in patients with stage 1 CTCL of either the unclassified or ALCL histology in contrast to the high sensitivity observed in patients with advanced-stage CTCL (34–36). The number of patients with other PTCL subtypes imaged with FDG-PET is too small to draw any meaningful conclusions.

There is general agreement that a staging FDG-PET/CT scan performed using current state-of-the-art PET/CT scanners and intravenous (i.v.) contrast provides at least equal but likely superior information to that provided by FDG-PET and a separately obtained i.v. contrast-enhanced CT (CECT) acquired using a dedicated CT scanner (8, 10, 12, 13). FDG-PET/CT scanning represents a functional-anatomical approach of lymphoma assessment which takes advantage of the strengths of both modalities, thereby minimizing the effects of shortcomings of either modality alone. PET provides functional/metabolic information lacking on CT images that may sometimes represent the only indication of disease in a particular organ or tissue (e.g., diffuse splenic uptake on a staging PET indicating splenic involvement or involvement of a normal-sized lymph node by CT). On the other hand, CT provides anatomic detail often lacking on PET enabling better lesion localization and, importantly, may identify relevant false-negative PET findings due to limited spatial resolution of current clinical PET scanners (in the order of 1 cm) or lack of FDG-avidity of some tumor lesions, as discussed above in the case of HL. CT also helps avoid misinterpretation of physiologic FDG uptake, for example, in the muscle and braun fat and, hence, reduces false-positive FDG-PET findings (37).

A recently published report supports the view that FDG-PET/CT performed using i.v. contrast with the CT portion is preferable to that performed without i.v. contrast (38). The investigators have compared the diagnostic performance of the typically acquired unenhanced low-dose FDG-PET/CT (80 mAs) with that of i.v. contrast-enhanced full-dose PET/CT acquired with up to 300 mAs. While no statistically significant difference was found between both imaging approaches, the authors observed that the enhanced full-dose FDG-PET/CT resulted in fewer indeterminate findings and a higher number of extranodal sites compared with unenhanced low-dose FDG-PET/CT, which the authors primarily attributed to the use of i.v. contrast rather than the high dose X-ray. Nevertheless, several studies suggest that a low-dose FDG-PET/CT performed even without i.v. contrast suffices as an alternative to separate CECT and PET scans notwithstanding the known limitations of the unenhanced CT in the assessment of the liver and spleen (27, 39, 40). This observation may be due to the reported exquisite sensitivity of PET in detecting splenic and hepatic lymphomatous involvement not seen even on CECT and the rarity of cases of non-FDG-avid splenic or hepatic involvement (27, 39, 40). Whether a low-dose unenhanced or low-dose CECT should be used in conjunction with FDG-PET currently remains a matter of controversy and this issue should probably be investigated further in a large prospective multicenter study. Until the results are conclusive, this author believes that a pretreatment FDG-PET/CT using low-dose i.v. contrast CT represents a reasonable choice of a single imaging modality for pretreatment assessment of patients with FDG-avid lymphomas such as HL, DLBCL, and FL (12, 13).

4. FDG-PET for Restaging

According to definitions used by the US CMS, the application of restaging is distinct from that of therapy monitoring in that the latter is performed during the planned course of therapy, for example, after two to three cycles of a six- to eight-cycle chemotherapy regimen, whereas restaging is performed after completion of treatment or to determine the extent of suspected or known recurrence (12, 13).

Response assessment at therapy conclusion, typically performed within 3–12 weeks of completing treatment, is currently undoubtedly the most routinely utilized application of restaging PET, particularly in patients with HL and DLBCL, consistent with the recently introduced revised response criteria for lymphoma (8, 9). Use of FDG-PET in this setting is clearly supported by the large body of evidence showing a high negative predictive value (NPV) of PET, exceeding 80% in virtually all reported studies for both HL and aggressive NHL, similar to that for spiral CT (8–15, 41–54). The 10–20% false-negative FDG-PET scans (depending on the lymphoma subtype and the efficacy of therapy) is related to the inability of PET to detect microscopic disease resulting in future relapse, a feature common to PET and CT or MRI.

The positive predictive value (PPV) of FDG-PET is substantially lower and considerably more variable than its NPV. In aggressive NHL, the PPV is probably in the range of 70–80% vs. only 60–70% in patients with HL, when using visual criteria for scan interpretation (8–15, 41–54). The somewhat lower PPV of PET in HL compared with aggressive NHL is most likely related to the substantial fraction of HL patients who received radiation therapy prior to undergoing FDG-PET, resulting in frequent occurrence of false-positive postradiation inflammatory changes, and the more frequent occurrence of thymic hyperplasia in the generally younger HL patients, a finding that can also lead to a false-positive interpretation (48).

Although only in the moderate range, the PPV of FDG-PET is substantially higher than that of CT with reported PPVs of about 40 and 20% in aggressive NHL and HL, respectively. This results in a considerably higher accuracy of FDG-PET for response assessment compared with CT (80% vs. 50%) (8–15, 41–54). The low accuracy of CT in this setting is clearly related to its inability to distinguish between viable tumor and necrosis or fibrosis in residual mass (es) (RM), a shortcoming that is largely overcome by FDG-PET, when FDG-PET scanning is performed at the appropriate timepoint (see below).

In HL, about two-thirds of patients have RMs by CT without any other clinical or biochemical evidence of disease and, of those, more than two-thirds are interpreted as negative by FDG-PET with relapse occurring in <10% of these patients (41–51, 53). These patients can, therefore, be safely observed. In aggressive NHL (e.g., DLBCL), only about one-third of patients have such RMs but here again more than two-thirds are interpreted as negative by FDG-PET with relapse occurring in <15–20% of these patients (10, 41–45, 52, 53). In both HL and aggressive NHL, the approximately one-third of patients with a positive FDG-PET are clearly at a higher risk of progression or relapse which occur in about 60–70% of patients. However, 30–40% of the patients with FDG-PET-positive RMs do not progress or relapse emphasizing the importance of histopathologic confirmation of the positive PET findings prior to administering salvage treatment (8–15, 41–53). False-positive FDG-PET findings at the site of RMs are almost invariably due to posttherapy inflammatory changes associated with necrosis. Figure 3 shows an example of a false-positive FDG-PET RM in patient with DLBCL treated with six cycles of R-CHOP. Other causes of false-positive FDG-PET scans, typically outside the site of RMs, are infectious or inflammatory process, such as granulomatous disease or sarcoidosis, brown fat, and rebound thymic hyperplasia in patients typically younger than 40 years (8, 9, 11–15). Figure 4 shows the typical uptake pattern of rebound thymic hyperplasia.

The IHP in Lymphoma which was convened to discuss harmonization of clinical trial parameters in lymphoma provided several important recommendations intended to decrease the rate of false-positive FDG-PET scans in the posttherapy setting (8, 9). These include that PET not be performed prior to at least 3 weeks following chemotherapy and 8–12 weeks after completion of RT. Another important recommendation of the IHP was the recommendation that RMs ≥2 cm in greatest transverse diameter (GTD) be only considered positive by FDG-PET-positive if their activity visually exceeds that of mediastinal blood pool; only RMs 1.1–1.9 cm are considered FDG-PET-positive with uptake exceeding surrounding background. The IHP consensus was also that visual assessment alone is adequate for determining whether FDG-PET

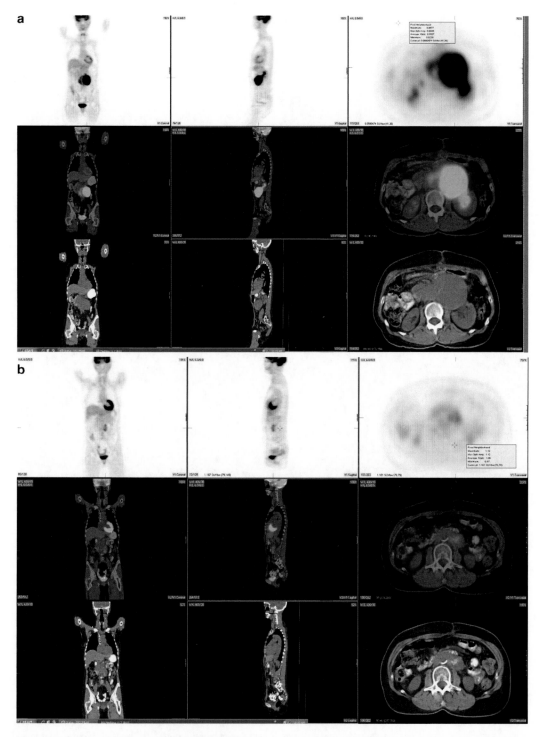

Fig. 3. Pre- and Posttherapy fused PET/CT images in a 62-year-old patient with diffuse large B-cell lymphoma (DLBCL). The pretherapy images (**a**) showed marked retroperitoneal lymphadenopathy. Posttherapy PET/CT (**b**) performed 1 month following completion of six cycles of R-CHOP showed tumor regression but still a PET-positive residual retroperitoneal mass. Biopsy was negative for lymphoma showing only tumor necrosis. Three follow-up PET/CT scans performed in 4–6 months intervals failed to show any evidence of tumor progression despite persistently positive PET.

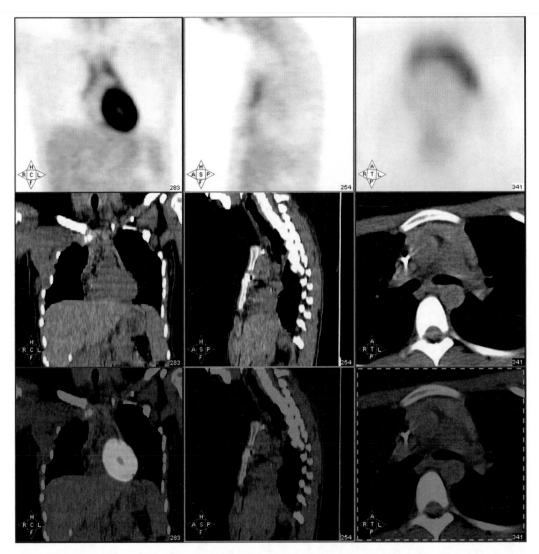

Fig. 4. Posttreatment PET/CT scan in a 20-year-old patient with Hodgkin lymphoma showing thymic hyperplasia with otherwise no PET evidence of disease.

is positive or negative for response assessment at the conclusion of therapy and that quantitative or semiquantitative approaches, for example, using the standardized uptake value (SUV), are not necessary in this setting. However, recent data by our group in 50 patients with treated aggressive NHL ($n = 24$) and HL ($n = 26$) show that the semiquantitative approaches result in a more reproducible and more accurate interpretation of FDG-PET findings at the site of residual masses compared with visually based interpretation (54). In this study, the NPV, PPV, and accuracy of FDG-PET/CT were 87, 64, and 82%, respectively, using the IHP-based visual interpretation criteria with two primary readers and an adjudicator in cases of disagreement. However, we found significant variability in study interpretation between three experienced nuclear medicine readers who independently interpreted the FDG-PET/CT scans resulting in a PPV for the three readers of 47–70% and accuracy of 74–84%. The NPVs were similar at 86–88%. In contrast, a cut-off SUV value of 2.5 resulted in NPV, PPV, and accuracy of 86, 75, and 84%, respectively. When the data were analyzed on a lesion-basis a more dramatic difference was found between the visual and semiquantitative evaluation. For the 60 RMs in 30 of the 50 patients, the PPV, NPV, and accuracy of the SUV-based approach using a cut-off of 2.5 were 92, 100, and 97%, respectively, with an area under the receiver operator characteristic (ROC) curve of 0.993. In contrast, the PPV for the three readers ranged from 67 to 81% and accuracy from 82 to 92%. The NPV was 100% for the three readers. The only limitation of the study was that FDG-PET scanning started at 90 min post-FDG injection rather than at 60 ± 10 min based on recommendations of the IHP Imaging Committee (9).

The higher accuracy of PET compared with CT in assessment of response in HL and aggressive NHL recently resulted in a revision of the primarily CT-based International Workshop Criteria (IWC) that are widely used for response assessment of NHL and, increasingly, also HL (1). For routinely FDG-avid lymphomas, such as HL and DLBCL, PET will now be incorporated into the definitions of the various response designations, such as complete response (i.e., CR), partial response (PR), stable disease (SD), unconfirmed complete (CRu), and progressive disease (PD) (9). Thus, the CR designation will now be primarily based on a negative PET in these patients: a posttherapy residual mass of any size is permitted as long as it is PET-negative. The CR designation also requires of course that there is otherwise complete disappearance of all detectable clinical and biochemical evidence of disease and that the BMB is negative. A PR still requires ≥50% decrease in sum of the product of the perpendicular diameters (SPD) of up to six of the largest dominant nodes or nodal masses with no new lesions but to be considered PR at least one of the residual lesions must now be PET-positive; otherwise, the patient is considered in CR (BMB must then be negative if positive prior to therapy). SD is less than a PR but not PD but also requires that at least one of the residual lesions be PET-positive. PD still requires ≥50% increase from nadir in the SPD of any previously involved nodes or other lesions (e.g., splenic or hepatic nodules) or appearance of any new lesion ≥1 cm in the short axis during or at the end of therapy. In this case, PET-positivity will be required only for new lesions ≥1.5 cm in diameter, approximately twice the spatial resolution of current PET systems, because moderately FDG-avid lymphomatous lesions below this size may be PET-negative. An interesting feature of the new criteria is that the CRu designation will now be eliminated; those responses will now be designated as CR if the

RM is PET-negative or PR if it is PET-positive. Using criteria very similar to those outlined here, Juweid et al. showed in a retrospective study of 54 patients with aggressive NHL (mostly DLBCL) who had been treated with an anthracycline-based regimen that PET not only doubled the number of CRs and eliminated the CRu's but significantly enhanced the difference in PFS between CR and PR (10). These findings provided the rationale for incorporating PET into revised criteria for routinely FDG-avid lymphomas, such as DLBCL and HL.

5. FDG-PET for Therapy Monitoring

FDG-PET for therapy monitoring, as defined above, is based on the premise that early or interim FDG-PET, typically performed after 1–4 cycles of chemo- or chemoimmunotherapy, provides accurate prediction of response to multicourse therapy and/or ultimate patient outcome. In fact, a large body of evidence supporting this premise, particularly with respect to the NPV of the test, reported to exceed 80% in patients with aggressive NHL and 90% in patients with HL (55–66).

In aggregate, published reports on interim FDG-PET demonstrate that interim FDG-PET scans are at least as accurate as end of therapy scans. The only exception here is the PPV of interim FDG-PET in early-stage HL where the PPV is in the range of only 30% albeit the NPV is very high exceeding 95% (55–66).

Interestingly, the PPV and, hence, accuracy of interim FDG-PET scans that are visually interpreted appears to depend on the "strictness" of the criteria used to define a scan as positive. There is evidence from several studies that a more "liberal" interpretation of PET findings at the site of RMs on interim PET scan results in higher PPV and accuracy without compromising the NPV. This liberal interpretation entails considering an FDG-PET scan as negative as long as it only shows minimal residual uptake that is similar or only slightly higher in intensity than normal liver uptake (59–66). For example, in a retrospective evaluation of 85 patients with HL who underwent FDG-PET after two or three cycles of first-line chemotherapy, Hutchings et al. showed that 94% (68/72) of patients with a "completely" negative FDG-PET (no uptake above background) or only minimal residual uptake (similar or only slightly higher than normal liver uptake) were progression-free after a median follow-up of 3.3 years compared to 39% (5/13) of patients with a clearly positive FDG-PET scan (60). A more stringent definition of FDG-PET-negativity during therapy did not enhance the difference in PFS between positive and negative studies; the opposite was true: 95% (60/63) of patients with a completely negative PET remained progression-free compared to 59% (14/22) of patients with any residual uptake above background (60). Using these liberal criteria for defining interim FDG-PET negativity, interim FDG-PET was at least as accurate for predicting patient outcome as end of therapy FDG-PET interpreted using strict criteria not allowing any residual uptake (60). Similar findings were subsequently reported in a prospective study by the same authors in patients with HL and in other studies in patients with aggressive NHL using similarly liberal visual criteria to interpret the interim FDG-PET scans (61–66). This suggests that a liberal visual interpretation of interim FDG-PET negativity is more accurate and, therefore, more appropriate in patients with HL and aggressive NHL. This may, at least in part be related to the posttherapy inflammatory nature of the minimal residual uptake in the vast majority of patients vs. minimal residual tumor that is apparently eradicated with subsequent treatment cycles.

There is some evidence that a semiquantitative SUV-based approach to interpreting interim FDG-PET may be more accurate that the dichotomous visual interpretation (i.e., positive vs. negative) used to date. For example, Lin et al. have shown an optimal cut-off value of 65.7% SUVmax reduction from baseline to post-two cycles of CHOP or CHOP-like regimen with or without rituximab resulted in an accuracy of 76.1% to predict event-free survival (EFS) in 92 patients with DLBCL (62, 63). In contrast, visual analysis using the so-called custom criteria allowing for minimal residual uptake at one residual site to be interpreted as negative resulted in an accuracy to predict EFS of only 65.2% (62, 63). Despite the liberal criteria used in the visual analysis, the PPV using the visual approach was far inferior to that using the SUV-based assessment (50% vs. 81.3%) with similar NPVs (74.1% vs. 75%). The use of a cutoff absolute SUVmax (based on body weight) of 5.0 resulted in a similar accuracy to that using %reduction in SUVmax from baseline to post-cycle 2 (62, 63). Interestingly, no significant difference was found between the SUV-based and visual assessments after four cycles of the same chemotherapy regimens in the same patient population perhaps suggesting that the semiquantitative assessment may be most useful early on following treatment (e.g., after 1–3 cycles of chemotherapy) (64). Obviously, if the SUV method is used for early prediction of prognosis or response in patients with HL and aggressive NHL, a standardized approach for SUV determination is critical, including strict adherence to predefined reconstruction algorithms and timing of PET imaging following FDG injection. Only such standardization will ensure comparability among various studies (8).

It is noteworthy that the vast majority of interim FDG-PET scans, at least as based on the published reports, appeared to have been performed because of the prognostic information provided with no indication that the results of these scans were actually used to alter treatment (55–66). As shown above, the prognostic power of a negative interim FDG-PET scan is remarkable and it is generally agreed that a negative FDG-PET scan after 1–4 cycles of chemo- or chemoimmunotherapy confers excellent prognosis in patients with HL and DLBCL. On the other hand, the limited PPV, at least using visual interpretation approaches, that extreme caution should be exercised in assessing prognosis in patients with positive interim FDG-PET. At this point, it is probably advisable to biopsy such findings if a change in treatment is contemplated (e.g., salvage chemotherapy with or without hematpoietic stem cell transplantation). In addition to the apparent influence of the criteria used to interpret the interim FDG-PET scans, the PPV of interim FDG-PET in predicting prognosis appears to depend on the disease stage in patients with HL. Based on two studies by the groups of Hutchings et al., the PPV of interim FDG-PET in patients with early-stage HL was only 25 compared to 94% in patients with advanced HL (60, 61). The high PPV of interim PET in advanced HL was recently confirmed by Gallamini et al. (66).

The high NPV of interim FDG-PET combined with the typically marked difference in outcome between patients with positive and negative interim FDG-PET scans led to increasing utilization of interim FDG-PET scanning in clinical trials in the context of risk-adjusted or "personalized" therapy (67, 68). The intention here is to either reduce the amount of therapy without compromising efficacy in patients with sensitive disease recognized as those with a negative interim FDG-PET or to improve outcome by early use of more aggressive therapy in patients with potentially resistant disease presumed to be the ones with positive interim FDG-PET. Examples of the use of interim FDG-PET in the former application are trials in patients with early-stage HL where patients with a negative FDG-PET (e.g., after two cycles) receive a reduced total number of chemotherapy (ABVD) cycles, whereas those with a positive PET would receive the full number of planned cycles or external beam radiation. An example of the use of interim FDG-PET in the second application is in advanced-stage HL patients where patients with a positive interim FDG-PET after two cycles of ABVD receive escalated BEACOPP, whereas those with a negative interim FDG-PET continue with their planned cycles of ABVD. These and similar trials have been or are currently being conducted by US and European Cooperative groups in patients with HL and aggressive NHL (66, 67). It is clear that the role of interim FDG-PET will dramatically increase in the clinical practice setting once these clinical trials demonstrate that the information provided by PET affect ultimate patient outcome.

6. FDG-PET for Posttherapy Surveillance

FDG-PET scanning for surveillance is performed following treatment in the absence of clinical, biochemical, or radiographic evidence of recurrent disease with the aim of early detection of recurrence. This FDG-PET application remains controversial, primarily because of the potential for a disproportionate fraction of false-positive findings, potentially resulting in increasing cost without proven benefit from earlier PET detection of disease compared to standard surveillance methods (69). This concern was dramatically demonstrated by the study of Jerusalem et al. where FDG-PET scanning was performed in 36 HL patients at the completion of therapy and every 4–6 months thereafter for 2–3 years. One patient with persistent tumor and four relapses were identified a few months prior to clinical, laboratory or CT evidence of disease. However, there were also six patients with false-positive PET studies requiring additional restaging procedures for further clarification, including subsequent PET scans performed several months later, all of which were then negative (69). Recently, Zinzani et al. reported a more extensive also clearly more positive experience with surveillance FDG-PET scanning in 421 lymphoma patients (160 HL, 183 aggressive NHL and 78 indolent NHL) who were imaged at 6, 12, 18, and 24 months then yearly following initial CR. In this study, the percent detection of proven relapses was higher with FDG-PET compared with CT or clinical assessment (signs and symptoms) in HL (32% vs. 23% and 22%, respectively), aggressive NHL (31% vs. 25% and 22%) and indolent NHL (60% vs. 49% and 38%) (70). There were 36 patients with inconclusive positive FDG-PET who then underwent biopsy. A lymphoma relapse was diagnosed in 24 (67%) but there were also 12 (33%) false-positive findings (nine lymph node reactive hyperplasia and three sarcoid-like granulomatosis) (70). Although this study is certainly more encouraging than that by Jerusalem et al., it still did not determine whether surveillance FDG-PET scanning was cost effective and whether the PET-derived information results in meaningful changes in patient management and, importantly, outcome. Until large prospective trials address these issues, surveillance FDG-PET scanning cannot be recommended outside of a clinical trial (68, 70).

7. FDG-PET for Assessment of Transformation

FDG-PET scanning may be used to confirm the clinical suspicion of transformation from an indolent lymphoma to an aggressive histology. FDG-PET is then not only expected to support the clinical suspicion by identifying lesions with unexpectedly high SUV (see below) but to also help select the optimal biopsy site for definitive histopathologic confirmation (i.e., the one with the highest SUV). Unfortunately, FDG-PET is unlikely to entirely replace biopsy for assessment of transformation because of the significant overlap in the degree of FDG uptake or SUV between indolent and aggressive lymphomas (71, 72). Yet, FDG-PET may be a useful alternative when a biopsy is not feasible because of inaccessibility or comorbidities. This is particularly the case when the SUVs of the "hottest" lesion fall in a range that is most consistent with aggressive or indolent histology, which according to the report by Schöder et al., are SUVmax of >13 and <6, respectively (72). It should be noted, however, that SUVmax ranges of >13 and <6 would comprise only about half of the patients of aggressive and indolent lymphomas assessed for transformation in either direction; the remaining half will have "intermediate" SUVs that are compatible with both indolent and aggressive lymphomas (72). On the other hand, F-18-fluorothymidine (FLT), an in vivo marker of proliferative activity, has been shown to be superior to FDG in differentiating between indolent and aggressive lymphomas and, hence, may prove superior to FDG in assessment of transformation particularly when the FDG-SUV is in the equivocal range (73).

References

1. Cheson, B.D., Horning, S.J., Coiffier, B., et al. (1999) Report of an international workshop to standardize response criteria for non-Hodgkin's lymphomas. *J Clin Oncol* **17(4)**, 1244–53.

2. Surbone, A., Longo, D.L., DeVita, V.T. Jr., et al. (1988) Residual abdominal masses in aggressive non-Hodgkin's lymphoma after combination chemotherapy. Significance and management. *J Clin Oncol* **6**, 832–7.

3. Canellos, G.P. (1988) Residual mass in lymphoma may not be residual disease. *J Clin Oncol* **6**, 931–3.

4. Kaplan, W.D., Jochelson, M.S., Herman, T.S., et al. (1990) Gallium-67 imaging: a predictor of residual tumor viability and clinical outcome in patients with diffuse large-cell lymphoma. *J Clin Oncol* **8**, 1966–70.

5. Front, D., Bar-Shalom, R., Mor, M., et al. (2000) Aggressive non-Hodgkin lymphoma: early prediction of outcome with ^{67}Ga scintigraphy. *Radiology* **214**, 253–7.

6. Vose, J.M., Bierman, P.J., Anderson, J.R., et al. (1996) Single-photon emission computed tomography gallium imaging versus computed tomography: predictive value in patients undergoing high-dose chemotherapy and autologous stem-cell transplantation for non-Hodgkin's lymphoma. *J Clin Oncol* **14**, 2473–9.

7. Janicek, M., Kaplan, W., Neuberg, D., et al. (1997) Early restaging gallium scans predict outcome in poor-prognosis patients with aggressive non-Hodgkin's lymphoma treated with high-dose CHOP chemotherapy. *J Clin Oncol* **15**, 1631–7.

8. Juweid, M.E., Stroobants, S., Hoekstra, O.S., et al. (2007) Use of positron emission tomography for response assessment of lymphoma: consensus of the Imaging Subcommittee of International Harmonization Project in Lymphoma. *J Clin Oncol* **25**, 571–8.

9. Cheson, B.D., Pfistner, B., Juweid, M.E., et al. (2007) Revised response criteria for malignant lymphoma. *J Clin Oncol* **25**, 579–86.

10. Juweid, M.E., Wiseman, G.A., Vose, J.M., et al. (2007) Response assessment of aggressive non-Hodgkin's lymphoma by integrated international workshop criteria and fluorine 18 fluorodeoxyglucose positron emission tomography. *J Clin Oncol* **23**, 4652–61.

11. Juweid, M.E., Cheson, B.D. (2005) Role of positron emission tomography in lymphoma. *J Clin Oncol* **23**, 4577–80.

12. Seam, P., Juweid, M.E., Cheson, B.D. (2007) The role of FDG-PET scans in patients with lymphoma. *Blood* **110(10)**, 3507–16.

13. Juweid, M.E. (2006) Utility of positron emission tomography (PET) scanning in managing patients with Hodgkin lymphoma. *Hematology Am Soc Hematol Educ Program* **259–65**, 510–1.

14. Juweid, M.E., Cheson, B.D. (2006) Positron emission tomography and assessment of cancer therapy. *N Engl J Med* **354**, 496–507.

15. Juweid, M.E. (2008) 18F-FDG PET as a routine test for posttherapy assessment of Hodgkin's disease and aggressive non-Hodgkin's lymphoma: where is the evidence. *J Nucl Med* **49(1)**, 9–12.

16. Friedberg, J.W., Fishman, A., Neuberg, D., et al. (2004) FDG-PET is superior to gallium scintigraphy in staging and more sensitive in the follow-up of patients with de novo Hodgkin lymphoma: a blinded comparison. *Leuk Lymphoma* **45**, 85–92.

17. Moog, F., Bangerter, M., Diederichs, C.G., et al. (1997) Lymphoma: role of whole-body 2-deoxy-2-[F-18]fluoro-D-glucose (FDG) PET in nodal staging. *Radiology* **203**, 795–800.

18. Moog, F., Bangerter, M., Diederichs, C.G., et al. (1998) Extranodal malignant lymphoma: detection with FDG PET versus CT. *Radiology* **206**, 475–81.

19. Buchmann, I., Reinhardt, M., Elsner, K., et al. (2001) 2-(fluorine-18)fluoro-2-deoxy-D-glucose positron emission tomography in the detection and staging of malignant lymphoma. A bicenter trial. *Cancer* **91**, 889–99.

20. Bangerter, M., Moog, F., Buchmann, I. (1998) Whole-body 2-[¹⁸F]-fluoro-2-deoxy-D-glucose positron emission tomography (FDG-PET) for accurate staging of Hodgkin's disease. *Ann Oncol* **9**, 1117–22.

21. Jerusalem, G., Beguin, Y., Fassotte, M.-F., et al. (2001) Whole-body positron emission tomography using ¹⁸F-fluorodeoxyglucose compared to standard procedures for staging patients with Hodgkin's disease. *Hematologica* **86**, 266–73.

22. Partridge, S., Timothy, A., O'Doherty, M.J., Hain, S.F., Rankin, S., Mikhaeel, G. (2000) 2-Fluorine-18-fluoro-2-deoxy-D glucose positron emission tomography in the pretreatment staging of Hodgkin's disease: influence on patient management in a single institution. *Ann Oncol* **11**, 1273–9.

23. Weihrauch, M.R., Re, D., Bischoff, S., et al. (2002) Whole-body positron emission tomography using 18F-fluorodeoxyglucose for initial staging of patients with Hodgkin's disease. *Ann Hematol* **81**, 20–5.

24. Menzel, C., Döbert, N., Mitrou, P., et al. (2002) Positron emission tomography for the staging of Hodgkin's lymphoma. *Acta Oncologica* **41**, 430–6.

25. Naumann, R., Beuthien-Baumann, B., Reiss, A., et al. (2004) Substantial impact of FDG PET imaging on the therapy decision in patients with early-stage Hodgkin's lymphoma. *Br J Cancer* **90**, 620–5.

26. Hutchings, M., Loft, A., Hansen, M., et al. (2006) Positron emission tomography with or without computed tomography in the primary staging of Hodgkin's lymphoma. *Haematologica* **91**, 482–9.

27. Schaefer, N.G., Hany, T.F., Taverna, C., et al. (2004) Non-Hodgkin lymphoma and Hodgkin disease: coregistered FDG PET and CT at staging and restaging – do we need contrast-enhanced CT. *Radiology* **232**, 823–9.

28. Moog, F., Bangerter, M., Kotzerke, J., Guhlmann, A., Frickhofen, N., Reske, S.N. (1998) 18-F-fluorodeoxyglucose-positron emission tomography as a new approach to detect lymphomatous bone marrow. *J Clin Oncol* **16**, 603–9.

29. Carr, R., Barrington, S.F., Madan, B., et al. (1998) Detection of lymphoma in bone marrow by whole-body positron emission tomography. *Blood* **91**, 3340–6.

30. Elstrom, R., Guan, L., Baker, G., et al. (2003) Utility of FDG-PET scanning in lymphoma by WHO classification. *Blood* **101**, 3875–6.

31. Pakos, E.E., Fotopoulos, A.D., Ioannidis, J.P.A. (2005) ¹⁸F-FDG PET for evaluation of bone marrow infiltration in staging of lymphoma: a meta-analysis. *J Nucl Med* **46**, 958–63.

32. Hoffmann, M., Kletter, K., Diemling, M., et al. (1999) Positron emission tomography with fluorine-18-2-fluoro-2-deoxy-D-glucose (F18-FDG) does not visualize extranodal B-cell lymphoma of the mucosa-associated lymphoid tissue (MALT)-type. *Ann Oncol* **10**, 1185–9.

33. Jerusalem, G., Beguin, Y., Najjar, F., et al. (2001) Positron emission tomography (PET) with ¹⁸F-fluorodeoxyglucose (¹⁸F-FDG) for the staging of low-grade non-Hodgkin's lymphoma (NHL). *Ann Oncol* **12**, 825–30.

34. Bishu, S., Quigley, J.M., Schmitz, J., et al. (2007) F-18-fluoro-deoxy-glucose (FDG) positron emission tomography (PET) in the

assessment of peripheral T-cell lymphomas. *Leuk Lymphoma* **48(8)**, 1531–8.

35. Kako, S., Izutsu, K., Ohta, Y., et al. (2007) FDG-PET in T-cell and NK-cell neoplasm. *Ann Oncol* **18**, 1685–90.

36. Juweid, M.E. (2007) Peripheral T-cell lymphomas: variably or routinely fluorodeoxyglucose-avid? Commentary in *Leuk Lymphoma* **48(8)**, 1455–67.

37. Allen-Auerbach, M., Quon, A., Weber, W.A., et al. (2004) Comparison between 2-deoxy-2-[(18)F]fluoro-D-glucose positron-emission tomography and positron-emission tomography/computed tomography hardware fusion for staging of patients with lymphoma. *Mol Imaging Biol* **6**, 411–6.

38. Rodríguez-Vigil, B., Gómez-León, N., Pinilla, I., et al. (2006) PET/CT in lymphoma: prospective study of enhanced full-dose PET/CT versus unenhanced low-dose PET/CT. *J Nucl Med* **47(10)**, 1643–8.

39. Elstrom, R.L., Leonard, J.P., Coleman, M., Brown, R.K. (2008) Combined PET and low-dose, noncontrast CT scanning obviates the need for additional diagnostic contrast-enhanced CT scans in patients undergoing staging or restaging for lymphoma. *Ann Oncol* **19(10)**, 1770–3.

40. Freudenberg, L.S., Antoch, G., Schütt, P., et al. (2004) FDG-PET/CT in re-staging of patients with lymphoma. *Eur J Nucl Med Mol Imaging* **31**, 325–9.

41. de Wit, M., Bumann, D., Beyer, W., et al. (1997) Whole-body positron emission tomography (PET) for diagnosis of residual mass in patients with lymphoma. *Ann Oncol* **8**, 57–60.

42. Jerusalem, G., Beguin, Y., Fassotte, M.F., et al. (1999) Whole-body positron emission tomography using ^{18}F-fluorodeoxyglucose for posttreatment evaluation in Hodgkin's disease and non-Hodgkin's lymphoma has higher diagnostic and prognostic value than classical computed tomography scan imaging. *Blood* **94**, 429–33.

43. Zinzani, P.L., Magagnoli, M., Chierichetti, F., et al. (1999) The role of positron emission tomography (PET) in the management of lymphoma patients. *Ann Oncol* **10**, 1181–4.

44. Bangerter, M., Moog, F., Griesshammer, M., et al. (1999) Positron emission tomography with 18-fluorodeoxyglucose in the staging and follow-up of lymphoma in the chest. *Acta Oncol* **38**, 799–804.

45. Mikhael, N.G., Timothy, A.R., Hain, S.F., O'Doherty, M.J. (2000) 18-FDG-PET for the assessment of residual masses on CT following treatment of lymphomas. *Ann Oncol* **11(1)**, 147–50.

46. de Wit, M., Bohuslavizki, K.H., Buchert, R., et al. (2001) [18]FDG-PET following treatment as valid predictor for disease-free survival in Hodgkin's lymphoma. *Ann Oncol* **12**, 29–37.

47. Naumann, R., Vaic, A., Beuthien-Baumann, B., et al. (2001) Prognostic value of positron emission tomography in the evaluation of post-treatment residual mass in patients with Hodgkin's disease and non-Hodgkin's lymphoma. *Br J Haematol* **115**, 793–800.

48. Weihrauch, M.R., Re, D., Scheidhauer, K., et al. (2001) Thoracic positron emission tomography using 18F-fluorodeoxyglucose for the evaluation of residual mediastinal Hodgkin disease. *Blood* **98**, 2930–4.

49. Dittman, H., Sokler, M., Kollmannsberger, C., et al. (2001) Comparison of 18FDG-PET with CT scans in the evaluation of patients with residual and recurrent Hodgkin's lymphoma. *Oncol Rep* **8**, 1393–9.

50. Spaepen, K., Stroobants, S., Dupont, P., et al. (2001) Can positron emission tomography with [(18)F]-fluorodeoxyglucose after first-line treatment distinguish Hodgkin's disease patients who need additional therapy from others in whom additional therapy would mean avoidable toxicity? *Br J Haematol* **115**, 272–8.

51. Hueltenschmidt, B., Sautter-Bihl, M.L., Lang, O., et al. (2001) Whole body positron emission tomography in the treatment of Hodgkin disease. *Cancer* **91**, 302–10.

52. Spaepen, K., Stroobants, S., Dupont, P., et al. (2001) Prognostic value of positron emission tomography (PET) with fluorine 18 Fluorodeoxyglucose ([18F]FDG) after first-line chemotherapy in non-Hodgkin's lymphoma: is [18F]FDG-PET a valid alternative to conventional diagnostic methods? *J Clin Oncol* **19**, 414–9.

53. Zijlstra, J.M., Linduer-vander Werf, G., Hoekstra, O.S., Hooft, L., Riphagen, I.I., Huijgens, P.C. (2006) ^{18}F-fluoro-deoxyglucose positron emission tomography for post-treatment evaluation of malignant lymphoma: a systematic review. *Haematologica* **91**, 522–9.

54. Thomas, D.L., Berbaum, K., Bushnell, D.L., Graham, M.M., Juweid, M.E. (2009) Reproducibility of the International Harmonization Project (IHP)-based interpretation of PET/CT in patients with Hodgkin's and aggressive non-Hodgkin's lymphoma. Presented at the Pan-Pacific Lymphoma Conference, June 22–26, 2009, Big Island, HI.

55. Römer, W., Hanauske, A.-R., Ziegler, S., et al. (1998) Positron emission tomography in non-Hodgkin's lymphoma: assessment of chemotherapy with Fluorodeoxyglucose. *Blood* **91**, 4464–71.

56. Jerusalem, G., Beguin, Y., Fassotte, M.F., et al. (2000) Persistent tumor 18F-FDG uptake after a few cycles of polychemotherapy is predictive of treatment failure in non-Hodgkin's lymphoma. *Haematologica* **85**, 613–8.

57. Spaepen, K., Stroobants, S., Dupont, P., et al. (2001) Early staging positron emission tomography (PET) with fluorine 18 fluorodeoxyglucose ([^{18}F]FDG) predicts outcome in patients with aggressive non-Hodgkin's lymphoma. *Blood* **98**, 726a.

58. Kostakoglu, L., Coleman, M., Leonard, J.P., et al. (2002) PET predicts prognosis after 1 cycle of chemotherapy in aggressive lymphoma and Hodgkin's disease. *J Nucl Med* **43**, 1018–27.

59. Mikhaeel, N.G., Timothy, A.R., O'Doherty, M.J., Hain, S., Maisey, M.N. (2000) 18-FDG-PET as a prognostic indicator in the treatment of aggressive non-Hodgkin's lymphoma-comparison with CT. *Leuk Lymphoma* **39**, 543–53.

60. Hutchings, M., Mikhaeel, N.G., Fields, P.A., Nunan, T., Timothy, A.R. (2005) Prognostic value of interim FDG-PET after two or three cycles of chemotherapy in Hodgkin lymphoma. *Ann Oncol* **16**, 1160–8.

61. Hutchings, M., Loft, A., Hansen, M., et al. (2006) FDG-PET after two cycles of chemotherapy predicts treatment failure and progression-free survival in Hodgkin Lymphoma. *Blood* **107**, 52–9.

62. Lin, C., Itti, E., Haioun, C., et al. (2007) Early 18F-FDG PET for prediction of prognosis in patients with diffuse large B-cell lymphoma: SUV-based assessment versus visual analysis. *J Nucl Med* **48(10)**, 1626–32.

63. Weber, W.A. (2007) 18-FDG PET in non-Hodgkin's lymphoma: qualitative or quantitative? *J Nucl Med* **48(10)**, 1580–2.

64. Itti, E., Lin, C., Dupuis, J., et al. (2009) Prognostic value of interim 18F-FDG PET in patients with diffuse large B-cell lymphoma: SUV-based assessment at 4 cycles of chemotherapy. *J Nucl Med* **50(4)**, 527–33.

65. Dupuis, J., Itti, E., Rahmouni, A., et al. (2009) Response assessment after an inductive CHOP or CHOP-like regimen with or without rituximab in 103 patients with diffuse large B-cell lymphoma: integrating 18fluorodeoxyglucose positron emission tomography to the International Workshop Criteria. *Ann Oncol* **20(3)**, 503–7.

66. Gallamini, A., Hutchings, M., Rigacci, L., et al. (2007) Early interim 2-[18F]fluoro-2-deoxy-D-glucose positron emission tomography is prognostically superior to international prognostic score in advanced-stage Hodgkin's lymphoma: a report from a joint Italian-Danish study. *J Clin Oncol* **25(24)**, 3746–52.

67. Horning, S.J., Juweid, M.E., Schoder, H., et al. 372 interim positron emission tomography (PET) in diffuse large B-cell lymphoma: independent expert nuclear medicine evaluation of ECOG 3404. Presented at the 50th ASH Annual Meeting and Exposition, December 6–9, 2008, San Francisco, CA.

68. Cheson, B. (2009) The case against heavy PETing. *J Clin Oncol* **27(11)**, 1742–3.

69. Jerusalem, G., Beguin, Y., Fassotte, M.F., et al. (2003) Early detection of relapse by whole-body emission tomography in the follow-up of patients with Hodgkin's disease. *Ann Oncol* **14**, 123–30.

70. Zinzani, P.L., Stefoni, V., Tani, M., et al. (2009) Role of [18F]fluorodeoxyglucose positron emission tomography scan in the follow-up of lymphoma. *J Clin Oncol* **27(11)**, 1781–7.

71. Lapela, M., Leskinen, S., Minn, H.R., et al. (1995) Increased glucose metabolism in untreated non-Hodgkin's lymphoma: a study with positron emission tomography and fluorine-18-fluorodeoxyglucose. *Blood* **86**, 3522–7.

72. Schöder, H., Noy, A., Gönen, M., et al. (2005) Intensity of ^{18}Fluorodeoxyglucose uptake in positron emission tomography distinguishes between indolent and aggressive non-Hodgkin's lymphoma. *J Clin Oncol* **23**, 4643–51.

73. Buck, A.K., Bommer, M., Stilgenbauer, S., et al. (2006) Molecular imaging of proliferation in malignant lymphoma. *Cancer Res* **66**, 11055–61.

Chapter 2

FDG PET Imaging of Head and Neck Cancers

Yusuf Menda and Michael M. Graham

Abstract

In initial staging of head and neck cancers, the addition of FDG PET to conventional imaging improves the accuracy for cervical nodal metastases. The sensitivity of FDG PET is, however, limited in nodes <1 cm and in completely necrotic nodes. In the posttherapy setting, PET scans obtained at least 10 weeks after radiotherapy have an excellent predictive value to rule out residual disease. Due to the limited positive predictive value of FDG PET after radiation therapy, a positive PET scan needs to be confirmed before management decisions are made.

Key words: F-18 Fluorodeoxyglucose, Positron emission tomography, Head and neck cancer

1. Introduction

Head and neck cancers are cancers involving all regions of the head and neck, except for the thyroid and central nervous system. Most of these cancers are squamous cell carcinomas. The most common sites are larynx, tongue, floor of the mouth, tonsils, and salivary glands, although these carcinomas can arise in almost any location in the nasopharynx, oropharynx, or hypopharynx. The estimated number of new cases in the USA for 2008 is 47,500, with approximately 11,000 deaths (1). The male:female ratio is about 2:1. Primary risk factors for virtually all head and neck cancers are tobacco and alcohol use. Early-stage head and neck tumors are treated with either surgery or radiotherapy with excellent prognosis. Locally advanced tumors without distant metastasis are typically treated with combination therapies with definitive chemoradiation therapy followed by salvage surgery (if necessary) or surgery and postoperative radiation therapy. Patients with distant metastatic disease have very poor prognosis and are usually referred for palliative chemotherapy or radiation.

Malik E. Juweid and Otto S. Hoekstra (eds.), *Positron Emission Tomography*, Methods in Molecular Biology, vol. 727,
DOI 10.1007/978-1-61779-062-1_2, © Springer Science+Business Media, LLC 2011

2. Diagnosis and Conventional Imaging

A working diagnosis of malignant tumor is usually obtained after history and careful clinical exam. Histologic characterization may be determined with fine needle aspiration (FNA) or biopsy. Flexible endoscopy with multiple biopsies is performed for tumors of the upper aerodigestive tract. Panendoscopy under general anesthesia, which includes laryngoscopy, esophagoscopy, and bronchoscopy, is performed in most patients to visualize and biopsy the primary tumor and to rule out synchronous tumors. CT of the neck with intravenous contrast is often the first-line imaging study to evaluate the extent of primary tumor and for cervical nodal metastasis. MRI may be complementary to CT in staging of primary tumors and is particularly helpful to evaluate for dural involvement of nasopharyngeal and sinonasal tumors. Evaluation for distant disease with chest CT is advised as part of the conventional workup of patients with locally advanced tumors with cervical nodal metastases.

3. FDG PET Imaging Technique of Head and Neck Cancer

FDG PET scans should not be performed if serum glucose level exceeds 200 mg/dl, since high glucose levels compete with FDG resulting in lower tumor uptake of FDG (2). Sedation with benzodiazepines during the uptake phase can be very helpful to reduce normal muscle uptake in the neck. This may be particularly helpful if the scan is not done on a hybrid PET/CT camera, because uptake in normal muscle may be difficult to distinguish from pathologic uptake in cervical lymph nodes. Muscle uptake can be particularly problematic following therapy when unilateral muscle uptake occurs in scalenes, longus colli, pterygoids, or one of the other numerous small muscles in the neck. Another important measure during the uptake phase is to prohibit speech, which results in increased uptake in peri-laryngeal muscles. Intense FDG uptake in brown fat uptake can be problematic, particularly in the supraclavicular fossa (3). This can be minimized by maintaining the uptake room at a relatively high temperature (≥24°C) (4).

The uptake period should be at least 60 min, and it may be advantageous to delay even longer to 90 or 120 min, since tumor to background ratio steadily increases with time (5). The resolution of the PET images can be improved by using a smaller pixel size than is routinely used for body imaging. The default voxel size for most PET-CT systems is approximately 4 mm. This means that the spatial resolution is about 10 mm. If the voxel size is reduced to 2 mm, a resolution of 5–6 mm can be obtained.

Interpretation of the PET images of head and neck is challenging and requires more experience that in most other areas of the body because many normal anatomic structures in the neck show elevated uptake of FDG compared to nearby soft tissue. These tissues include the salivary glands, lingual, palatine, and pharyngeal tonsils, base of the tongue, floor of the mouth and the laryngeal, pterygoid and strap muscles of the neck. Many of these are demonstrated in an atlas of head and neck PET imaging published in the Seminars of Nuclear Medicine (6).

4. Staging of Head and Neck Cancers

Head and neck cancers are staged according to the TNM classification (7). Although the description of T-stage varies with the site of the primary tumor, generally tumors <2 cm are staged as T1, 2–4 cm as T2, >4 cm as T3, and tumors invading into adjacent neck structures are staged as T4. Cervical nodes are staged as N1 for a single ipsilateral node <3 cm, N2 indicates single or multiple nodes between 3 and 6 cm, and N3 refers to node(s) >6 cm in greatest dimension. Metastatic disease, which is most commonly seen in the lungs, bone, and liver, results in an M1 designation.

Involvement of neck nodes is an important prognostic factor and therapeutic determinant for all head and neck cancers. Thus, it is important to have a solid understanding of the nodal anatomy and the standard system for describing the location of nodes to be able to effectively communicate with the referring surgeons (8). Level IA nodes are submental nodes close to midline and Level IB are more lateral and anterior to the posterior edge of the submandibular glands. These nodes receive drainage from the anterior oral cavity. Level II nodes are between the base of the skull and the inferior margin of the hyoid bone. They are further classified into IIA and IIB nodes. Level IIA nodes are anterior to the posterior aspect of the internal jugular vein and IIB nodes are posterior to the vein. Level III nodes are between the inferior border of the hyoid and inferior border of the cricoid cartilage. Level II and Level III nodal metastases are seen with tumors of the oral cavity, pharynx, and larynx. Level IV nodes are inferior to the cricoid and extend to the level of the clavicle. Metastatic disease in level IV nodes is usually associated with tumors of the hypopharynx, larynx, cervical esophagus, or thyroid. Level V nodes are in the posterior triangle and are between the posterior border of the sternocleidomastoid muscle and the trapezius muscle. Level V nodes are classified as VA if they are between the skull base and the inferior border of the cricoid cartilage and VB if they are between the cricoid and clavicle. Level V nodes are at highest risk for metastases from nasopharynx, oropharynx, and posterior scalp. Level VI nodes are the anterior compartment nodes, medial to the common carotid artery and extend from the hyoid to the manubrium. Metastatic disease at level VI is commonly associated with thyroid cancer, larynx, hypopharynx, and cervical esophagus.

Diagnostic criteria for cervical nodal metastases with CT or MRI are based primarily on nodal size. The nodes are considered to be metastatic if >15 mm for jugulodigastric nodes and >10 mm for other neck nodes. In addition, round shape with central necrosis, presence of more than three nodes or presence of extracapsular invasion also indicates metastatic disease. However, >40% of metastatic nodes are <10 mm in size (5) and many larger nodes simply represent reactive inflammatory lymph nodes. FDG uptake in a lymph node is significantly more accurate in predicting nodal metastases. PET-CT scan of a patient with cervical nodal metastases from a tonsillar cancer is shown in Fig. 1. In comparative studies, sensitivity and specificity of PET in detection of nodal metastases was found between 70–100% and 82–94%, respectively, compared to 58–85% and 58–96% for CT/MRI (9–12). FDG PET may be falsely negative in small nodes <1 cm in diameter or in completely necrotic nodes. False-positive FDG uptake in cervical nodes can be due to inflammation. Because of significant overlap between inflammatory and metastatic nodes, quantitation of uptake using standardized uptake values (SUV) does not appear to significantly improve the interpretation accuracy of FDG PET in cervical lymph nodes.

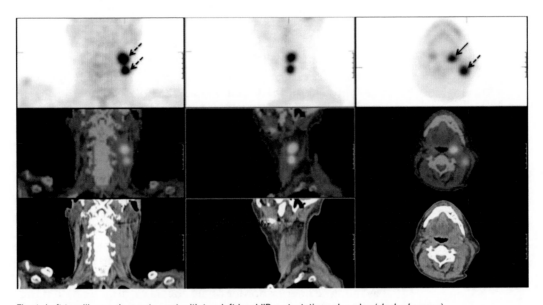

Fig. 1. Left tonsillar carcinoma (*arrow*) with two left level IIB metastatic neck nodes (*dashed arrows*).

The clinically negative neck (N0 neck) is particularly challenging. Only 25–30% of patients with N0 neck are found to have metastatic neck nodes at surgery. This means that the majority of patients with N0 neck undergoing a potentially morbid neck dissection are unlikely to benefit from this procedure. In three studies totaling 48 patients, where a sentinel node biopsy with immunohistochemistry was used as the gold standard, the detection rate of PET for nodal involvement in clinically N0 patients was limited between 0 and 30% (13–15). Integrated PET-CT may improve the accuracy in clinically N0 neck, with a reported sensitivity and specificity of 67 and 85%; however, this is still not sufficient to replace surgical staging in these patients (16). Sentinel node biopsy with immunohistochemistry appears significantly more accurate in patients with clinical N0 neck.

A major advantage of FDG PET over conventional imaging in pretherapy staging of head and neck cancer is its ability to detect synchronous and/or metastatic disease in the chest and abdomen (17). A PET scan in the initial staging is most helpful with in patients with advanced local disease (Stage III or IV). Several studies suggest that PET finds unexpected distant metastasis in approximately 10% of patients with locally advanced head and neck cancer (18–21).

5. Carcinoma of Unknown Primary

Squamous cervical nodal metastases from an unknown primary tumor constitute approximately 2% of newly diagnosed head and neck cancers. The most common sites of the primary tumor are tonsil and base of tongue (22). These patients are routinely treated with wide-field radiation therapy, which includes the entire pharynx, larynx, and bilateral neck. The wide-field irradiation definitely reduces the risk of tumor recurrence; however, it causes significant morbidity particularly in terms of xerostomia (23). Correct localization of the primary tumor substantially reduces the complications associated with radiotherapy by decreasing the size of the radiation portal and may also improve survival (22). The initial conventional workup of patients with a squamous cell nodal metastasis with unknown primary includes CT of the neck followed by endoscopy and directed biopsies. Even after such an extensive workup the detection rate of the primary tumor is <50%.

The current FDG PET literature on carcinoma of unknown primary includes a number of small single-center studies with variable diagnostic workup before the PET scan. In a meta-analysis which included 16 studies with PET in 302 patients, the average detection rate of the primary tumor with FDG PET was 24.5% with additional regional metastases found in 15.9% and distant metastases in 11.2 % of patients (24). The detection rate of the primary tumor with PET is not different in studies where FDG PET is only performed after a negative endoscopy and conventional imaging (25–30). It seems therefore reasonable to obtain an FDG PET as the initial imaging study in patients with carcinoma of unknown primary. If the FDG PET scan is negative, a primary tumor is found subsequently only in 12% of patients (24).

6. Detection of Residual and Recurrent Disease After Treatment

Early detection of recurrent head and neck cancer is important because the disease-free survival after salvage surgery is highly dependent on the stage of the recurrent tumor. The 2-year disease-free survival is 67–73% for stage I or II recurrent tumor compared to 22–33% for stage III and IV disease (31). Diagnosis of recurrence is difficult with CT or MRI because of the loss of symmetry and inflammation associated with healing from surgery and with radiotherapy. Routine biopsy of treated areas is also not recommended because of increased risk of bleeding and infection in irradiated tissue and potential false-negative biopsies due to sampling errors. FDG PET is more sensitive and specific than CT or MRI in detection of residual or recurrent disease (32).

The role of PET in the follow-up of head and neck cancer was reviewed in a meta-analysis by Isles et al. (33). The mean pooled sensitivity and specificity of FDG PET for recurrent disease at primary site following radiotherapy or chemoradiation therapy was 94 and 82%, respectively. For diagnosis of recurrent disease in neck nodes, the mean sensitivity was 74% and mean specificity was 84%, with a positive predictive value of 49% and a negative predictive value of 96% (33). A true positive FDG PET-CT for recurrent tumor is demonstrated in Fig. 2. The largest single-center study regarding PET for recurrent disease included 188 patients, who were imaged for suspected recurrence within 12 months of completion of definitive treatment with surgery and radiation therapy or combined chemoradiation therapy (34). The sensitivity and specificity for FDG PET in the assessment of the treatment response in the neck was 86 and 97%, respectively. Patients with positive post-RT PET findings had significantly worse 3-year overall survival and disease-free survival (34).

Many patients with locally advanced head and neck cancer, particularly originating from larynx and hypopharynx, are treated with initial radiation and chemotherapy, which results in functional preservation. These patients may subsequently undergo salvage surgery if residual disease is present and PET-CT seems to be the most accurate way to make that determination. Greven et al. reported a sensitivity and specificity of 100 and 90% in

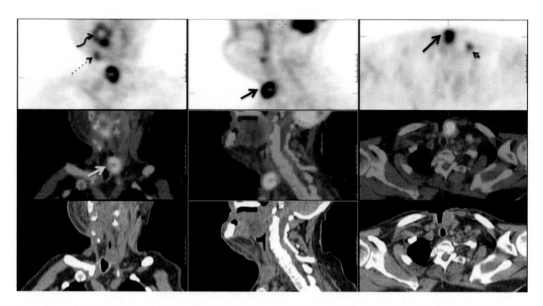

Fig. 2. Supraglottic malignancy treated with surgery, chemotherapy, and radiation, which was completed 3 months prior to the FDG PET-CT scan. PET-CT shows a large necrotic tumor in the right base of the tongue (*curved arrow*), as well as recurrent tumor adjacent to the tracheostomy (*solid arrow*) and a metastatic right level III neck node (*dashed arrow*). The uptake in the lower left neck is in the left anterior scalene muscle and is benign (*arrowhead*).

28 patients with head and neck cancer who were imaged 4 months after completion of radiotherapy (35). Yao et al. found a similar high negative predictive value in 53 patients who were imaged with FDG PET at 3 months posttreatment (100%); however, the specificity was lower at 43% (36). A negative FDG PET study after chemoradiation has a very high negative predictive value even when there is residual nodal enlargement on follow-up CT. Comparing PET studies obtained at a median of 3 months after treatment with histology from salvage surgery in 39 patients with residual nodal enlargement after chemoradiation, Porceddu et al. have reported a negative predictive value of 97% for PET and a positive predictive value of 71% (37). Although there is general agreement that a 3-month postradiation PET scan has an acceptable accuracy, earlier PET imaging may be desirable, as many surgeons prefer to perform the salvage surgery within 6–8 weeks after radiation, before postradiation fibrotic changes develop in the neck (38). At least two studies have shown that 1-month posttherapy PET has an unacceptably low sensitivity. Greven et al. have reported that the sensitivity of 1-month PET for detection of residual disease was only 59% compared to 100% for 4-month posttherapy PET (35). In another study, Rogers et al. have reported a sensitivity of 45% for a 1-month posttherapy FDG PET in comparison to the 6–8 week posttreatment surgical histopathology (39). Data for accuracy of FDG PET scans obtained between 1 and 3 months after therapy is limited; however,

in a recent meta-analysis the sensitivity of PET was significantly lower if performed earlier than 10 weeks after completion of radiation therapy (33). In summary, a PET scan performed 10–12 weeks months after radiation or chemoradiation therapy has a high negative predictive value so that patients with negative studies can be safely followed up without intervention. A positive PET finding needs to be confirmed before management decisions are made as postradiation changes lower the specificity of FDG PET.

False-positive FDG uptake in the posttherapy setting is seen secondary to reactive inflammatory changes from treatment, infection, or osteoradionecrosis. There is a significant overlap in SUV between recurrent tumors and posttherapy changes and no SUV cutoff has been found to outperform visual analysis by an experienced reader. If the initial biopsy after a positive PET scan fails to demonstrate tumor, a follow-up PET scan is suggested in 2–3 months (40, 41). Tumor is very unlikely if the uptake on the follow-up PET scan is decreased (consistent with healing), whereas repeat biopsy is usually necessary if the SUV is unchanged or has increased in the interval.

7. Radiotherapy Planning with PET-CT

FDG PET-CT is beginning to be used frequently as an adjunct to radiotherapy treatment planning. One of the most obvious uses is to include all sites that are identified as FDG avid tumor in the radiation field since tumors with high FDG uptake have a high recurrence rate and poor prognosis (42). The FDG PET data needs to be imported into the treatment planning computer and co-registered with the treatment planning CT scan to be able to incorporate it into the radiation treatment planning. For precise co-registration, the same immobilization head mask should be used for the treatment planning CT and the PET or PET/CT scan. In a pilot study by Ciernik et al., the co-registration of PET/CT with the planning CT images was highly successful with average deviations of 1.2 ± 0.8 mm in the x-axis, 1.5 ± 1.2 mm in the y-axis, and 2.1 1.1 mm in the z-axis (43). Paulino et al. were able to consistently obtain a co-registration error of <5 mm (44). Incorporation of FDG PET into radiotherapy planning may significantly alter the target gross tumor volume (GTV). The GTV may be increased because a metabolically active tumor can be detected in normal sized nodes. The PET-based GTV may be smaller than CT-based GTV in some patients because the tumor may not be metabolically active in its entirety or because of benign enlarged nodes that are not hypermetabolic.

Paulino et al. compared the CT-based and PET-CT-based GTV in 40 patients who underwent intensity-modulated radiation therapy (IMRT) for squamous cell carcinoma of the head and neck (44). They found that the PET-based GTV was significantly smaller compared to CT-based GTV and furthermore metabolically active tumor would have been underdosed in approximately 25% of patients if only CT-based GTV was used for IMRT. Heron et al. found that the nodal target volume was approximately 43% higher with PET-based GTV compared with CT-based GTV as PET identified additional hypermetabolic nodal metastases that were too small to detect using CT (45). In addition to treatment volume, FDG PET can also change the intent from curative to palliative therapy by identification of distant metastases (46). Although the use of PET is gaining more acceptance in the radiation oncology community, issues remain that need to be addressed before PET/CT is used as a routine tool for radiotherapy planning in head and neck cancer (47). Contouring the tumor volume with PET is not standardized; the target volume on PET will be significantly overestimated with an increased window level and can be underestimated by lowering the PET window. 50% of the tumor/image maximum intensity has been used by some groups (48), while others have used intensity of liver uptake (45) or standardized uptake value (SUV) of 2.5 for their threshold standard (49). So far, there have been no studies showing that the changes in treatment volume actually improve outcome.

References

1. Jemal, A., Siegel, R., Ward, E., et al. (2008) Cancer statistics, 2008. *CA Cancer J Clin* **58**, 71–96.

2. Lindholm, P., Minn, H., Leskinen-Kallio, S., Bergman, J., Ruotsalainen, U., Joensuu, H. (1993) Influence of the blood glucose concentration on FDG uptake in cancer–a PET study. *J Nucl Med* **34**, 1–6.

3. Yeung, H.W., Grewal, R.K., Gonen, M., Schoder, H., Larson, S.M. (2003) Patterns of (18)F-FDG uptake in adipose tissue and muscle: a potential source of false-positives for PET. *J Nucl Med* **44**, 1789–96.

4. Garcia, C.A., Van Nostrand, D., Atkins, F., et al. (2006) Reduction of brown fat 2-deoxy-2-[F-18]fluoro-D-glucose uptake by controlling environmental temperature prior to positron emission tomography scan. *Mol Imaging Biol* **8**, 24–9.

5. Brink, I., Klenzner, T., Krause, T., et al. (2002) Lymph node staging in extracranial head and neck cancer with FDG PET – appropriate uptake period and size-dependence of the results. *Nuklearmedizin* **41**, 108–13.

6. Graham, M.M., Menda, Y. (2005) Positron emission tomography/computed tomography imaging of head and neck tumors: an atlas. *Semin Nucl Med* **35**, 220–52.

7. Greene F., Fleming, I.D. (2002) *AJCC (American Joint Committee on Cancer) Cancer Staging Manual* 6th edn, Springer-Verlag, New York.

8. Robbins, K.T., Clayman, G., Levine, P.A., et al. (2002) Neck dissection classification update: revisions proposed by the American Head and Neck Society and the American Academy of Otolaryngology-Head and Neck Surgery. *Arch Otolaryngol Head Neck Surg* **128**, 751–8.

9. Di Martino, E., Nowak, B., Krombach, G.A., et al. (2000) Results of pretherapeutic lymph node diagnosis in head and neck tumors. Clinical value of 18-FDG positron emission tomography (PET). *Laryngorhinootologie* **79**, 201–6.

10. Hannah, A., Scott, A.M., Tochon-Danguy, H., et al. (2002) Evaluation of 18 F- fluorodeoxyglucose positron emission tomography and computed tomography with histopathologic correlation in the initial staging of head and neck cancer. *Ann Surg* **236**, 208–17.

11. Kresnik, E., Mikosch, P., Gallowitsch, H.J., et al. (2001) Evaluation of head and neck

cancer with 18 F-FDG PET: a comparison with conventional methods. *Eur J Nucl Med* **28**, 816–21.

12. Stuckensen, T., Kovacs, A.F., Adams, S., Baum, R.P. (2000) Staging of the neck in patients with oral cavity squamous cell carcinomas: a prospective comparison of PET, ultrasound, CT and MRI. *J Craniomaxillofac Surg* **28**, 319–24.

13. Civantos, F.J., Gomez, C., Duque, C., et al. (2003) Sentinel node biopsy in oral cavity cancer: correlation with PET scan and immunohistochemistry. *Head Neck* **25**, 1–9.

14. Hyde, N.C., Prvulovich, E., Newman, L., Waddington, W.A., Visvikis, D., Ell, P. (2003) A new approach to pre-treatment assessment of the N0 neck in oral squamous cell carcinoma: the role of sentinel node biopsy and positron emission tomography. *Oral Oncol* **39**, 350–60.

15. Stoeckli, S.J., Steinert, H., Pfaltz, M., Schmid, S. (2002) Is there a role for positron mission tomography with 18 F-fluorodeoxyglucose in the initial staging of nodal negative oral and oropharyngeal squamous cell carcinoma. *Head Neck* **24**, 345–9.

16. Schoder, H., Carlson, D.L., Kraus, D.H., et al. (2006) 18 F-FDG PET/CT for detecting nodal metastases in patients with oral cancer staged N0 by clinical examination and CT/MRI. *J Nucl Med* **47**, 755–62.

17. Kim, S.Y., Roh, J.L., Yeo, N.K., et al. (2007) Combined 18 F-fluorodeoxyglucose-positron emission tomography and computed tomography as a primary screening method for detecting second primary cancers and distant metastases in patients with head and neck cancer. *Ann Oncol* **18**, 1698–703.

18. Goerres, G.W., Schmid, D.T., Gratz, K.W., von Schulthess, G.K., Eyrich, G.K. (2003) Impact of whole body positron emission tomography on initial staging and therapy in patients with squamous cell carcinoma of the oral cavity. *Oral Oncol* **39**, 547–51.

19. Schwartz, D.L., Rajendran, J., Yueh, B., et al. (2003) Staging of head and neck squamous cell cancer with extended-field FDG-PET. *Arch Otolaryngol Head Neck Surg* **129**, 1173–8.

20. Sigg, M.B., Steinert, H., Gratz, K., Hugenin, P., Stoeckli, S., Eyrich, G.K., et al. (2003) Staging of head and neck tumors: [18 F]fluorodeoxyglucose positron emission tomography compared with physical examination and conventional imaging modalities. *J Oral Maxillofac Surg* **61**, 1022–9.

21. Teknos, T.N., Rosenthal, E.L., Lee, D., Taylor, R., Marn, C.S. (2001) Positron emission tomography in the evaluation of stage III and IV head and neck cancer *Head Neck* **23**, 1056–60.

22. Mendenhall, W.M., Mancuso, A.A., Parsons, J.T., Stringer, S.P., Cassisi, N.J. (1998) Diagnostic evaluation of squamous cell carcinoma metastatic to cervical lymph nodes from an unknown head and neck primary site. *Head Neck* **20**, 739–44.

23. Mendenhall, W.M., Mancuso, A.A., Amdur, R.J., Stringer, S.P., Villaret, D.B., Cassisi, N.J. (2001) Squamous cell carcinoma metastatic to the neck from an unknown head and neck primary site. *Am J Otolaryngol* **22**, 261–7.

24. Rusthoven, K.E., Koshy, M., Paulino, A.C. (2004) The role of fluorodeoxyglucose positron emission tomography in cervical lymph node metastases from an unknown primary tumor. *Cancer* **101**, 2641–9.

25. Fogarty, G.B., Peters, L.J., Stewart, J., Scott, C., Rischin, D., Hicks, R.J. (2003) The usefulness of fluorine 18-labelled deoxyglucose positron emission tomography in the investigation of patients with cervical lymphadenopathy from an unknown primary tumor. *Head Neck* **25**, 138–45.

26. Greven, K.M., Keyes, J.W., Jr., Williams, D.W., III, McGuirt, W.F., Joyce, W.T., III. (1999) Occult primary tumors of the head and neck: lack of benefit from positron emission tomography imaging with 2-[F-18] fluoro-2-deoxy-D-glucose. *Cancer* **86**, 114–8.

27. Johansen, J., Eigtved, A., Buchwald, C., Theilgaard, S.A., Hansen, H.S. (2002) Implication of 18 F-fluoro-2-deoxy-D-glucose positron emission tomography on management of carcinoma of unknown primary in the head and neck: a Danish cohort study. *Laryngoscope* **112**, 2009–14.

28. Jungehulsing, M., Scheidhauer, K., Damm, M., et al. (2000) 2[F]-fluoro-2-deoxy-D-glucose positron emission tomography is a sensitive tool for the detection of occult primary cancer (carcinoma of unknown primary syndrome) with head and neck lymph node manifestation. *Otolaryngol Head Neck Surg* **123**, 294–301.

29. Kole, A.C., Nieweg, O.E., Pruim, J., et al. (1998) Detection of unknown occult primary tumors using positron emission tomography. *Cancer* **82**, 1160–6.

30. Wong, W.L., Saunders, M. (2003) The impact of FDG PET on the management of occult primary head and neck tumours. *Clin Oncol (R Coll Radiol)* **15**, 461–6.

31. Goodwin, W.J., Jr. (2000) Salvage surgery for patients with recurrent squamous cell carcinoma of the upper aerodigestive tract: when

do the ends justify the means. *Laryngoscope* **110**, 1–18.

32. Klabbers, B.M., Lammertsma, A.A., Slotman, B.J. (2003) The value of positron emission tomography for monitoring response to radiotherapy in head and neck cancer. *Mol Imaging Biol* **5**, 257–70.

33. Isles, M.G., McConkey, C., Mehanna, H.M. (2008) A systematic review and meta-analysis of the role of positron emission tomography in the follow up of head and neck squamous cell carcinoma following radiotherapy or chemoradiotherapy. *Clin Otolaryngol* **33**, 210–22.

34. Yao, M., Smith, R.B., Hoffman, H.T., et al. (2009) Clinical significance of postradiotherapy [18 F]-fluorodeoxyglucose positron emission tomography imaging in management of head-and-neck cancer – a long-term outcome report. *Int J Radiat Oncol Biol Phys* **74**, 9–14.

35. Greven, K.M., Williams, D.W., III, McGuirt, W.F., Sr., et al. (2001) Serial positron emission tomography scans following radiation therapy of patients with head and neck cancer. *Head Neck* **23**, 942–6.

36. Yao, M., Smith, R.B., Graham, M.M., et al. (2005) The role of FDG PET in management of neck metastasis from head-and-neck cancer after definitive radiation treatment. *Int J Radiat Oncol Biol Phys* **63**, 991–9.

37. Porceddu, S.V., Jarmolowski, E., Hicks, R.J., et al. (2005) Utility of positron emission tomography for the detection of disease in residual neck nodes after (chemo)radiotherapy in head and neck cancer. *Head Neck* **27**, 175–81.

38. Kutler, D.I., Patel, S.G., Shah, J.P. (2004) The role of neck dissection following definitive chemoradiation. *Oncology (Williston Park)* **18**, 993–8; discussion 999, 1003–4, 1007.

39. Rogers, J.W., Greven, K.M., McGuirt, W.F., et al. (2004) Can post-RT neck dissection be omitted for patients with head-and-neck cancer who have a negative PET scan after definitive radiation therapy. *Int J Radiat Oncol Biol Phys* **58**, 694–7.

40. Schoder, H., Yeung, H.W. (2004) Positron emission imaging of head and neck cancer, including thyroid carcinoma. *Semin Nucl Med* **34**, 180–97.

41. Terhaard, C.H., Bongers, V., van Rijk, P.P., Hordijk, G.J. (2001) F-18-fluoro-deoxy-glucose positron-emission tomography scanning in detection of local recurrence after radiotherapy for laryngeal/pharyngeal cancer. *Head Neck* **23**, 933–41.

42. Allal, A.S., Slosman, D.O., Kebdani, T., Allaoua, M., Lehmann, W., Dulguerov, P. (2004) Prediction of outcome in head-and-neck cancer patients using the standardized uptake value of 2-[18 F]fluoro-2-deoxy-D-glucose. *Int J Radiat Oncol Biol Phys* **59**, 1295–300.

43. Ciernik, I.F., Dizendorf, E., Baumert, B.G., et al. (2003) Radiation treatment planning with an integrated positron emission and computer tomography (PET/CT): a feasibility study. *Int J Radiat Oncol Biol Phys* **57**, 853–63.

44. Paulino, A.C., Koshy, M., Howell, R., Schuster, D., Davis, L.W. (2005) Comparison of CT- and FDG-PET-defined gross tumor volume in intensity-modulated radiotherapy for head-and-neck cancer. *Int J Radiat Oncol Biol Phys* **61**, 1385–92.

45. Heron, D.E., Andrade, R.S., Flickinger, J., et al. (2004) Hybrid PET-CT simulation for radiation treatment planning in head-and-neck cancers: a brief technical report. *Int J Radiat Oncol Biol Phys* **60**, 1419–24.

46. Dietl, B., Marienhagen, J., Kuhnel, T., Schreyer, A., Kolbl, O. (2008) The impact of FDG-PET/CT on the management of head and neck tumours: the radiotherapist's perspective. *Oral Oncol* **44**, 504–8.

47. Paulino, A.C., Johnstone, P.A. (2004) FDG-PET in radiotherapy treatment planning: Pandora's box. *Int J Radiat Oncol Biol Phys* **59**, 4–5.

48. Scarfone, C., Lavely, W.C., Cmelak, A.J., et al. (2004) Prospective feasibility trial of radiotherapy target definition for head and neck cancer using 3-dimensional PET and CT imaging. *J Nucl Med* **45**, 543–52.

49. Wang, D., Schultz, C.J., Jursinic, P.A., et al. (2006) Initial experience of FDG-PET/CT guided IMRT of head-and-neck carcinoma. *Int J Radiat Oncol Biol Phys* **65**, 143–51.

Chapter 3

PET and PET-CT of Lung Cancer

Hans C. Steinert

Abstract

Accurate staging is essential to offer the patient the most effective available treatment and the best estimate of prognosis. In non-small cell lung cancer (NSCLC), surgical resection offers the best chance of cure in the early stages, either alone or in combination with chemo- or radiotherapy at the more advanced stages. However, many patients present with metastatic disease at the time of diagnosis.

Both computed tomography (CT) and positron emission tomography (PET) using fluorodeoxyglucose (FDG) play an important role in the diagnosis and staging of lung cancer. CT provides excellent morphologic information but has significant limitations in differentiating between benign and malignant lesions either in an organ or in lymph nodes. FDG-PET is highly accurate in the detection of mediastinal lymph node metastases as well as extratharacic metastases. However, due to the poor anatomic information provided by PET, additional morphologic information is needed to properly locate a lesion. Imaging with PET integrated with computed tomography (PET/CT) offers essential advantages in comparison to PET alone, CT alone, or visual correlation of separate PET and CT. A combined PET/CT system provides PET and CT images perfectly coregistered so that lesions can be exactly localized.

Key words: Lung cancer, Staging, Positron emission tomography, Computed tomography, Image fusion

1. Introduction

Lung cancer is currently the leading cause of cancer deaths in both men and women in the USA and Europe. Deaths from lung cancer in woman surpassed those of breast cancer in 1987. The incidence of lung cancer is higher in men than in women, but at present the incidence is decreasing in men and increasing in women. Lung cancer is mostly caused by smoking. Heavy smoking is combined with a 20- to 30-fold increase in lung cancer risk compared to nonsmokers. About 25% of lung cancers in nonsmokers are attributed to second-hand smoke. Squamous cell carcinomas, small cell lung carcinoma, large cell carcinoma, and

Malik E. Juweid and Otto S. Hoekstra (eds.), *Positron Emission Tomography*, Methods in Molecular Biology, vol. 727,
DOI 10.1007/978-1-61779-062-1_3, © Springer Science+Business Media, LLC 2011

to a lesser extent adenocarcinoma have an increased incidence with increased number of cigarettes smoked per day. Chronic obstructive lung disease is another risk factor for developing lung cancer, independent of smoking. Decreased clearance of inhaled carcinogens and epithelial metaplasia result in an increased cancer risk. Genetic lesions play an important role in the development of lung cancer. Genetic alterations include abnormalities of tumor suppressor gene inactivation and overactivity of growth-promoting oncogenes. Mutations may occur during adult life as a result of cigarette smoking, but some of them may be acquired during the embryonic development of the bronchial epithelium.

Both the cell type of the tumor and the tumor extent affect the prognosis and survival following treatment. An important distinction is to separate non-small cell lung cancer (NSCLC) from small cell lung cancer (SCLC). The management strategies of both forms are significantly different. In NSCLC, surgical resection offers the best chance of cure in the early stages either alone or in combination with chemo- or radiotherapy at the more advanced stages. However, most patients present with metastatic disease at the time of diagnosis. Patients with small cell lung cancer (SCLC) initially respond well to chemotherapy and radiation treatment and generally do not undergo surgery. However, their long-term prognosis is poor.

2. Non-Small Cell Lung Cancer

Squamous cell carcinoma is strongly associated with cigarette smoking and accounts for about 30% of lung cancer cases. Squamous cell carcinoma typically arises within the main bronchi near the center of the chest (65%). In this central location, tumor growth results in bronchial obstruction of the bronchial lumen. Atelectasis and consolidation are common. Only about 30% of squamous cell carcinoma present in the lung periphery as a lung nodule. Central necrosis and cavitation are more common than with other cell types. Squamous cell carcinoma is the most common cause of Pancoast tumors. These occur typically at the apex of the lung and are associated with Horner's syndrome and bone destruction.

Adenocarcinoma is the most common cell type of lung cancer and accounts for 30–35% of lung cancer cases. They are most common in women and in nonsmokers. Adenocarcinoma most commonly arises in the lung periphery from epithelial cells and is characterized by glandular differentiation and production of mucus. Early metastases particularly to the central nervous system and adrenal glands are common. Seventy-five percent of adenocarcinomas present as a peripheral lung nodule most commonly in the upper lobes. They frequently have an irregular and spiculated margin due to associated lung fibrosis.

Bronchioalveolar carcinoma (BAC) is a well-differentiated subtype of adenocarcinoma. BACs typically grow along the alveolar spaces without invasion of the stroma. It is the most common type of lung cancer in never-smokers. BAC grows along the alveolar spaces without invasion of the stroma. Typically, the nonmucinous subtype of BAC presents as a solitary nodule (60%). This subtype has an excellent prognosis. In 40% of cases, BAC presents as a pneumonia-like consolidation or as multiple nodules throughout the lung. This appearance is typical for the mucinous subtype of BAC and carries a poor prognosis.

Large cell carcinoma is a more poorly differentiated form. Distinction of poorly differentiated squamous cell and adenocarcinoma can be difficult. Large cell carcinomas that express neuroendocrine tumor markers are less responsive to chemotherapy. They account for 10% of lung cancers and typically present as a large peripheral mass. More than 60% are larger than 4 cm at presentation. Large cell carcinoma metastasizes early and has a poor prognosis. It is strongly associated with smoking. Other cell types represent only a small minority of all lung carcinomas.

Carcinoid tumors originate from neuroendocrine cells in the bronchial wall. These tumors are classified as typical and atypical carcinoid tumors. The typical carcinoid is a low-grade malignancy. Metastases are relatively uncommon. The atypical carcinoid is a more aggressive variant and has a poorer prognosis.

3. Small Cell Lung Cancer

Small cell lung cancer (SCLC) accounts for about 20% of all lung cancer cases and represents the most aggressive lung cancer. SCLC is characterized by rapid growth and early metastases, which are present in 60–80% at the time of diagnosis. SCLC is associated with a poor survival prognosis, and it has a very strong association with cigarette smoking. It is considered to be a type of neuroendocrine carcinoma. SCLC is a common cause of paraneoplastic syndromes. SCLC typically occurs in the main bronchi and is commonly associated with bulky mediastinal lymph node metastases. SCLC generally not considered amenable to surgery.

4. Staging

Appropriate staging is critical in the selection of treatment and in the evaluation of prognosis in patients with lung cancer. The knowledge of the current staging system for lung cancer is essential to understand the role of imaging in the assessment of these patients.

Both CT and PET using F-18 FDG play an important role in the diagnosis and staging of patients with lung cancer. CT provides excellent morphological information, but has significant limitations in differentiating between benign and malignant lesions either in an organ or in lymph nodes. Whole-body PET improves the rate of detection of mediastinal lymph node metastases as well as extrathoracic metastases when compared to CT, MRI, ultrasound (US), or bone scanning. Since good PET scanners have a fairly high resolution (<6 mm), even small lesions can be detected. Limitations are that F-18 FDG is not specific for malignant tissue and that F-18 FDG-PET provides little information on the exact anatomic localization of lesions.

It has been shown that integrated PET-CT provides more than the sum of PET and CT (1–3). In particular it improves T staging. Due to precise CT correlation with the extent of F-18 FDG uptake, the location of the primary tumor can be exactly defined, and thereby diagnosis of chest wall infiltration by the tumor is improved.

5. Classification

After a tissue diagnosis of lung cancer has been established or in patients in whom the clinical suspicion of a lung cancer is high, the determination of the extent of tumor disease is the next step. For choosing the appropriate treatment strategy and to predict survival, it is essential to determine which patients have localized disease and benefit of resection, and alternatively which patients have extensive disease not amenable to surgical resection.

The TNM staging system is widely used to classify NSCLC, which is based on a combination of findings: the location and extent of the primary tumor (T), the presence or absence of intrapulmonary, hilar, or mediastinal lymph node metastases (N), and the presence or absence of extrathoracic metastases (M) (4, 5).

Patients with SCLC have a poor prognosis regardless of tumor stage. SCLC should be regarded as a systemic disease regardless of stage. SCLC is generally classified as either limited (LD) or extensive disease (ED). LD is present, when the disease is confined to one hemithorax, mediastinum, and supraclavicular nodes, which can be targeted with a single radiation portal field. Disease extension outside the thorax or the existence of malignant pleural effusion is considered as ED. Patients with SCLC are generally not candidates for surgery. Patients with ED receive chemotherapy alone. In patients with LD, a combined radiation and chemotherapy approach is used.

6. TNM-Classification of Non-Small Cell Lung Cancer

6.1. Primary Tumor

T1 lung cancer presents as a small peripheral nodule which is surrounded by the lung or visceral pleura. T1 tumors are divided into T1a ($\leq$2 cm) and T1b (>2 to $\leq$3 cm). These tumors are easily resectable.

T2 tumors are divided into T2a (>3 to $\leq$5 cm) and T2b (>5 to $\leq$7 cm). T2 carcinomas may invade the visceral pleura or are associated with atelectasis or obstructive pneumonitis that extends to the hilar region.

T3 lung cancer is a tumor >7 cm or invading the chest wall, diaphragma, mediastinal pleura, or parietal pericardium, or a tumor involving the main bronchus less than 2 cm from the carina or associated with atelectasis or obstructive pneumonitis of the entire lung. Additional nodes in the same lobe as primary tumors are classified as T3.

T4 lung cancer is a tumor invading the mediastinum, heart, great vessels, trachea, esophagus, vertebral body, carina, or a tumor with pleural or pericardial effusion. Additional nodes in another ipsilateral lobe present T4 carcinoma.

6.2. Nodal Disease

N1 disease refers to peribronchial and ipsilateral hilar metastases including direct extension. All N1 nodes lie distal to the mediastinal pleural reflection and within the visceral pleura. These patients are considered respectable. However, the presence of ipsilateral hilar lymph node metastases decreases the overall survival rate.

N2 disease refers to ipsilateral paratracheal and/or subcarinal lymph node metastases. These patients have potentially resectable disease. Today, at our institution, most patients with N2 disease receive neoadjuvant chemotherapy for reduction of the tumor mass before surgery.

N3 disease refers to contralateral mediastinal nodal metastases, contralateral hilar nodal metastases, and ipsilateral or contralateral scalene or supraclavicular nodal metastases. N3 disease is considered unresectable.

6.3. Distant Metastases

Distant metastases are present in about 10–40% of patients with newly diagnosed NSCLC and carry a poor prognosis. They are most common with adenocarcinoma and large cell carcinoma. Most frequent sites of extrathoracic metastases are adrenal glands, liver, bone, and brain.

Adrenal metastases occur in about 20% of patients with NSCLC and are often the only site of extrathoracic spread. Liver metastases are present in 5–10% of patients. Isolated liver metastases are uncommon. Bone metastases are present at diagnosis in approximately 10% of cases. Osteolytic lesions are most common with squamous cell carcinoma and large cell carcinoma. Adenocarcinoma produces combined osteolytic and osteoblastic bone metastases. Most commonly are involved with the vertebrae, pelvis, and proximal extremities. Brain metastases are the most frequent site of extrathoracic metastasis in patients without lymph node involvement. They occur in about 15% of patients and are often symptomatic.

Recently, M category was subclassified into two groups. M1a status represents contralateral lung metastases or pleural dissemination. M1b disease refers to extrathoracic metastases.

6.4. Staging Groups

NSCLC is also classified into four stages (4–6). Stage I and II tumors are usually treated by surgical resection. Stage I is subgrouped into stage Ia (T1 N0 M0) and stage Ib (T2a N0 M0). Stage II is divided into stage IIa (T1 N1 M0, T2a N1 M0, T2b N0 M0) and stage IIb (T2b N1 M0, T3 N0 M0). Stage III is divided into stage IIIA (T1-T2 N2 M0, T3 N1-N2 M0, T4 N0-N1 M0) and stage IIIB (T1-T3 N3 M0). Stage IIIa tumors are often treated by chemotherapy followed by surgery, while stage IIIB is considered unresectable and treated by radiation or chemotherapy, or both. Stage IV includes those patients with evidence of distant metastasis. These patients are treated by chemotherapy.

7. Imaging in the Evaluation and Staging of Lung Cancer

7.1. Solitary Lung Nodule

Lung masses have been evaluated traditionally by using planar chest X-rays, CT, and more recently MRI. Some radiographic parameters such as calcifications and smooth margins of a lesion may indicate a lower likelihood that a solitary nodule is malignant, although a substantial portion remains radiographically indeterminate. Factors that increase the probability of malignancy include size, absence of calcification, and irregular margins. Unchanged radiographic appearance of a nodule at follow-up examinations over a 2-year period implies that the lesion is benign. Definite diagnoses are established with invasive techniques such as bronchoscopy, mediastinoscopy, and biopsy. If the lesion is benign, nondiagnostic biopsy results are not uncommon.

The ability of PET to separate between benign and malignant lesions is high but not perfect. For benign lesions, Patz et al. (7) demonstrated a very high specificity for F-18 FDG-PET. Gupta et al. (8) showed that F-18 FDG-PET is highly accurate in differentiating malignant from benign solitary pulmonary nodules for sizes from 6 to 30 mm when radiographic findings are indeterminate. In a series of 61 patients, PET had a sensitivity of 93% and a specificity of 88% for detecting malignancy. However, F-18

FDG-PET may show negative results for pulmonary carcinoids and BAC (9, 10).

PET is clinically useful in patients with a solitary pulmonary nodule less than 3 cm in diameter, especially where biopsy may be risky or where there is a low risk for malignancy based on the history or radiographic findings. Lesions with low F-18 FDG uptake can be considered to be benign and monitored with chest radiographs. Lesions with increased F-18 FDG uptake should be considered malignant, although false-positive results have been reported in cases of inflammatory and infectious processes, such as histoplasmosis, aspergillosis, or active tuberculosis. With integrated PET-CT, additional certainty to the presence or absence of F-18 FDG uptake in the pulmonary nodule can be achieved because morphologic CT criteria and functional CT criteria are available simultaneously.

7.2. T Staging

CT is an important imaging modality for the evaluation of the primary tumor. However, the low accuracy of chest CT in the evaluation of invasion of the chest wall or involvement of the mediastinum and the correct differentiation between tumor and peritumoral atelectasis is often limiting precise T staging with CT (11). A disadvantage of PET is the limited anatomical resolution which makes the assessment of tumor extension unreliable, particularly if the tumor infiltrates the chest wall or the mediastinum.

It has been demonstrated that integrated PET-CT is a useful tool for the detection of tumor invasion into the chest wall (1–3). Due to the exact anatomic correlation to the F-18 FDG uptake, the delineation of the primary tumor can be defined precisely. Therefore the diagnosis of chest wall infiltration and mediastinal invasion by the tumor is improved. Lesions with chest wall infiltration are classified as Stage T3 and are potentially resectable. Surgical treatment requires en bloc resection of the primary tumor and the contiguous chest wall. Particularly in patients with poor cardio-pulmonary reserve, the preoperative determination of chest wall infiltration is desirable in order to avoid extended en bloc resection.

Integrated PET-CT provides important information on mediastinal infiltration as well. Contrast-enhanced CT to evaluate infiltration of hilar and vessels have a relatively low sensitivity, specificity, and accuracy (12). Our experience suggests that unenhanced PET-CT imaging is unable to identify direct invasion of the walls of vital mediastinal structures. Therefore, we currently use contrast-enhanced CT in most patients receiving an integrated PET-CT scan.

It has been shown that F-18 FDG-PET is a useful tool for the differentiation between tumor and peritumoral atelectasis. This is particularly important for the planning of radiotherapy in patients with lung cancer associated with an atelectasis.

7.3. N Staging

Accurate mediastinal staging is particularly important, as the status of these nodes will in many cases determine whether surgical resection of lung cancer is possible.

Surgical resection is the treatment of choice for early stages of NSCLC. Patients with ipsilateral mediastinal lymph node metastases (N2 disease) are considered to have potentially resectable disease (Fig. 1). If contralateral mediastinal lymph node metastases (N3 disease) are present, surgery is generally not indicated. CT and MRI have substantial limitations in depicting

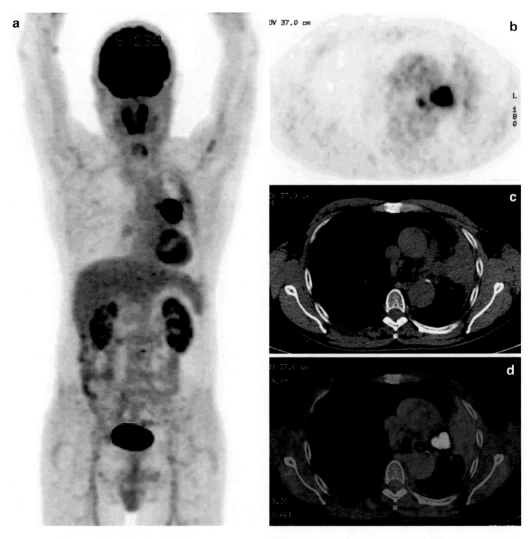

Fig. 1. A 60-year-old man with a histologically proven adenocarcinoma in the left central lung. PET/CT was performed for staging. The images include a MIP scan (**a**), a transaxial PET section (**b**), a corresponding transaxial low-dose and nonenhanced CT section (**c**), and a corresponding transaxial PET/CT section (**d**). Diagnosis based on coregistered PET/CT imaging: Central lung tumor in the left lung, with a lymph node metastasis in the aortopulmonary window. No extrathoracic lesions. Induction chemotherapy was planned on the basis of this information.

mediastinal lymph node metastases. The only CT and MR criteria for tumor involvement are morphologic; that is, the criteria rely on the size and shape of the lymph nodes. However, normal-sized regional lymph nodes may prove to have metastases upon histologic examination, and nodal enlargement can be due to reactive hyperplasia or other nonmalignant conditions. The sensitivity and specificity of identifying mediastinal lymph node metastases of NSCLC by CT is 51% (95% confidence interval, 47–54%) and 85% (95% confidence interval, 84–88%), respectively (13).

Several studies have demonstrated that F-18 FDG-PET is significantly more accurate than CT in the determination of nodal status (14–16). Since good PET scanners have a fairly high resolution (<6 mm), even small lesions with an increased F-18 FDG uptake can be detected. This represents a critical advantage of PET over CT and MRI. For PET scanning, the sensitivity and specificity for identifying mediastinal lymph node metastases are 74% (95% confidence interval, 69–79%) and 85% (95% confidence interval, 82–88%) (13). Corresponding positive and negative likelihood ratios for mediastinal staging with PET scanning are 4.9 and 0.3, respectively. Even PET scanning is more accurate than CT scanning for mediastinal staging, it is not perfect.

Some studies have demonstrated that the accuracy of PET imaging in the mediastinum is dependent on the size of the nodal involvement. PET scanning is more sensitive but less specific when CT imaging identifies enlarged nodes. A median sensitivity and specificity of PET scans of 100 and 78%, respectively, in patients with enlarged lymph nodes has been reported (13). It has been concluded that PET scanning is very accurate in identifying malignant nodal involvement when nodes are enlarged.

Conversely, PET scanning is less sensitive but more specific in patients with normal-sized mediastinal nodes by CT scanning. It has been shown that CT scanning of the mediastinum is falsely negative in about 20% of patients with normal-sized nodes but malignant involvement.

Gould et al. reported a median sensitivity and specificity in these patients of 82 and 93%, respectively (17). These data indicate that nearly 20% of patients with normal-sized nodes but with malignant involvement had falsely negative PET scans. Most likely, the negative PET results are due to microscopic or inhomogeneous tumor involvement of the nodes.

With either imaging test, pathological findings must be confirmed by tissue biopsy to ensure accurate staging. The findings of PET-CT guide the pneumologists and surgeons to the suspicious lymph nodes. In general, the biopsy of the lymph node with the highest stage by endoscopic bronchial ultrasound (EBUS) or mediastinoscopy is sufficient for further treatment decisions.

However, not all mediastinal lymph nodes are routinely reachable by EBUS or mediastinoscopy (paraaortic region, aortopulmonary window). The limited view through the mediastinoscope and the single direction approach of the biopsy prevent 100% accuracy. The accuracy of mediastinoscopy is approximately 90% and surgeon dependent (18). Recently, it has been demonstrated that PET assists mediastinoscopy. Due to the PET information, mediastinoscopy revealed additional mediastinal disease in 6% of patients (19). F-18 FDG-PET may reduce the necessity for mediastinoscopy if the primary tumor is localized in the periphery of the lung and the mediastinum is PET negative. This approach would reduce the need for mediastinoscopy by 12%.

There is an ongoing controversy whether a negative PET scan can be used to obviate further invasive mediastinal staging. Microscopic foci of metastases within normal-sized lymph nodes cannot be detected with any imaging modality. In our institution, in patients with negative PET scan but with enlarged mediastinal lymph nodes by CT scan further evaluation by EBUS or mediastinoscopy will be performed. While PET scanning samples all mediastinal lymph node groups, it is less sensitive in nodes <8 mm. While mediastinoscopy cannot sample all mediastinal nodal groups, it can reveal microscopic involvement even in small lymph nodes.

In our experience, integrated PET-CT imaging will become the new standard of mediastinal staging. The high reliability of integrated PET-CT in the exact localization of extrathoracic vs. intrathoracic and mediastinal vs. hilar lymph nodes might have very important therapeutic implications.

7.4. M Staging

Despite radical surgical treatment of potentially curable NSCLC the overall 5-year survival rate remains low (20–40%). One reason for this is undetected extrathoracic metastases, which cause underestimation of the tumor stage. Whole-body F-18 FDG-PET is an excellent method to screen for extrathoracic metastases with exception of the brain (20) (Fig. 2). In a meta-analysis of 581 patients, sensitivity, specificity, and accuracy of F-18 FDG-PET were 94, 97, and 96%, respectively (21). Current imaging methods are inadequate for accurate M staging of patients. PET detects unexpected extrathoracic metastases in 10–20% of patients and changes therapeutic management in about 20% of patients. F-18 FDG-PET is more accurate than CT in the evaluation of adrenal metastases (22, 23). Marom et al. (24) compared the accuracy of F-18 FDG-PET to conventional imaging in 100 patients with newly diagnosed NSCLC. Comparing bone scintigraphy and F-18 FDG-PET for the detection of bone metastases, the accuracy was 87 and 98%, respectively. All hepatic metastases were correctly identified with PET and CT. With CT, however,

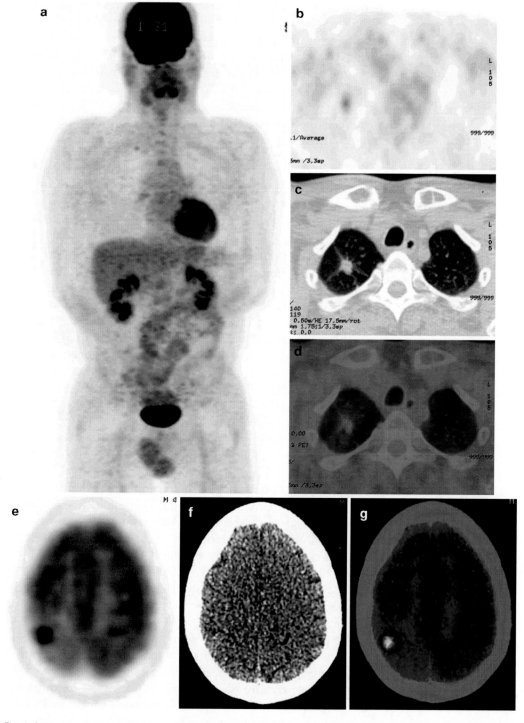

Fig. 2. A 50-year-old man with a suspicious lesion in the right upper lobe. The man was a heavy smoker. PET/CT was performed for staging. The images include a MIP scan (**a**), axial PET sections (**b, e**), corresponding axial low-dose and nonenhanced CT sections (**c, f**), and corresponding axial PET/CT sections (**d, g**). Diagnosis based on integrated PET/CT imaging: Lung tumor in the right upper lobe. No mediastinal metastases. Single brain metastasis. Surgical resection of the primary tumor and of the brain metastasis were performed.

benign liver lesions were over-staged as metastases, thus accuracy of PET was superior to CT in the diagnosis of liver metastases. The advantage of integrated PET-CT imaging is the exact localization and classification of a hot spot on PET, especially when no morphological alterations are seen on CT images (1–3). Due to the physiological F-18 FDG uptake in the brain, the detection of brain metastases by PET is poor. Therefore, in patients with neurological symptoms a MRI of the brain should be performed.

7.5. False-Negative and False-Positive F-18 FDG-PET Results

False-negative F-18 FDG-PET results have been reported in pulmonary carcinoid tumors and in BACs (9, 10). Typical carcinoid tumors are highly differentiated and are low-grade malignant carcinomas. These factors might result in a lower sensitivity of F-18 FDG-PET.

Spatial resolution limitations of PET also can be responsible for false-negative results. PET cannot detect lymph node metastases smaller than 4–6 mm. The detection of micrometastases is not possible with any imaging modality. It has been reported that F-18 FDG-PET after induction therapy is less accurate in mediastinal staging than in staging of untreated NSCLC (25). PET overstaged nodal status in 33% of patients, understaged nodal status in 15%, and was correct in 52%. Future studies have to be required to correlate F-18 FDG-PET before and after treatment with the degree of pathologic response.

False-positive results can be due to the lack of specificity of F-18 FDG with regard to inflammatory lesions. Lung empysema, tuberculosis, eosinophilic lung disease, histoplasmosis, aspergillosis, and other infections may have a significant uptake of F-18 FDG (26). Occult lung infarction may induce false interpretation of F-18 FDG accumulation in PET imaging (27). Therefore, lesions with an increased F-18 FDG accumulation should be histologically confirmed. However, most chronic inflammatory processes do not significantly take up F-18 FDG.

It is well known that active muscles accumulate F-18 FDG. In some patients with lung cancer an intense focal F-18 FDG accumulation is seen in the lower anterior neck just lateral to the midline. Coregistered PET-CT images revealed that this focal F-18 FDG uptake is frequently localized in the internal laryngeal muscles (28). This finding was a result of compensatory laryngeal muscle activation caused by contralateral recurrent laryngeal nerve palsy due to direct nerve invasion by lung cancer of the left mediastinum or lung apices. This is also found with surgically induced lesions of the recurrent nerve. The knowledge of this finding is important to avoid false-positive PET results.

Our own group assessed the incidence and etiology of solitary extrapulmonary lesions with an increased F-18 FDG accumulation

(29). In the study population of 350 patients, PET-CT revealed extrapulmonary lesions in 110 patients. In 72 patients solitary lesions were present. Histopathological correlation revealed in approximately 50% of patients with solitary extrapulmonary lesions metastases of NSCLC, in 25 % of patients unknown second primary, and in 25% of patients benign lesions as acute fracture, colon adenoma, or Warthin's tumor.

8. Recurrent Lung Cancer

Despite radical therapy, the overall 5-year survival rate for patients with NSCLC remains low. Progression of disease may occur as intrathoracic recurrence or metastases. The differentiation of recurrent lung cancer and posttherapeutic changes remains a problem for radiological imaging. Thus, some patients may undergo a biopsy to determine tumor viability, although invasive procedures including transthoracic needle biopsy and open lung biopsy carry associated risks. Furthermore, due to sampling errors, these procedures do not always provide a definitive answer. A high accuracy of F-18 FDG-PET or PET-CT in distinguishing recurrent disease from benign treatment effects has been reported (30–32). PET-CT is helpful to select biopsy sites to confirm recurrent disease. Patients should be evaluated a minimum of 2 months after completion of therapy. Otherwise, posttherapeutic healing processes or radiation pneumonitis may result in false-positive F-18 FDG findings. These abnormal findings return to normal at variable times without further intervention.

9. Therapy Monitoring

The early prediction of tumor response is of high interest in patients with advanced NSCLC. Tumor progression during first-line chemotherapy occurs in approximately one-third of the patients. Thus a significant percentage of patients undergo several weeks of toxic and costly therapy without benefit. It has been shown that effective chemotherapy cause a rapid reduction of the SUV in the primary tumor during the course of therapy (33). In patients without metabolic response, the drug regimen may be changed to second-line therapy, thereby reducing the morbidity and costs from ineffective therapy (Figs. 3 and 4). PET has also been evaluated to assess the response after radiation treatment in patients with NSCLC (34). In this study, PET scans were performed at a median of 70 days after completion of radiation

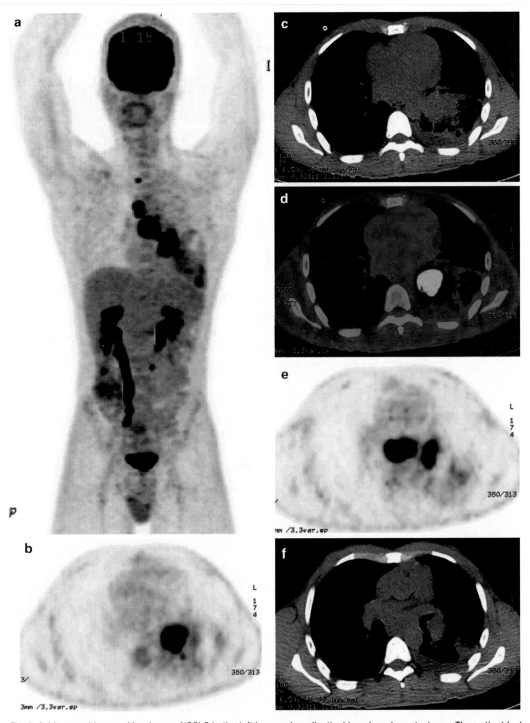

Fig. 3. A 36-year-old man with a known NSCLC in the left lung and mediastinal lymph node metastases. The patient lost 15 kg of weight in 10 weeks. PET/CT was performed for staging, especially for the extent of mediastinal metastases and for distant metastases. The images include a MIP scan (**a**), axial PET sections (**b, e, h, k, n**), corresponding axial low-dose and nonenhanced CT sections (**c, f, i, l, o**), and corresponding axial PET/CT sections (**d, g, j, m, p**). Diagnosis based on integrated PET/CT imaging: Lung tumor in the left lung with poststenotic atelectasis. Subcarinal and multilevel contralateral mediastinal metastases. No extrathoracic metastases. Chemotherapy was started.

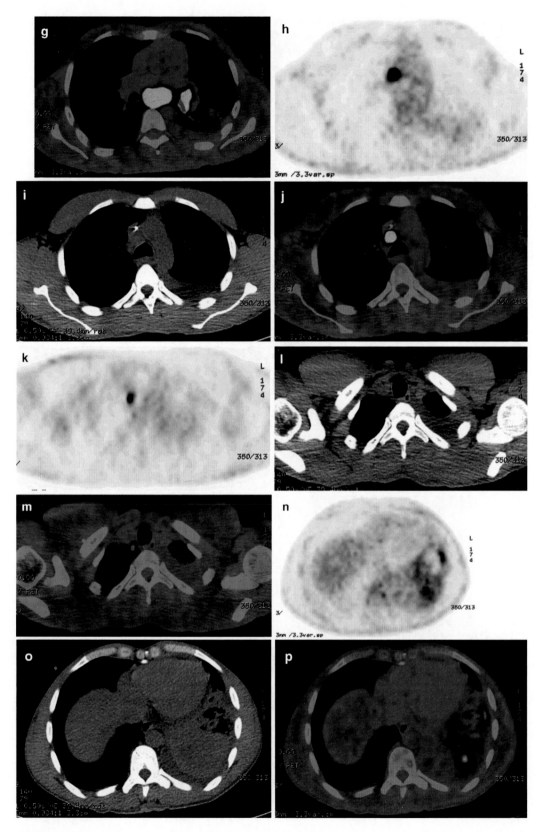

Fig. 3. (continued)

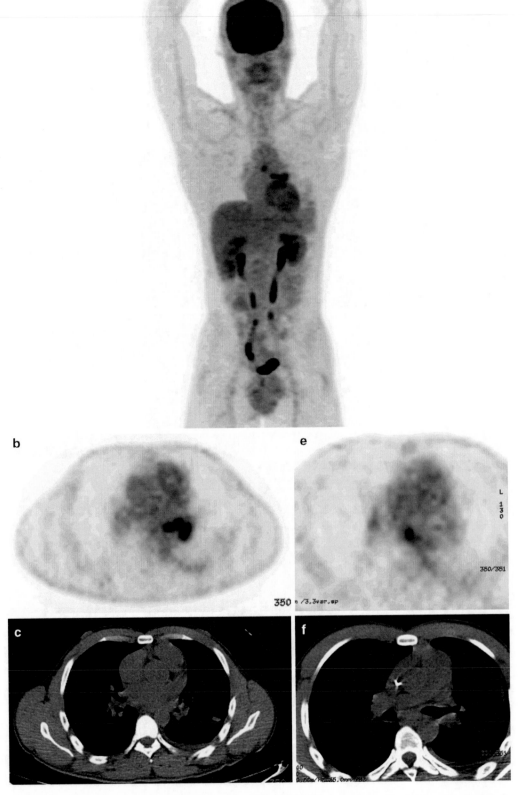

Fig. 4. Same patient as in Fig. 3, after 2 months of chemotherapy. PET/CT was performed for treatment evaluation. The images include a MIP scan (**a**), axial PET sections (**b**, **e**), corresponding axial low-dose and nonenhanced CT sections

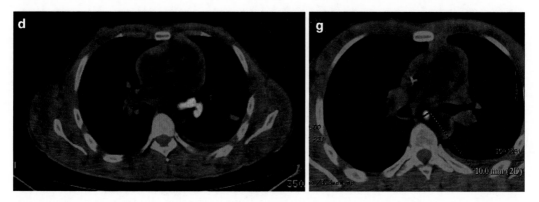

Fig. 4. (continued) (**c, f**), and corresponding axial PET/CT sections (**d, g**). PET/CT imaging demonstrated a partial response on chemotherapy. The contralateral mediastinal lymph node metastases showed a complete metabolic response. Chemotherapy was continued.

treatment. PET imaging allowed differentiation of viable tumor or fibrotic tissue. PET response was significantly associated with survival duration. PET and PET-CT may have a wide application in measuring treatment response in patients with NSCLC. Because prognostic information can be obtained at an early time point, therapies could be modified depending on the PET response.

10. Effectiveness

Gambhir et al. demonstrated that a combined CT- and PET-based strategy is cost-effective in the staging of patients with NSCLC (35). The study evaluated the expected costs and projected life expectancy. The combined CT and PET strategy showed savings of more than 1,000 USD per patient without loss of life expectancy compared with the alternate strategy using CT alone. The major advantage of F-18 FDG-PET is the cost savings that result from a patient with unresectable disease not undergoing unnecessary surgery. The cost savings are the result of improved staging of lung carcinoma before deciding on surgery. In a subsequent study, five decision strategies of selecting potential surgical candidates were compared (36); one was based on thoracic CT alone, while the other four used chest CT plus PET. For all possible outcomes of each strategy, the expected cost and projected life expectancy were compared. A strategy that uses PET after a negative CT study was shown to be a cost-effective alternative to the CT-alone strategy (25,286 US $ per life-year saved). Dietlein et al. demonstrated that the implementation of whole-body F-18 FDG-PET using a dedicated PET scanner in the preoperative staging of patients with NSCLC and normal-sized lymph nodes is clearly cost-effective (37). However, patients with nodal-positive PET results should not be excluded from biopsy. A randomized controlled trial in patients with suspected NSCLC, who were scheduled for surgery after conventional workup, was performed to test whether F-18 FDG-PET reduces the numbers of thoracotomies (38). Patients were followed up for 1 year. Thoracotomy was regarded as futile if the patient had benign disease, explorative thoracotomy, pathological stage IIIA-N2/IIIB, or postoperative relapse or death within 12 months of randomization. The investigators found that addition of PET to standard workup in routine clinical practice improved selection of surgically curable patients and prevented unnecessary surgery in 20% of patients with suspected NSCLC.

References

1. Lardinois, D., Weder, W., Hany, T.F., et al. (2003) Staging of non-small-cell lung cancer with integrated positron-emission tomography and computed tomography. *N Engl J Med* **348**, 2500–7.

2. Antoch, G., Stattaus, J., Nemat, A.T., et al. (2003) Non small cell lung cancer: dual-modality PET-CT in preoperative staging. *Radiology* **229**, 526–33.

3. Sung, S.S., Kyung, S.L., Byung-Tae, K., et al. (2005) Non-small cell lung cancer: prospective comparison of integrated FDG PET-CT and CT alone for preoperative staging. *Radiology* **236**, 1011–19.

4. Mountain, C.F. (2000) The international system for staging lung cancer. *Semin Surg Oncol* **18**, 106–15.

5. Rami-Porta, R., Crowley, J.J., Goldstraw, P. (2009) The revised TNM staging system for lung cancer. *Ann Thorac Cardivasc Surg* **15**, 4–9.

6. Goldstraw, P., Crowley, J.J., Chansky, K., et al. (2007) The IASLC lung cancer staging project: proposals for the revision of the TNM stage groupings in the forthcoming (seventh) edition of the TNM classification of malignant tumors. *J Thorac Oncol* **2**, 706–14.

7. Patz, E.F., Lowe, J.M., Hoffmann, J.M., et al. (1993) Focal pulmonary abnormalities: Evaluation with F-18 fluorodeoxyglucose PET scanning. *Radiology* **188**, 487–90.

8. Gupta, N.C., Maloof, J., Gunel, E. (1996) Probability of malignancy in solitary pulmonary nodules using flurine-18-FDF and PET. *J Nucl Med* **37**, 943–8.

9. Higashi, K., Ueda, Y., Seki, H., et al. (1998) Fluorine-18-FDG imaging is negative in bronchioloalveolar lung carcinoma. *J Nucl Med* **39**, 1016–20.

10. Erasmus, J.J., McAdams, H.P., Patz, E.F., Coleman, R.E., Ahuma, V., Goodman, P.C. (1998) Evaluation of primary pulmonary carcinoid tumors using positron emission tomography with 18F-fluorodeoxyglucose. *AJR Am J Roentgenol* **170**, 1369–73.

11. Webb, W.R., Gatsonis, C., Zerhouni, E., et al. (1991) CT and MR imaging in staging non-small cell bronchogenic carcinoma: Report of the Radiology Diagnostic Oncology Group. *Radiology* **178**, 705–13.

12. Rendina, E.A., Bognolo, D.A., Mineo, T.C., et al. (1987) Computer tomography for the evaluation of intrathoracic invasion by lung cancer. *J Thorac Cardiovasc Surg* **94**, 57–63.

13. Toloza, E., Harpole, L., McCrory, D.C. (2003) Noninvasive staging of non-small cell lung cancer: a review of the current evidence. *Chest* (suppl), 137s–46s.

14. Steinert, H.C., Hauser, M., Allemann, F., et al. (1997) Non-small cell lung cancer: nodal staging with FDG PET versus CT with correlative lymph node mapping and sampling. *Radiology* **202**, 441–6.

15. Vansteenkiste, J.F., Stroobants, S.G., De Leyn, P.R., et al. (1998) Lymph node staging in non-small cell lung cancer with FDG PET scan: a prospective study on 690 lymph node stations from 68 patients. *J Clin Oncol* **16**, 2142–9.

16. Pieterman, R.M., van Putten, J.W.G., Meuzelaar, J.J., et al. (2000) Preoperative staging of non-small-cell lung cancer with positron-emission tomography. *N Engl J Med* **343**, 254–61.

17. Gould, M.K., Kuschner, W.G., Rydzak, C.E., et al. (2003) Test performance of positron emission tomography and computed tomography for mediastinal staging in patients with non-small lung cancer: a meta-analysis. *Ann Intern Med* **139**, 879–92.

18. Patterson, G.A., Ginsberg, R.J., Poon, P.Y., et al. (1987) A prospective evaluation of magnetic resonance imaging, computed tomography, and mediastinoscopy in the preoperative assessment of mediastinal node status in bronchogenic carcinoma. *J Thorac Cardiovasc Surg* **94**, 679–84.

19. Kernstine, K.H., McLaughlin, K.A., Menda, Y., et al. (2002) Can-FDG PET reduce the need for mediastinoscopy in potentially resectable nonsmall cell lung cancer. *Ann Thorac Surg* **73**, 394–402.

20. Weder, W., Schmid, R., Bruchhaus, H., Hillinger, S., von Schulthess, G.K., Steinert, H.C. (1998) Detection of extrathoracic metastases by positron emission tomography in lung cancer. *Ann Thorac Surg* **66**, 886–93.

21. Hellwig, D., Ukena, D., Paulsen, F., Bamberg, M., Kirsch, C.M. (2001) Metaanalyse zum Stellenwert der Positronen-Emissions-Tomographie mit F-18-Fluorodesoxyglucose (FDG-PET) bei Lungentumoren. *Pneumologie* **55**, 367–77.

22. Lamki, L.M. (1997) Positron emission tomography, bronchogenic carcinoma, and the adrenals. *AJR Am J Roentgenol* **168**, 1361–2.

23. Erasmus, J.J., Patz, E.F., McAdams, H.P., et al. (1997) Evaluation of adrenal masses in patients with bronchogenic carcinoma using 18F-fluorodeoxyglucose positron emission tomography. *AJR Am J Roentgenol* **168**, 1357–62.

24. Marom, E.M., McAdams, H.P., Erasmus, J.J. (1999) Staging non-small cell lung cancer with whole-body PET. *Radiology* **212**, 803–9.

25. Akhurst, T., Downey, R.J., Ginsberg, M.S., et al. (2002) An initial experience with FDG-PET in the imaging of residual disease after induction therapy for lung cancer. *Ann Thorac Surg* **73**, 259–66.

26. Strauss, L.G. (1996) Fluorine-18 deoxyglucose and false-positive results: a major problem in the diagnosis of oncological patients. *Eur J Nucl Med* **23**, 1409–14.

27. Kamel, E.M., McKee, T.A., Calcagni, M.L., et al. (2005) Occult lung infarction may induce false interpretation of F-18 FDG PET in primary staging of pulmonary malignancies. *Eur J Nucl Med Mol Imaging* **32**, 641–6.

28. Kamel, E., Goerres, G.W., Burger, C., von Schulthess, G.K., Steinert, H.C. (2002) Detection of recurrent laryngeal nerve palsy in patients with lung cancer using PET-CT image fusion. *Radiology* **224**, 153–6.

29. Lardinois, D., Weder, W., Roudas, M., et al. (2005) Etiology of solitary extrapulmonary positron emission tomography and computed tomography findings in patients with lung cancer. *J Clin Oncol* **23**, 6846–53.

30. Inoue, T., Kim, E., Komaki, R., et al. (1995) Detecting recurrent or residual lung cancer with FDG-PET. *J Nucl Med* **36**, 788–93.

31. Hicks, R.J., Kalff, V., MacManus, M.P., et al. (2001) The utility of F-18 FDG PET for suspected recurrent non-small cell lung cancer after potentially curative therapy: impact on management and prognostic stratification. *J Nucl Med* **42**, 1605–13.

32. Keidar, Z., Haim, N., Guralnik, L., et al. (2004) PET-CT using F-18 FDG in suspected lung cancer recurrence: diagnostic value and impact on patient management. *J Nucl Med* **45**, 1640–6.

33. Weber, W.A., Peterson, V., Schmidt, B., et al. (2003) Positron emission tomography in non-small cell lung cancer: prediction of response to chemotherapy by quantitative assessment to glucose use. *J Clin Oncol* **21**, 2651–7.

34. MacManus, M.P., Hicks, R.J., Matthews, J.P., et al. (2003) Positron emission tomography is superior to computed tomography for response-assessment after radical radiotherapy or chemoradiotherapy in patients with non-small cell lung cancer. *J Clin Oncol* **21**, 1285–92.

35. Gambhir, S.S., Hoh, C.K., Phelps, M.E., Madar, I., Maddahi, J. (1996) Decision tree sensitivity analysis for cost-effectiveness of FDG-PET in the staging and management of non-small-cell lung carcinoma. *J Nucl Med* **37**, 1428–36.

36. Scott, W.J., Shepherd, J., Gambhir, S.S. (1998) Cost-effectiveness of FDG-PET for staging non-small cell lung cancer: a decision analysis. *Ann Thorac Surg* **66**, 1876–85.

37. Dietlein, M., Weber, K., Gandjour, A., et al. (2000) Cost-effectiveness of FDG-PET for the management of potentially operable non-small cell lung cancer: priority for a PET-based strategy after nodal-negative CT results. *Eur J Nucl Med* **27**, 1598–609.

38. Van Tinteren, H., Hoekstra, O.S., van den Bergh, J.H., et al. (2002) Effectiveness of positron emission tomography in the preoperative assessment of patients with suspected non-small-cell lung cancer: the PLUS multicentre randomised trial. *Lancet* **359**, 1388–92.

Chapter 4

PET-CT in Radiotherapy for Lung Cancer

Dirk De Ruysscher

Abstract

For NSCLC, F-18 FDG-PET scans allow more thorough staging, thus avoiding unnecessary treatments. It reduces radiation treatment volumes because of the avoidance of mediastinal lymph nodes that are PET negative and hence reduces toxicity with the same radiation dose or enables radiation dose escalation with the same toxicity. Further research is needed to assess the effect of PET on survival. PET also reduces interobserver variability for delineating tumors and opens perspective for more automated delineation parts in radiation planning.

F-18 FDG-PET-CT scans can already at present be used in routine clinical practice. It is of paramount importance that the necessary calibrations have been done and that strictly standardized protocols for every step in the treatment and planning chain are implemented. For the delineation of target volumes, a combination of PET-CT images, auto-delineation tools, and last not but least manual editing of the target volumes is necessary. The latter is needed because of resolution deficiencies of PET and any other imaging modality as well as the incorporation of other that image information (e.g., know patterns of tumor spread according to pathological studies, knowledge of endoscopic findings, and other tumor and patient factors) to come to target volume definitions that have proven their clinical efficacy.

Key words: Lung cancer, NSCLC, SCLC, Molecular imaging, PET, Combined modality treatment, Chemotherapy, Radiotherapy

1. Introduction

Radiotherapy is a key treatment modality in the curative treatment of patients with both non-small-cell lung cancer (NSCLC) and small-cell lung cancer (SCLC). Recent progress in combined modality treatments incorporating radio-chemotherapy, with or without surgery, as well as the technical advances in radiation delivery, have all led to significant improvements in treatment outcomes. Careful staging and patient selection is important to achieve the maximal chance of long-term survival with acceptable side effects. Similarly, accurate delineation of target volumes is

Malik E. Juweid and Otto S. Hoekstra (eds.), *Positron Emission Tomography*, Methods in Molecular Biology, vol. 727, DOI 10.1007/978-1-61779-062-1_4, © Springer Science+Business Media, LLC 2011

crucial for preventing geographical misses. An incorrect definition of the gross tumor volume (GTV) (i.e., detectable tumor) or clinical target volume (CTV) (tumor plus a margin for microscopic extension) is a source of systematic errors, which can lead to under-treatment and reduce the probability of tumor control. An overview of the definitions of frequently used target volumes in radiotherapy is depicted in Figure 1.

As the overwhelming majority of the clinical relevant work has been done with F18-deoxyglucose (F-18 FDG), the only PET isotope that is widely available, in the rest of this section, by PET, F-18 FDG-PET is meant unless otherwise stated.

In contrast with diagnostic questions, which basically go down to dichotomous outcomes, i.e., cancer yes/no, in radiotherapy, also the volume and shape of the tumor volumes is of importance. Moreover, uncertainties, for example, due to tumor movements should be tackled.

Although covered in other sections, it should directly be stressed that as with any other imaging and therapeutic modality, also PET in radiotherapy should be calibrated thoroughly as well as used in strict clinical protocols. Indeed, the influence of technical factors in the measurement of the Standardized Uptake Value cannot be overemphasized. Volume assessment with PET is crucially dependent on technical factors and huge mistakes can only be avoided by sticking to well-established protocols (1).

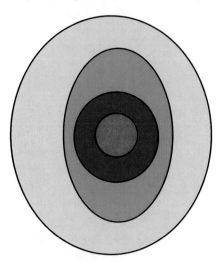

Fig. 1. Terminology used for defining target volumes in radiation oncology. *Red*: GTV (gross tumor volume): the volume encompassing all recognized tumor volume. *Blue*: CTV (clinical target volume): the GTV volume and an extra margin for potential microscopic tumor extension and inaccuracies in target definition; this margin can be symmetrical around the tumor (typically 5 mm), or asymmetrical, for example, lesser margins in the direction of an adjacent bony structure. *Green*: ITV (internal target volume): the CTV volume and an extra margin to account for intrafractional movement of lung tumors and pathological nodes. *Yellow*: PTV (planning target volume): the CTV or ITV plus an extra margin for planning and patient setup inaccuracy. The PTV is the volume used for treatment planning.

The following questions will be addressed:

1. Does PET scanning allow accurate tumor delineation? Does PET scanning change gross tumor volume (GTV), clinical target volume, and/or the planning target volume (PTV), both for the primary tumor and the local and regional lymph nodes?

2. Does PET scanning allow improvement of treatment outcome?

2. PET for Defining Tumor Volumes in NSCLC

2.1. Nodal Target Volumes

Accurate identification of nodal metastases is crucial for planning curative radiotherapy, particularly as routine elective nodal irradiation is no longer recommended in NSCLC (2). In several planning studies, it was shown that PET or PET-CT influences the GTV (reviewed in (3)). The PET volumes were in general smaller than with CT, thus leading to a decreased radiation exposure of the lungs and the esophagus sufficiently as to allow for radiation dose escalation (4, 5). A prospective clinical trial using this approach reported isolated nodal failures in only 1 of 44 patients (6). These results were subsequently confirmed in another, similar prospective study from the Netherlands Cancer Institute (7) but not in a US retrospective series (8). The latter may be due to the absence of a clearly defined PET-delineation protocol.

Although PET-defined mediastinal radiotherapy fields appears to be safe, because of a false-positive rate of approximately 30%, depending on the patient population, ideally, pathological confirmation of PET-positive mediastinal nodes should be obtained by mediastinoscopy or endoscopic ultrasound-guided fine needle aspiration (EUS-FNA).

2.2. Target Volumes for Primary NSCLC

At present, F-18 FDG-PET scans offer little additional advantage over CT or MRI scans for staging of the primary tumor because of its lack of precise anatomical localization. The spatial resolution of modern CT scanners (typically about 1 mm) is far superior to that of current PET scanners (6–8 mm), so that the extra gain with fusion is expected to be not large, unless PET scans can reliably address tumor delineation caused by atelectasis or intratumor heterogeneity.

Nevertheless, PET scans reduce the interobserver variability compared to CT alone (9). Integrated PET-CT scans further improved delineation variability (10). The next step is to use the PET signal to construct automatic delineation of the tumor and to offer the radiation oncologist a solution that only needs contour editing. This method was on its turn to be less prone to variability than PET-CT (11).

As PET acquisition takes several minutes, tumor motion due to respiration or cardiac action results in PET "GTVs" that incorporate at least some effects of this motion. Respiration-gated PET acquisition techniques have been developed (12) and are at present evaluated in clinical studies.

2.3. Clinical Target Volume

In view of the relatively poor spatial resolution of PET scans, it does not come as a surprise that at the time of writing, no clear advantage of PET to define the microscopic extensions of the tumor were reported. The development of new methods may change this picture in the future (13).

3. Do PET Scans Change the Outcome of Patients with NSCLC Treated with Radiotherapy?

PET scans have shown to detect distant metastases in up to 30% of the patients with stage III NSCLC who were M0 with conventional staging (14, 15). This clearly affects patient outcome for it spares toxic therapy in individuals who will not benefit from it.

The incorporation of PET in radiotherapy planning has previously shown the potential to allow radiation dose escalation without increasing side effects, this is because of the reduction of radiation fields (4, 5). In a phase I/II trial, it was shown that this pre-requisite is indeed true (16). Whether this radiation dose increase will ultimately lead to higher cure rates is a matter of current research. PET scans may also allow the identification of therapy-resistant areas within the tumor that could be given a higher radiation dose and hence lead to a better outcome (17).

4. PET Scan for Radiotherapy for Limited Disease Small-Cell Lung Cancer

Literature is sparse on the role of PET in limited disease small-cell lung cancer (LD-SCLC). A planning study suggests a decrease of geographical miss compared to CT (18), but more research is clearly needed.

5. Can Diagnostic PET-CT Scans Be Used for Radiotherapy Planning Purposes?

Using diagnostic PET-CT scans for radiotherapy treatment planning is attractive, for it saves time and resources. However, disadvantages are the influence of time delay between the diagnosis and referral for radiotherapy on tumor volume and tracer uptake, the effects of induction systemic therapy on F-18 FDG uptake, the differences in patient position and immobilization devices between diagnostic and therapeutic sets, calibration and SUV measurement issues, and breathing (4D) information that has now become standard in radiotherapy treatment for lung cancer and is not regularly available from diagnostic images. Although many issues can be solved (19), especially breathing and positioning differences support the use of a new PET-CT scan specifically designed for radiotherapy planning (20).

6. New PET Tracers

Although F-18 FDG has been extremely useful for lung cancer radiotherapy and new applications still emerge, new tracers are of interest, for they may be more specific for tumor characteristics such as proliferation and hypoxia. The proliferation-related marker [18 F]-fluorothymidine (FLT) has been tested for diagnostic purposes, but to the best of our knowledge, it has not been used in the process of radiotherapy for lung cancer. In contrast, hypoxia tracers such as the nitro-imidazole [18 F]-fluoromisonidazole are at present in use in clinical trials because early results suggest that its uptake may be of prognostic value and they hold the premise to select patients for hypoxic sensitizers (21).

References

1. Nestle, U., Kremp, S., Schaefer-Schuler, A., et al. (2005) Comparison of different methods for delineation of F-18 FDG PET-positive tissue for target volume definition in radiotherapy of patients with non-Small cell lung cancer. *J Nucl Med* **46**, 1342–8.

2. Senan, S., De Ruysscher, D., Giraud, P., Mirimanoff, R., Budach, V. Radiotherapy Group of European Organization for Research and Treatment of Cancer.(2004) Literature-based recommendations for treatment planning and execution for high-precision radiotherapy in lung cancer *Radiother Oncol* **71**, 139–46.

3. Nestle, U., Kremp, S., Grosu, A.L. (2006) Practical integration of [18 F]-FDG-PET and PET-CT in the planning of radiotherapy for non-small cell lung cancer (NSCLC): the technical basis, ICRU-target volumes, problems, perspectives. *Radiother Oncol* **81**, 209–25.

4. van Der Wel, A., Nijsten, S., Hochstenbag, M., et al. (2005) Increased therapeutic ratio by [18]FDG-PET-CT planning in patients with clinical CT stage N2/N3 M0 non-small cell lung cancer (NSCLC): A modelling study. *Int J Radiat Oncol Biol Phys* **61**, 648–54.

5. De Ruysscher, D., Wanders, S., Minken, A., et al. (2005) Effects of radiotherapy planning with a dedicated combined PET-CT-simulator of patients with non-small cell lung cancer on dose limiting normal tissues and radiation dose-escalation: Results of a prospective study. *Radiother Oncol* **77**, 5–10.

6. De Ruysscher, D., Wanders, S., van Haren, E., et al. (2005) Selective mediastinal node irradiation on basis of the FDG-PET scan in patients with non-small cell lung cancer: A prospective clinical study. *Int J Radiat Oncol Biol Phys* **62**, 988–94.

7. Belderbos, J.S., Heemsbergen, W.D., De Jaeger, K., Baas, P., Lebesque, J.V. (2006)

Final results of a Phase I/II dose escalation trial in non-small-cell lung cancer using three-dimensional conformal radiotherapy. *Int J Radiat Oncol Biol Phys* **66**, 126–34.

8. Sura, S., Greco, C., Gelblum, D., Yorke, E.D., Jackson, A., Rosenzweig, K.E. (2008) (18) F-fluorodeoxyglucose positron emission tomography-based assessment of local failure patterns in non-small-cell lung cancer treated with definitive radiotherapy. *Int J Radiat Oncol Biol Phys* **70**, 1397–1402.

9. Mah, K., Caldwell, C.B., Ung, Y.C., et al. (2002) The impact of (18)FDG-PET on target and critical organs in CT-based treatment planning of patients with poorly defined non-small-cell lung carcinoma: a prospective study. *Int J Radiat Oncol Biol Phys* **52**, 339–50.

10. Steenbakkers, R.J., Duppen, J.C., Fitton, I., et al. (2006) Reduction of observer variation using matched CT-PET for lung cancer delineation: a three-dimensional analysis. *Int J Radiat Oncol Biol Phys* **64**, 435–48.

11. van Baardwijk, A., Bosmans, G., Boersma, L., et al. (2007) PET-CT-based auto-contouring in non-small-cell lung cancer correlates with pathology and reduces interobserver variability in the delineation of the primary tumor and involved nodal volumes. *Int J Radiat Oncol Biol Phys* **68**, 771–8.

12. Nehmeh, S.A., Erdi, Y.E. (2008) Respiratory motion in positron emission tomography/computed tomography: a review. *Semin Nucl Med* **38**, 167–76.

13. Stroom, J., Blaauwgeers, H., van Baardwijk, A., et al. (2007) Feasibility of pathology-correlated lung imaging for accurate target definition of lung tumors. *Int J Radiat Oncol Biol Phys* **69**, 267–75.

14. Hicks, R.J., Kalff, V., MacManus, M.P., et al. (2001) F-18 FDG PET provides high-impact and powerful prognostic stratification in staging newly diagnosed non–small cell lung cancer. *J Nucl Med* **42**, 1596–1604.

15. Mac Manus, M.P., Hicks, R.J., Matthews, J.P., Wirth, A., Rischin, D., Ball, D.L. (2001) High rate of detection of unsuspected distant metastases by PET in apparent stage III non-small-cell lung cancer: implications for radical radiation therapy. *Int J Radiat Oncol Biol Phys* **50**, 287–93.

16. van Baardwijk, A., Bosmans, G., Boersma, L., et al. (2008) Individualized radical radiotherapy of non-small-cell lung cancer based on normal tissue dose constraints: a feasibility study. *Int J Radiat Oncol Biol Phys* **71**, 1394–1401.

17. Aerts, H.J., Bosmans, G., van Baardwijk, A.A., et al. (2008) Stability of (18) F-Deoxyglucose uptake locations within tumor during radiotherapy for NSCLC: A prospective study. *Int J Radiat Oncol Biol Phys* **71**, 1402–7.

18. van Loon, J., Offermann, C., Bosmans, G., et al. (2008) 18FDG-PET based radiation planning of mediastinal lymph nodes in limited disease small cell lung cancer changes radiotherapy fields: a planning study. *Radiother Oncol* **87**, 49–54.

19. Öllers, M., Bosmans, G., van Baardwijk, A., et al. (2008) The integration of PET-CT scans from different hospitals into radiotherapy treatment planning. *Radiother Oncol* **87**, 142–6.

20. Grgic, A., Nestle, U., Schaefer-Schuler, A., Kremp, S., Kirsch, C.M., Hellwig, D. (2009) FDG-PET-based radiotherapy planning in lung cancer: optimum breathing protocol and patient positioning-an intraindividual comparison *Int J Radiat Oncol Biol Phys* **73(1)**, 103–11.

21. Gagel, B., Reinartz, P., Demirel, C., et al. (2006) [18 F] fluoromisonidazole and [18 F] fluorodeoxyglucose positron emission tomography in response evaluation after chemo-/radiotherapy of non-small-cell lung cancer: a feasibility study. *BMC Cancer* **6**, 51.

Chapter 5

PET and PET–CT in Esophageal and Gastric Cancer

Hinrich A. Wieder, Bernd J. Krause, and Ken Herrmann

Abstract

Esophageal cancer ranks among the ten most common malignancies in the world and is a frequent cause of cancer-related death. Almost all therapeutic modalities for esophageal cancer are associated with considerable mortality and morbidity. Consequently, there has been growing concern regarding effective management of esophageal cancer. Imaging plays an important role in the initial selection of patients. 18F-fluorodeoxyglucose positron emission tomography (18F-FDG-PET) is playing an increasing role in the management of esophageal cancer. The role of FDG-PET in diagnosis, preoperative staging, monitoring of response to neoadjuvant therapy, and detection of disease recurrence is evaluated in this chapter.

Key words: Esophageal cancer, PET/CT, Staging, Recurrence, Therapy monitoring

1. Introduction

Esophageal cancer ranks among the ten most common malignancies in the world and is a frequent cause of cancer-related death. However, carcinomas of the esophagus are a heterogeneous group of tumors in terms of etiology, histopathology, and epidemiology.

In the upper two-thirds of the esophagus, squamous cell carcinomas (SCCs) predominate, with alcohol and smoking being the main risk factors. Carcinomas of the distal esophagus/esophagogastric junction (AEG), on the other hand, are mostly adenocarcinomas. The primary etiological factors for adenocarcinomas are gastroesophageal reflux disease and obesity, whereas alcohol and smoking seem to play no major roles. Adenocarcinomas arise from metaplastic epithelial cells at the esophagogastric junction, which have been transformed into an intestinal-type mucus layer in response to prolonged irritation from gastric juice. In Western countries, the incidence and prevalence of esophageal adenocarcinomas have increased over the past 25 years paralleled

Malik E. Juweid and Otto S. Hoekstra (eds.), *Positron Emission Tomography*, Methods in Molecular Biology, vol. 727,
DOI 10.1007/978-1-61779-062-1_5, © Springer Science+Business Media, LLC 2011

by a shift from SCCs to adenocarcinomas. Adenocarcinomas of the esophagus (–gastric junction) are among the carcinomas with the highest increase in incidence per year. Depending on the tumor stage, the available therapeutic options for esophageal cancer are endoscopic mucosal resection, primary esophagectomy, neoadjuvant or palliative chemotherapy/radiotherapy followed by surgery, and palliative resection. Most of the therapeutic modalities are associated with substantial morbidity and mortality. Accurate pretherapeutic staging is crucial to select the appropriate type of therapy. Primarily, it is important to distinguish between patients with locoregional and systemic disease, because for patients with distant lymph node metastasis or organ metastasis, there is no curative therapeutic option; these patients are candidates for palliative treatment regimens. Palliative resections should only be considered based on individual decision for relief of symptoms or after response to chemotherapy or chemoradiotherapy in metastatic disease.

After exclusion of distant metastasis, the choice of therapeutic approach depends on the T-stage. In case of a localized stage (T1/T2), there is a high probability of complete (R0) resection. In these cases, patients are mostly offered primary esophagectomy as the most important and frequently only therapeutic procedure. Patients with T3 and T4 tumors may undergo neoadjuvant chemotherapy or chemoradiotherapy. These therapeutic modalities have been employed in an attempt to increase the rate of complete resections by downsizing the primary tumor in order to improve local tumor control and to prevent distant metastatic spread. However, so far, clinical trials have not shown better survival through neoadjuvant chemotherapy compared with surgery alone. Nevertheless, numerous studies have provided evidence that patients undergoing neoadjuvant treatment and showing an objective tumor response have a better prognosis compared to those undergoing surgical treatment alone. The problem associated with neoadjuvant therapy is that only 30–40% of the patients respond to neoadjuvant chemotherapy. Sixty percent or even more undergo several months of toxic therapy without obvious benefit, which in turn may compromise overall survival due to delayed surgery, may result in therapy-associated side effects, or may even result in selection of biologically more aggressive tumors. In line with these observations, prognosis for patients with nonresponding tumor seems to be even worse than for patients treated by surgery alone in a neoadjuvant setting. Therefore, a diagnostic test that allows prediction of response is considered to be crucial for the use of neoadjuvant chemotherapy in patients with esophageal cancer. For recurrent esophageal cancer, the available therapeutic approaches are radical and palliative re-resection, stenting, laser thermocoagulation, brachytherapy, chemotherapy, and/or radiotherapy. The choice of the specific therapeutic modality depends on the location and the extent of the recurrence. In 30% of patients, the recurrence is located in the prior surgical bed. However, in the majority of cases, distant recurrence occurs, underlining the systemic character of the disease.

2. Initial Staging

2.1. Primary Cancer and Regional Lymph Node Involvement

Several studies report a high sensitivity of F-18 FDG-PET for staging SCC and adenocarcinomas of the esophagus. Detection rates for the primary tumor range from 69 to 100% (1–7). In most studies, F-18 FDG-PET is more sensitive than CT. Rasanen et al. investigated 42 patients who had undergone F-18 FDG-PET and CT before esophagectomy (8). They found that the primary tumor was correctly detected in 35 (83%) of 42 patients by F-18 FDG-PET and in 28 (67%) patients by CT. Furthermore, Heeren et al. reported that the primary tumor was visualized in 95% (70/74 patients) with F-18 FDG-PET but only in 84% (62/74 patients) with CT (2). False-negative F-18 FDG-PET findings in SCC are often due to a small tumor size. This is a consequence of the limited spatial resolution of F-18 FDG-PET which is approximately 5–8 mm in studies of the chest or abdomen. Interestingly, approximately one-third of gastric cancer patients, even those with locally advanced tumors, shows a limited or absent F-18 FDG accumulation regardless of tumor size. This seems to be related to the growth type: limited or absent F-18 FDG-uptake has been found in diffusely growing and/or mucus producing and/or signet-ring cell containing subtypes. In a recent study, Herrmann et al. (9) compared the accuracy of fluorothymidine (FLT)-PET and F-18 FDG-PET for the detection of locally advanced gastric cancer in 45 patients. In all patients, focal FLT-uptake was detectable in the primary tumor. In contrast, 14 primary tumors were negative for F-18 FDG-PET. FLT-PET was more sensitive than F-18 FDG-PET, and might therefore prove useful as a diagnostic adjunct reflecting the proliferative activity of the tumor.

Locoregional lymph node metastases are important prognostic factors in patients with esophageal cancer. Not only the number and location of regional metastatic lymph nodes, but also the lymph node size is predictive of the patients' outcome. Despite the importance of regional lymph node staging, noninvasive staging is still limited for this purpose. Depending on the criteria used for the detection of regional lymph node involvement, the values for sensitivity and specificity vary substantially between different studies.

In a metaanalysis, Westreenen et al. analyzed 12 studies concerning the diagnostic accuracy of F-18 FDG-PET in staging the locoregional lymph node status (10). The pooled sensitivity and

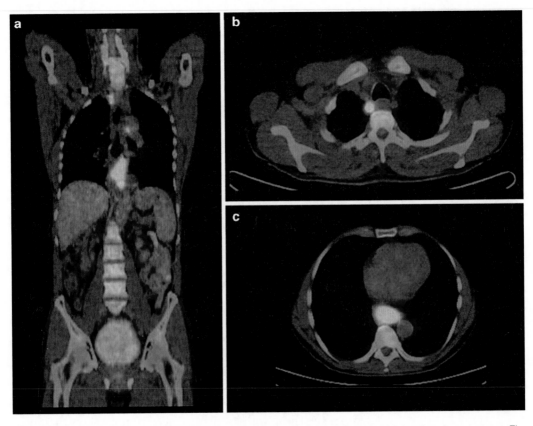

Fig. 1. Coronal (**a**) and axial (**b, c**) PET–CT fusion images of a patient with AEG type 1 with lymph node metastases. The primary tumor as well as lymph node metastases shows a high-F-18 FDG-uptake.

specificity of F-18 FDG-PET in detecting locoregional lymph node involvement was 51 and 84%, respectively (Fig. 1a, b). Flamen et al. prospectively studied 74 patients with esophageal cancer with regard to lymph node staging (1). Endoscopic ultrasound (EUS) was more sensitive (81 vs. 33%) but less specific (67 vs. 89%) than F-18 FDG-PET for the detection of regional lymph node metastasis. Compared with the combined use of CT and EUS, F-18 FDG-PET had a higher specificity (98 vs. 90%) and a similar sensitivity (43 vs. 46%) for the assessment of regional and distant lymph node involvement. Choi et al. compared the diagnostic accuracy of F-18 FDG-PET and CT/EUS in 61 consecutive patients (11). Forty-eight patients (13 excluded because of nonsurgical treatment) underwent transthoracic esophagectomy with lymph node dissection, with 382 lymph nodes being dissected, 100 of which were malignant on histologic examination (in 32 patients). On a patient basis, N-staging was correct in 83% of the patients on F-18 FDG-PET, whereas it was correct in only 60% on CT and in 58% by using EUS ($p < 0.05$). However, in the neighborhood of the primary tumor, the authors report a low sensitivity of PET in detecting metastatic lymph nodes related to the limited spatial resolution of PET and scatter effects arising from F-18 FDG accumulation in the primary tumor. In contrast to other tumor types, regional lymph node metastases in esophageal cancer are frequently located very close to the primary tumor resulting in the difficulty to differentiate lymph node metastasis from the primary tumor on F-18 FDG-PET. Lerut et al. prospectively included 42 patients for staging of esophageal carcinoma (12). All patients underwent F-18 FDG-PET, CT, and EUS. For the diagnosis of regional lymph node metastasis, F-18 FDG-PET was not considered useful because of a lack of sensitivity which was 22% compared to 83% for CT and EUS. The authors assign the low sensitivity of F-18 FDG-PET to difficulties in discriminating regional lymph nodes from the primary tumor.

Yuan et al. evaluated the additional value of PET–CT over PET in the assessment of locoregional lymph nodes in esophageal SCC (13). Forty-five patients underwent F-18 FDG-PET–CT before surgery. The sensitivity, specificity, and accuracy for PET–CT were 94, 92, and 92%, respectively, whereas those of F-18 FDG-PET were 82, 87, and 86%, respectively. The differences in sensitivity ($p < 0.032$) and accuracy ($p < 0.006$) were statistically significant. This additional value of combined F-18 FDG-PET–CT over F-18 FDG-PET was mainly related to the capability to determine the precise location of pathologic F-18 FDG-uptake in the vicinity of the primary tumor.

Kim et al. (14) included 73 patients with gastric cancer in their prospective study and assessed the diagnostic accuracy of F-18 FDG-PET with respect to lymph node metastasis. F-18 FDG-PET was able to detect primary lesions in 70 of the 73 cases. The sensitivity, specificity, positive predictive value, and negative predictive value of F-18 FDG-PET for lymph node metastasis were 40, 95, 91, and 56%, respectively. Signet-ring cell carcinoma was associated with the lowest sensitivity (15%), whereas other cell types could be detected with moderate sensitivity (30–71%) and high specificity (93–100%). CT was superior to PET in terms of sensitivity ($p < 0.0001$), and PET was superior to CT in terms of specificity ($p < 0.0001$) and positive predictive value ($p = 0.05$). F-18 FDG-PET exhibits good specificity for lymph node staging of gastric cancer. F-18 FDG-uptake in the primary tumor is significantly related to the accuracy of F-18 FDG-PET.

3. Distant Metastasis

CT of the chest and the abdomen currently presents the standard noninvasive test for evaluating distant metastasis in esophageal cancer with a sensitivity of 37–66%. However, CT is entirely dependent on structural characteristics for diagnosis. In esophageal cancer, metastatic involvement is often found in normal-sized nodes (limitations in diagnostic sensitivity) and, on the other hand, unspecific lymph node enlargement is commonly observed in the cervical and mediastinal area (limitations in diagnostic specificity). F-18 FDG-PET offers the advantage over CT that unspecific lymph node enlargement does not lead to increased F-18 FDG-uptake per se and the F-18 FDG-uptake may already be increased in metastatic lymph nodes that are not enlarged.

Van Westreenen et al. included 12 studies in a metaanalysis in patients with newly diagnosed cancer of the esophagus (10). Pooled sensitivity and specificity for the detection of distant metastasis were 67 and 97%, respectively. Flamen et al. evaluated 74 patients with potentially respectable esophageal cancer in a prospective study and compared the diagnostic accuracy for F-18 FDG-PET, CT, and EUS (1). For the detection of distant metastases, the sensitivities for F-18 FDG-PET, CT, and EUS were 74, 41, and 42% and the corresponding specificities were 90, 83, and 94%, respectively. The diagnostic accuracy of F-18 FDG-PET was 82% while it was only 64% for a combination of CT and EUS mainly by virtue of a superior sensitivity. These findings changed patient management in 22% of the studied patients by upstaging 11 patients (15%) and downstaging 5 patients (7%). In two patients, F-18 FDG-PET falsely understaged disease because of false-negative PET findings with regard to supradiaphragmatic lymph nodes. Heeren et al. compared F-18 FDG-PET with a combination of CT/EUS in pretherapeutic staging for distant node lymph metastasis and distant organ metastasis in 74 patients (2). F-18 FDG-PET identified distant nodal disease in 17 of 24 (71%) patients compared to only 7 of 24 patients (29%) for CT/EUS. The sensitivity for the detection of distant metastasis was also significantly higher for F-18 FDG-PET (70%) than for the combined use of CT and EUS (30%). PET correctly upstaged 15 patients (20%) who were missed on CT/EUS and correctly downstaged 4 patients (5%). However, in this study, PET also misclassified 8 of the 74 patients (11%) by false upstaging in five (7%) and false downstaging in three patients (4%). There are several sources for false-positive findings in F-18 FDG-PET: inflammatory reactions (e.g., inflammatory infiltrates in the lung), benign tumors (e.g., benign thyroid adenoma or Warthin's tumor of the parotid gland), and increased F-18 FDG-uptake in brown fat or skeletal muscles. However, all these causes are rare in patients with esophageal cancer. In all studies published so far, the diagnostic accuracy of F-18 FDG-PET for the detection of distant metastasis of esophageal cancer was found to be higher compared to that of morphological imaging techniques such as CT or EUS. This seems to apply to both, detection of distant lymph node and organ metastases. F-18 FDG-PET excels by an outstanding sensitivity

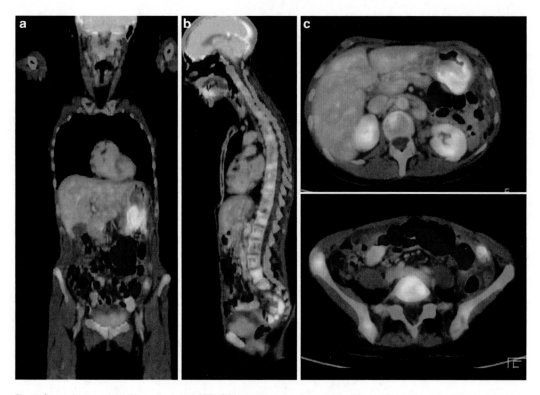

Fig. 2. Coronal (**a**), sagittal (**b**), and axial (**c**) PET–CT fusion images of a patient with gastric cancer with distant metastasis. The primary tumor as well as the bone marrow infiltration and the peritoneal carcinomatosis show a high glucose metabolism.

for bone metastases and appears to have a higher specificity than CT for the detection of lung metastases and liver metastases (Fig. 2a–c). CT, on the other hand, appears to have a higher sensitivity for lung metastases.

In summary, the value of F-18 FDG-PET for staging esophageal carcinoma mainly resides in better characterization of distant metastases (lymph nodes and organs). However, F-18 FDG-PET should be regarded a supplemental procedure (e.g., in addition to CT), as it does not accurately determine the local tumor extent and locoregional lymph node involvement.

4. Recurrence

Kato et al. studied 55 patients with thoracic SCC who had undergone radical esophagectomy (15). Twenty-seven of the 55 patients had recurrent disease in a total of 37 organs. The accuracy of F-18 FDG-PET and CT in detecting recurrences during follow-up was calculated by using the first scan suggesting the presence of recurrent disease. F-18 FDG-PET showed 100% sensitivity,

75% specificity, and 84% accuracy for detecting locoregional recurrence. The corresponding values for CT were 84, 86, and 85% respectively. The specificity of F-18 FDG-PET was lower because of unspecific F-18 FDG-uptake in the gastric tube and in thoracic lymph nodes of the lung hilum or the pretracheal region. Distant recurrence was observed in 15 patients in 18 organs. Most of the recurrences were located in liver, lung, and bone. The sensitivity, specificity, and accuracy for F-18 FDG-PET were 87, 95, and 93% vs. 87, 98, and 95%, respectively, for CT. The diagnostic accuracy of F-18 FDG-PET for distant recurrence was similar to that of CT. The sensitivity of PET in detecting bone metastasis was higher than that of CT. The sensitivity for lung metastasis was higher on CT due to the higher spatial resolution and high tumor-to-tissue contrast in lung. Similar sensitivities for F-18 FDG-PET and CT were observed for both liver and distant lymph node metastasis.

Flamen et al. used F-18 FDG-PET in 41 symptomatic patients for diagnosis and staging of disease recurrence after radical esophagectomy (16). All patients underwent a whole-body F-18 FDG-PET and a conventional diagnostic workup including a combination of CT and EUS. Recurrent disease was present in 33 patients (40 locations). Nine lesions were located at the anastomotic site, 12 at regional, and 19 at distant sites. For the diagnosis of disease recurrence at the anastomotic site, no significant difference between PET and CT/EUS was found. The sensitivity, specificity, and accuracy of F-18 FDG-PET were 100, 57, and 74% vs. 100, 93, and 96% for conventional diagnostic workup. A reason for the high incidence of false-positive PET findings at the perianastomotic region might have been progressive benign anastomotic strictures in these patients, requiring repetitive endoscopic dilatation. Probably the dilatation-induced trauma resulted in an inflammatory reaction. For the diagnosis of regional and distant recurrence, F-18 FDG-PET showed 94% sensitivity, 82% specificity, and 87% accuracy vs. 81, 84, and 81% for CT/EUS, respectively. On a patient basis, PET provided additional information in 27% (11/41) of the patients. In summary, F-18 FDG-PET is associated with a clinical benefit in restaging esophageal carcinoma. However, the perianastomotic site often remains equivocal, as an unspecific increase or metabolic activity may be present owing to inflammatory or reparative processes. Figure 3a–c shows the PET–CT examination of a patient with histological proven recurrence of an SCC of the esophagus.

De Potter et al. (17) studied 33 patients who had received surgical treatment for gastric cancer with curative intent and who had subsequently undergone F-18 FDG-PET for suspected recurrence. Results were compared with a gold standard, consisting of histological confirmation or radiological and clinical follow-up. The gold standard established disease recurrence in 20/33

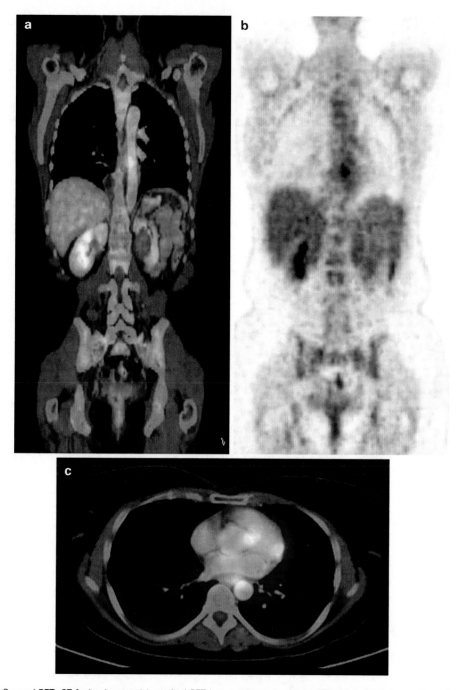

Fig. 3. Coronal PET–CT fusion images (**a**), sagittal PET images (**b**), and axial (**c**) PET–CT fusion images of a patient after esophagectomy of a squamous cell carcinoma of the esophagus. The F-18 FDG-PET scan shows locoregional recurrent cancer.

patients (prevalence 61%). Sensitivity and specificity of F-18 FDG-PET for the diagnosis of recurrence were 70% (14/20) and 69% (9/13), respectively. Positive and negative predictive values were 78% (14/18) and 60% (9/15), respectively. Of the six false-negative cases, all had intraabdominal lesions (three had generalized abdominal metastases, one liver metastasis, one local recurrence, and one ovarian metastasis). In the subgroup with previous signet-cell differentiation of the primary tumor ($n = 13$, disease prevalence 62%), sensitivity was 62% (5/8) and specificity was 60% (3/5). In the patient group with proven recurrence ($n = 20$), the mean survival for the PET-negative group was 18.5 (±12.5) months, as compared with 6.9 (±6.5) months for the PET-positive group ($p = 0.05$). The authors pointed out that because of its poor sensitivity and low-negative predictive value, F-18 FDG-PET is not suited for screening purposes in the follow-up of treated gastric cancer. However, F-18 FDG-PET appears to provide important additional information concerning the prognosis of recurrent gastric cancer. In a recent study by Park et al. (18), 105 patients with clinical or radiologic suspicion of recurrence of gastric cancer underwent PET–CT. Of all 105 patients, 75 patients were confirmed to have true recurrence with 108 recurrence sites. The sensitivity, specificity, positive predictive value, negative predictive value, and accuracy for diagnosing true recurrence on a per-person basis were 75, 77, 89, 55, and 75%, respectively. On a per-lesion basis, 75 (69%) of 108 true recurrences showed positive F-18 FDG-uptake, while 75 (89%) of 84 positive F-18 FDG-uptake was confirmed to have true recurrence. In this study, PET–CT was relatively accurate in detecting recurrence in postoperative patients with gastric cancer. PET–CT might be helpful in confirming the presence of recurrence particularly in patients who are highly suspicious of recurrence because of its high positive predictability.

5. Therapy Monitoring

Response rates to neoadjuvant chemotherapy and/or radiotherapy in esophageal cancer are below 50% for all carcinoma types as measured by histopathological examination of the surgical specimen (after termination of therapy). A common criterion for histopathological response to therapy is the presence of no or only scattered tumor cells (<10% viable tumor cells) in the resected specimen (19–21). In a neoadjuvant setting, the overall survival of patients is strongly dependent on whether histopathological response is achieved or not (19). However, due to the heterogeneity of response within the tumor and heterogeneity of the tumor after neoadjuvant therapy, small biopsies of the tumor tissue are not representative of the whole tumor mass. A complete tumor resection and a histopathological examination of the whole tumor including adjacent tissue are needed to definitely determine the histopathological tumor response. In contrast to pre- or posttherapeutic biopsies used for histopathologic analysis, the whole tumor mass can be analyzed noninvasively by imaging techniques such as contrast enhanced CT or EUS. However, morphological changes are not always representative of tumor response, as large tumor masses may remain despite response or therapy-induced fibrosis, and edema may mimic residual tumor, and shrinking tumors may still contain vital tumor cells. The overall accuracy for response assessment is relatively low when posttherapeutic T-stage or comparing pre- and posttherapeutic T-stage are determined by morphological imaging. Thus, following chemotherapy or chemoradiotherapy, tumor response cannot reliably be assessed by computed tomography or EUS. Despite these limitations, changes in tumor size have been used to assess tumor response in patients with esophageal cancer. According to criteria of the World Health Organization (WHO), the size of the tumor is to be measured in two perpendicular diameters. In 2000, Therasse et al. (22) published newer guidelines so called Response Evaluation Criteria for Solid Tumors (RECIST). RECIST characterized target lesions and nontarget lesions, which are used to extrapolate an overall response to treatment. In addition, the bidimensional measurements required by the WHO criteria have been replaced by unidimensional measurements. RECIST defines response as 30% decrease of the largest diameter of the tumor. For a spherical lesion, this is equivalent to a 50% decrease of the product of two diameters. Metaanalyses combining the results of several large phase II and phase III studies have shown that the tumor response according to WHO or RECIST criteria is correlated with patient survival for some tumor types (23). However, there is a considerable variability between individual studies and the same response rate can be associated with completely different survival rates in different studies (24). For some tumor types, metaanalyses found no or only very weak correlation with patient survival (25, 26).

FDG accumulation in esophageal tumors has been shown to be reproducible at repeated examinations (27). The interstudy variability of repeated F-18 FDG measurements within 3 weeks is less than 20% (27). In other words, during therapy, any change in tumor F-18 FDG-uptake greater than ±20% between baseline PET and follow-up PET must be considered a true one. The metabolic response to a neoadjuvant chemotherapy/radiochemotherapy can be assessed during and after treatment. Late evaluation in the course of a treatment and after completion of treatment may predict the amount of residual viable tumor cells, histopathological tumor response, and survival. However, the therapeutic relevance of this prognostic information is limited, as it does not allow changing the therapeutic strategy.

6. Late Response Assessment

In a metaanalysis, Westerterp et al. in 2005 (28) compared the diagnostic accuracy of CT, EUS, and F-18 FDG-PET for the assessment of response to neoadjuvant therapy in patients with esophageal cancer. Four studies with CT, 13 with EUS, and 7 with F-18 FDG-PET met the inclusion criteria. The ROC analysis showed maximum joint values for sensitivity and specificity of 54% for CT, 86% for EUS, and 85% for F-18 FDG-PET. Accuracy of CT was significantly lower compared to that of F-18 FDG-PET ($p<0.006$) and of EUS ($p<0.003$). Accuracy of F-18 FDG-PET and of EUS was similar ($p=0.839$). However, the authors stated that the assessment of response by EUS may be limited due to postradiation esophagitis, luminal stenosis, and compression of the tumor by the endoscope. EUS could not be performed in 6% of the patients and was suboptimal in 14% of the patients.

In 2001, Brücher et al. were the first to report on a study evaluating F-18 FDG-PET for the assessment of a late metabolic response after completion of chemoradiotherapy in patients with advanced SCC of the esophagus (29). Twenty-seven patients underwent a PET scan prior to therapy and another PET 3–4 weeks after completion of therapy. Therapy-induced reduction of tumor F-18 FDG-uptake was significantly higher for histopathologic responders ($72 \pm 11\%$) than for nonresponders ($42 \pm 22\%$). At a threshold of 52% decrease of metabolic activity, the sensitivity for detecting histopathological response was 100%, with a corresponding specificity of 55%, respectively. Metabolic tumor response was also a strong prognostic parameter. PET-responders had a median survival of 23 months, compared to only 9 months for PET-nonresponders. Similar results were confirmed by Flamen et al. who studied 36 patients with esophageal cancer before and 3–4 weeks after completion of chemoradiotherapy (30). In contrast to Brucher et al., PET response was assessed using a visual analysis. Patients were classified as PET-responders if they showed a complete or almost complete normalization of the F-18 FDG-uptake at the primary site of the tumor and a complete normalization of all lymph node metastases seen on the prior to therapy PET scan. Complete and subtotal histopathologic response was detected with a sensitivity of 78% and a specificity of 82% by F-18 FDG-PET. However, the sensitivity and the positive predictive value of the PET scan for the diagnosis of a complete histopathologic response was only 67 and 50%, respectively. The authors stated that the underestimation of complete histopathological response by PET was mainly based on false-positive findings at the primary tumor site. An influx of leucocytes and macrophages due to inflammatory and scavenging reactions may increase the F-18 FDG-uptake, resulting in an underestimation of therapeutic efficacy. Again, metabolic response was also correlated with overall survival. The median overall survival for patients without a PET response was 6.4 months, whereas it was 16.4 months for patients classified as PET responders. Port et al. compared F-18 FDG-PET response with clinical response for the prediction of pathological downstaging and disease-free survival in 62 patients with esophageal carcinoma (31). A reduction of SUV max of more than 50% compared to baseline was more significantly associated with improved disease-free survival compared to clinical response. With respect to the prediction of pathological downstaging, both methods appeared of equivalent accuracy. However, Port et al. showed that a complete absence of residual F-18 FDG-uptake is not equivalent of a complete histopathological response (31). This observation confirmed an earlier study published by Swisher et al. in 103 patients, showing that F-18 FDG-PET failed to rule out residual microscopic disease by showing that F-18 FDG-uptake in the tumor bed was not different for patients with no residual viable tumor cells compared to patients with up to 10% viable tumor cells (32). Swisher et al. also investigated the prognostic relevance of F-18 FDG-uptake after completion of neoadjuvant chemoradiation, claiming that a residual uptake of $SUV > 4$ was the best long-term survival predictor (hazard ratio 3.5, $p = 0.04$). Accuracy of $[^{18}F]$-FDG-PET for the prediction of histopathological response was comparable to that of CT and ultrasound. In contrast to these results, Smithers et al. found no correlation between F-18 FDG-PET response and histopathological response in 45 patients undergoing neoadjuvant chemotherapy or chemoradiation (33). These conflicting reported results underline the need for randomized multicenter studies with standardized imaging protocols such as that recently launched by the EORTC (34).

Future approaches will combine metabolic information determined by F-18 FDG-PET with biological markers. For an example Westerterp et al. assessed F-18 FDG-uptake as well as stained biopsy tissue samples immunohistochemical for angiogenic markers (VEGF, CD31), glucose transporter-1 (Glut-1), hexokinase (HK) isoforms, for proliferation marker (Ki67), for macrophage marker (CD68), and for apoptosis marker (cleaved caspase-3) in 26 patients (35). The only parameters that showed a correlation with the F-18 FDG-uptake were Glut-1 expression and tumor size.

7. Early Response Assessment

Using quantitative measurements of tumor F-18 FDG-uptake, it is possible not only to assess tumor response late after onset of therapy but also to predict response early during chemotherapy.

In a study by Weber et al., 40 consecutive patients with an AEG, according to Siewert et al. (36), had PET scans prior and on day 14 of the first chemotherapy cycle (20). The reduction of tumor F-18 FDG-uptake after 14 days of therapy was significantly different between tumors that showed a clinical and histopathological response and those which showed no response. Optimal differentiation was achieved by a cut-off value of 35% reduction of initial F-18 FDG-uptake. Applying this cut-off value as a criterion for a metabolic response predicted clinical response with a sensitivity and specificity of 93 and 95%, respectively. Histopathologically complete or subtotal tumor regression was observed in 53% of the patients with a metabolic response but in only 5% of the patients without a metabolic response. Patients with a metabolic response were also characterized by a significantly longer time to progression/recurrence and longer overall survival. Ott et al. evaluated this 35% SUV mean decrease cut-off in a prospective study in 65 patients (37). PET predicted histopathological responders with a sensitivity of 80% and a specificity of 95%. Metabolic response was also characterized by an improved 3-year survival rate. In the subgroup of completely resected (R0) patients, multivariate analysis revealed metabolic response as the only factor predicting recurrence.

Based on the findings by Weber et al. (20), the recently published MUNICON trial was the first in which treatment was tailored to the individual patient in dependence of the F-18 FDG-PET results (38). A total of 119 patients with locally advanced adenocarcinoma of AEG type 1 (distal esophageal adenocarcinoma) or type 2 (gastric cardia adenocarcinoma) were recruited into this prospective, single-center study. All patients were assigned to 2 weeks of platinum-based induction chemotherapy (evaluation period). Metabolic responders continued to receive chemotherapy after 2 weeks of induction chemotherapy for a maximum of 12 weeks before undergoing surgery, whereas metabolic nonresponders discontinued chemotherapy and were immediately referred to surgery after only 2 weeks of chemotherapy. In the MUNICON trial, 110 patients were evaluable for metabolic response and 49% were classified as metabolic responders after 2 weeks of induction chemotherapy; 104 patients underwent tumor resection. Histopathological response was achieved in 58% of the metabolic responders, but in none of the metabolic nonresponders. After a median follow-up of 2.3 years, survival analysis revealed better event-free and overall survival for metabolic responders than for nonresponders (29.7 vs. 14.1 months $p=0.002$; and not reached vs. 25.8; $p=0.015$). This study confirmed prospectively the usefulness of early metabolic response evaluation, and shows the feasibility of an F-18 FDG-PET-guided treatment algorithm. The findings might enable tailoring of multimodal treatment in accordance with individual tumor biology in future randomized trials.

As noted above, up to one third of gastric carcinomas are F-18 FDG-nonavid. Recently published long-term results claim that in locally advanced gastric cancer three different metabolic groups exist (39). Metabolic responders had a higher histopathological response rate (69%) than metabolic nonresponders (17%) and initially nonFDG-avid patients (24%). Survival of nonFDG-avid patients was not significantly different from that of F-18 FDG-avid nonresponders (36.7 vs. 24.1 months; $p=0.46$), whereas for F-18 FDG-avid responders median overall survival was not reached yet. Ott et al. therefore assumed that even though metabolic response assessment is not possible in F-18 FDG-nonavid tumors, a therapy modification might be considered in this patient subgroup. Another group investigated a different time point and cut-off value in 41 patients with gastric cancer (40). In this retrospective study, a decrease of more than 45% of the initial SUV after 35 days revealed to be the best criterion for predicting response and prognosis to neoadjuvant chemotherapy. Metabolic response was significantly correlated with histopathological response (less than 50% residual tumor; $p=0.007$) and disease-free survival ($p=0.01$).

Radiotherapy/chemoradiotherapy often causes local inflammatory reactions in the esophagus. Uptake of F-18 FDG in inflammatory lesions is a commonly known phenomenon. Increased F-18 FDG-uptake due to radiation-induced inflammation may limit the use of F-18 FDG-PET for metabolic monitoring of esophageal carcinomas as observed in late response assessment with F-18 FDG-PET (see above). Therefore, it has been recommended that F-18 FDG-PET should be further postponed and only be performed several weeks or even months after completion of radiotherapy in order to assess tumor response. However, these recommendations are not based on systematic clinical data, but only on theoretical considerations and a few case reports. Wieder et al. studied the time course of changes in tumor F-18 FDG-uptake in 38 patients with locally advanced SCCs of the esophagus during neoadjuvant chemoradiotherapy (21). Patients underwent PET scans prior to chemoradiotherapy 2 weeks after the initiation of therapy and 3–4 weeks after the completion of chemoradiotherapy, i.e., before surgery. None of the serial PET scans demonstrated a relevant increase in tumor F-18 FDG-uptake, indicating that radiation-induced inflammation is too small to outweigh the decrease in F-18 FDG-uptake due to therapy-induced loss of viable tumor cells. Furthermore, radiation-induced esophagitis often involves a long segment of the esophagus and, in most cases, its F-18 FDG-uptake pattern is markedly different from tumoral uptake. Therefore, in most cases, it is possible to differentiate between residual tumor tissue and radiation-induced inflammation. The reduction of tumor F-18 FDG-uptake after 14 days of chemoradiotherapy was significantly higher in histopathologic responding tumors ($44 \pm 15\%$, Fig. 4a, b) than in nonresponders ($21 \pm 14\%$, Fig. 5a, b). The ROC analysis

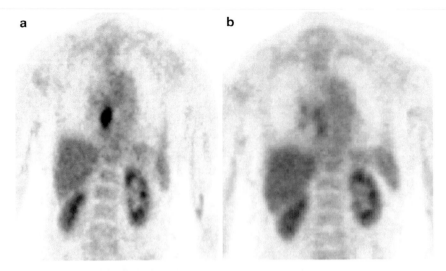

Fig. 4. (**a**, **b**) Coronal PET images of a patient with locally advanced AEG. Already 14 days after the initiation of neoadjuvant chemotherapy, there is a marked decrease in tumor metabolic activity (>35%). After completion of chemotherapy, no viable tumor cells were found in the resected specimen.

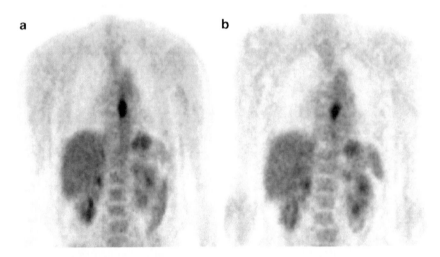

Fig. 5. (**a**, **b**) Coronal PET images of a patient with locally advanced AEG. Fourteen days after the initiation of neoadjuvant chemotherapy, there is a marginal decrease in tumor metabolic activity (<35%). After the completion of chemotherapy, >50% tumor cells were found in the resected specimen.

demonstrated that the highest accuracy for differentiation of subsequently responding and nonresponding tumors was achieved by applying a cutoff of a 30% decrease in tumor F-18 FDG-uptake from baseline values. Applying this cut-off value as a criterion for metabolic response allowed the prediction of histopathologic response with a sensitivity and a specificity of 93 and 88%, respectively. Metabolic responders were also characterized by a significantly longer overall survival. The median overall survival for patients with a decrease in F-18 FDG-uptake by more than 30% was more than 38 months, whereas it was only 18 months for nonresponders. Thus, response prediction is clearly feasible with F-18 FDG-PET early in the course of chemoradiotherapy.

References

1. Flamen, P., Lerut, A., Van Cutsem, E., et al. (2000) Utility of positron emission tomography for the staging of patients with potentially operable esophageal carcinoma. *J Clin Oncol* **18**, 3202–10.

2. Heeren, P.A., Jager, P.L., Bongaerts, F., van Dullemen, H., Sluiter, W., Plukker, J.T. (2004) Detection of distant metastases in esophageal cancer with (18)F-FDG PET. *J Nucl Med* **45**, 980–7.

3. Kato, H., Kuwano, H., Nakajima, M., et al. (2002) Usefulness of positron emission tomography for assessing the response of neoadjuvant chemoradiotherapy in patients with esophageal cancer. *Am J Surg* **184**, 279–83.

4. Kim, K., Park, S.J., Kim, B.T., Lee, K.S., Shim, Y.M. (2001) Evaluation of lymph node metastases in squamous cell carcinoma of the esophagus with positron emission tomography. *Ann Thorac Surg* **71**, 290–4.

5. McAteer, D., Wallis, F., Couper, G., et al. (1999) Evaluation of F-18 FDG positron emission tomography in gastric and oesophageal carcinoma. *Br J Radiol* **72**, 525–9.

6. Meltzer, C.C., Luketich, J.D., Friedman, D., et al. (2000) Whole-body FDG positron emission tomographic imaging for staging esophageal cancer comparison with computed tomography. *Clin Nucl Med* **25**, 882–7.

7. Yoon, Y.C., Lee, K.S., Shim, Y.M., Kim, B.T., Kim, K., Kim, T.S. (2003) Metastasis to regional lymph nodes in patients with esophageal squamous cell carcinoma: CT versus FDG PET for presurgical detection prospective study. *Radiology* **227**, 764–70.

8. Rasanen, J.V., Sihvo, E.I., Knuuti, M.J., et al. (2003) Prospective analysis of accuracy of positron emission tomography, computed tomography, and endoscopic ultrasonography in staging of adenocarcinoma of the esophagus and the esophagogastric junction. *Ann Surg Oncol* **10**, 954–60.

9. Herrmann, K., Ott, K., Buck, A.K., et al. (2007) Imaging gastric cancer with PET and the radiotracers 18F-FLT and F-18 FDG: A comparative analysis. *J Nucl Med* **48**, 1945–50.

10. van Westreenen, H.L., Westerterp, M., Bossuyt, P.M., et al. (2004) Systematic review of the staging performance of 18F-fluorodeoxyglucose positron emission tomography in esophageal cancer. *J Clin Oncol* **22**, 3805–12.

11. Choi, J.Y., Lee, K.H., Shim, Y.M., et al. (2000) Improved detection of individual nodal involvement in squamous cell carcinoma of the esophagus by FDG PET. *J Nucl Med* **41**, 808–15.

12. Lerut, T., Flamen, P., Ectors, N., et al. (2000) Histopathologic validation of lymph node staging with FDG-PET scan in cancer of the esophagus and gastroesophageal junction: A prospective study based on primary surgery with extensive lymphadenectomy. *Ann Surg* **232**, 743–52.

13. Yuan, S., Yu, Y., Chao, K.S., et al. (2006) Additional value of PET-CT over PET in assessment of locoregional lymph nodes in thoracic esophageal squamous cell cancer. *J Nucl Med* **47**, 1255–9.

14. Kim, S.K., Kang, K.W., Lee, J.S., et al. (2006) Assessment of lymph node metastases using F-18 FDG PET in patients with advanced gastric cancer. *Eur J Nucl Med Mol Imaging* **33**, 148–55.

15. Kato, H., Miyazaki, T., Nakajima, M., Fukuchi, M., Manda, R., Kuwano, H. (2004) Value of positron emission tomography in the diagnosis of recurrent oesophageal carcinoma. *Br J Surg* **91**, 1004–9.

16. Flamen, P., Lerut, A., Van Cutsem, E., et al. (2000) The utility of positron emission tomography for the diagnosis and staging of recurrent esophageal cancer. *J Thorac Cardiovasc Surg* **120**, 1085–92.

17. De Potter, T., Flamen, P., Van Cutsem, E., et al. (2002) Whole-body PET with FDG for the diagnosis of recurrent gastric cancer. *Eur J Nucl Med Mol Imaging* **29**, 525–9.

18. Park, M.J., Lee, W.J., Lim, H.K., Park, K.W., Choi, J.Y., Kim, B.T. (2009) Detecting recurrence of gastric cancer: The value of FDG PET-CT. *Abdom Imaging* **34**, 441–7.

19. Mandard, A.M., Dalibard, F., Mandard, J.C., et al. (1994) Pathologic assessment of tumor regression after preoperative chemoradiotherapy of esophageal carcinoma clinicopathologic correlations. *Cancer* **73**, 2680–6.

20. Weber, W.A., Ott, K., Becker, K., et al. (2001) Prediction of response to preoperative chemotherapy in adenocarcinomas of the esophagogastric junction by metabolic imaging. *J Clin Oncol* **19**, 3058–65.

21. Wieder, H.A., Brucher, B.L., Zimmermann, F., et al. (2004) Time course of tumor metabolic activity during chemoradiotherapy of esophageal squamous cell carcinoma and response to treatment. *J Clin Oncol* **22**, 900–8.

22. Therasse, P., Arbuck, S.G., Eisenhauer, E.A., et al. (2000) New guidelines to evaluate the response to treatment in solid tumors. *J Natl Cancer Inst* **92**, 205–16.

23. Buyse, M., Piedbois, Y., Piedbois, P., Gray, R. (2000) Tumour site, sex, and survival in colorectal cancer. *Lancet* **356**, 858.

24. Bruzzi, P., Del Mastro, L., Sormani, M.P., et al. (2005) Objective response to chemotherapy as a potential surrogate end point of survival in metastatic breast cancer patients. *J Clin Oncol* **23**, 5117–25.

25. Goffin, J., Baral, S., Tu, D., Nomikos, D., Seymour, L. (2005) Objective responses in patients with malignant melanoma or renal cell cancer in early clinical studies do not predict regulatory approval. *Clin Cancer Res* **11**, 5928–34.

26. Ratain, M.J. (2005) Phase II oncology trials: Let's be positive. *Clin Cancer Res* **11**, 5661–2.

27. Weber, W.A., Ziegler, S.I., Thodtmann, R., Hanauske, A.R., Schwaiger, M. (1999) Reproducibility of metabolic measurements in malignant tumors using FDG PET. *J Nucl Med* **40**, 1771–7.

28. Westerterp, M., van Westreenen, H.L., Reitsma, J.B., et al. (2005) Esophageal cancer: CT, endoscopic US, and FDG PET for assessment of response to neoadjuvant therapy – systematic review. *Radiology* **236**, 841–51.

29. Brucher, B.L., Weber, W., Bauer, M., et al. (2001) Neoadjuvant therapy of esophageal squamous cell carcinoma: Response evaluation by positron emission tomography. *Ann Surg* **233**, 300–9.

30. Flamen, P., Van Cutsem, E., Lerut, A., et al. (2002) Positron emission tomography for assessment of the response to induction radiochemotherapy in locally advanced esophageal cancer. *Ann Oncol* **13**, 361–8.

31. Port, J.L., Lee, P.C., Korst, R.J., et al. (2007) Positron emission tomographic scanning predicts survival after induction chemotherapy for esophageal carcinoma. *Ann Thorac Surg* **84**, 393–400; discussion.

32. Swisher, S.G., Maish, M., Erasmus, J.J., et al. (2004) Utility of PET, CT, and EUS to identify pathologic responders in esophageal cancer. *Ann Thorac Surg* **78**, 1152–60; discussion 60.

33. Smithers, B.M., Couper, G.C., Thomas, J.M., et al. (2008) Positron emission tomography and pathological evidence of response to neoadjuvant therapy in adenocarcinoma of the esophagus. *Dis Esophagus* **21**, 151–8.

34. Lordick, F., Ruers, T., Aust, D.E., et al. (2008) European Organisation of Research and Treatment of Cancer (EORTC) Gastrointestinal Group: Workshop on the role of metabolic imaging in the neoadjuvant treatment of gastrointestinal cancer. *Eur J Cancer* **44**, 1807–19.

35. Westerterp, M., Sloof, G.W., Hoekstra, O.S., et al. (2008) 18FDG uptake in oesophageal adenocarcinoma: Linking biology and outcome. *J Cancer Res Clin Oncol* **134**, 227–36.

36. Siewert, J.R., Stein, H.J., Sendler, A., Fink, U. (1999) Surgical resection for cancer of the cardia. *Semin Surg Oncol* **17**, 125–31.

37. Ott, K., Weber, W.A., Lordick, F., et al. (2006) Metabolic imaging predicts response, survival, and recurrence in adenocarcinomas of the esophagogastric junction. *J Clin Oncol* **24**, 4692–8.

38. Lordick, F., Ott, K., Krause, B.J., et al. (2007) PET to assess early metabolic response and to guide treatment of adenocarcinoma of the oesophagogastric junction: The MUNICON phase II trial. *Lancet Oncol* **8**, 797–805.

39. Ott, K., Herrmann, K., Lordick, F., et al. (2008) Early metabolic response evaluation by fluorine-18 fluorodeoxyglucose positron emission tomography allows in vivo testing of chemosensitivity in gastric cancer: Long-term results of a prospective study. *Clin Cancer Res* **14**, 2012–8.

40. Shah, M.A., Yeung, H.W., Coit, D., Trocola, R., Ilson, D., Randazzo, J. (2007) A phase II study of preoperative chemotherapy with irinotecan (CPT) and cisplatin (CIS) for gastric cancer (NCI 5917): FDG-PET-CT predicts patient outcome. *J Clin Oncol* **25**, 18S.

Chapter 6

FDG PET and PET/CT for Colorectal Cancer

Dominique Delbeke and William H. Martin

Abstract

The evaluation of patients with known or suspected recurrent colorectal carcinoma is now an accepted indication for positron emission tomography using ^{18}F-fluorodeoxyglucose (FDG-PET) imaging. PET and CT are complimentary, and therefore, integrated PET/CT imaging should be performed where available. FDG-PET/CT is indicated as the initial test for diagnosis and staging of recurrence, and for preoperative staging (N and M) of known recurrence that is considered to be resectable. FDG-PET imaging is valuable for the differentiation of posttreatment changes from recurrent tumor, differentiation of benign from malignant lesions (indeterminate lymph nodes, hepatic, and pulmonary lesions), and the evaluation of patients with rising tumor markers in the absence of a known source. The addition of FDG-PET/CT to the evaluation of these patients reduces overall treatment costs by accurately identifying patients who will and will not benefit from surgical procedures. This new powerful technology provides more accurate interpretation of both CT and FDG-PET images and therefore more optimal patient care. PET/CT fusion images affect the clinical management by guiding further procedures (biopsy, surgery, and radiation therapy), excluding the need for additional procedures, and changing both inter- and intra-modality therapy.

Key words: Colorectal carcinoma, Positron emission tomography, Computed tomography

1. Introduction

Colorectal cancer is the third most common cause of cancer in men and women, and the incidence rate has been decreasing for most of the last two decades partially due to an increase in screening. The American Cancer Society estimates that there are approximately 149,000 new cases of colorectal cancer per year in the USA and approximately 50,000 patients per year die from this disease in the USA, representing 10% of new cases of cancers and 8% of all cancer deaths. Approximately 70–80% of patients are treated with curative intent. Surgery is the most common treatment.

Malik E. Juweid and Otto S. Hoekstra (eds.), *Positron Emission Tomography*, Methods in Molecular Biology, vol. 727, DOI 10.1007/978-1-61779-062-1_6, © Springer Science+Business Media, LLC 2011

Chemotherapy alone, or in combination with radiation (for rectal cancer), is given before or after surgery to most patients whose cancer has penetrated the bowel wall or spread to lymph nodes. The overall survival at 1 and 5 years is 82% and 64%, respectively. The 5-year survival is 90% for localized stage, 68% when there is regional spread, and 10% when there are distant metastases (1).

2. Screening and Diagnosis of Colorectal Carcinoma

The diagnosis of colorectal carcinoma is based on colonoscopy and biopsy. The American Cancer Society recommends screening for colorectal cancer with yearly fecal occult blood test and flexible sigmoidoscopy every 5 years after the age of 50 for asymptomatic individuals (2).

In 2008, the American College of Radiology (ACR), the American Cancer Society (ACS), and the US Multisociety Task Force on Colorectal Cancer (composed of the three gastroenterology societies: the American Gastroenterology Association, American Society for Gastrointestinal Endoscopy, and American College of Gastroenterology) reviewed a broad range of modalities for screening for colorectal cancer including stool tests, flexible sigmoidoscopy, colonoscopy, barium enema, and computed tomographic (CT) colonography (3). Tests used primarily to detect cancer are the stool tests, including guaiac–fecal occult blood tests, fecal immunochemical tests, and stool DNA tests. Tests with a higher potential for cancer prevention help detect both precancerous polyps and early asymptomatic cancer and include flexible sigmoidoscopy, colonoscopy, barium enema examination, and CT colonography. Examinations designed to both prevent and detect cancer are recommended and include either colonoscopy or CT colonography (virtual colonoscopy).

Although FDG PET is not routinely used for screening or diagnostic purposes, it is not uncommon to incidentally detect colorectal carcinoma on whole body studies performed for other indications.

A study of 110 patients demonstrated that precancerous adenomatous polyps can be detected incidentally on whole body images performed for other indications with a sensitivity of 24% (24/59). The positivity rate increased to 90% for polyps larger than 13 mm in diameter, and the false-positive rate was 5.5% (6/10) (4). Agress et al. (5) reviewed FDG PET studies of 1,750 patients referred for evaluation of known or suspected malignancies. The authors found 58 unexpected focal areas of FDG uptake not related to the known primary in 53 (3.3%)

patients. Forty-two lesions were pathologically confirmed and 30/42 (71%) were malignant or premalignant, including 18 colonic adenomas and three colon carcinoma. Similar data was published by Kamel et al. on a review of 3,281 patients (6), Gutman et al. on a review of 1,716 patients (7), and Israel et al. on a review of 4,390 patients (8). The clinical history, physical examination, pattern of uptake, and correlation with anatomy are more helpful in avoiding false-positive interpretations than semi-quantitative evaluation by the standard uptake value (SUV). The sensitivity of FDG PET is highly dependent of both the size of the lesion, reaching 72% sensitivity for lesions greater than 1 cm, and the degree of dysplasia reaching 89% for carcinomas, 76% for high-grade, and 36% for low-grade dysplasia (9). The sensitivity is more limited for flat premalignant lesions (10). FDG uptake normally present in the gastrointestinal tract can occasionally be difficult to differentiate from a malignant lesion. Incidental colonic FDG uptake in 27 patients without colorectal carcinoma has been correlated with colonoscopic and/or histolopathologic findings (11). Diffuse uptake in eight patients was normal and associated with a normal colonoscopy. Segmental uptake was due to colitis in 5/6 patients. Focal uptake in seven patients was associated with benign adenomas.

Accurate interpretation of FDG PET images requires knowledge of the normal physiological distribution of FDG. Uptake in the gastrointestinal tract is variable from patient to patient. For example, FDG uptake along the esophagus is common, especially in the distal portion and at the gastroesophageal junction and in the presence of esophagitis. The wall of the stomach is usually faintly seen and can be used as an anatomical landmark, but occasionally the uptake can be relatively intense. There is uptake in the cecum of many patients probably related to abundant lymphoid tissue in the intestinal wall, among other factors. When marked activity is present in the bowel, evaluation for recurrence at the anastomotic site can be masked. Mild to moderate uptake is also usually seen at colostomy sites.

Although PET is not recommended for detection or screening for precancerous or malignant colonic neoplasms, the identification of focal colon uptake should not be ignored. Figure 1 illustrates the incidental finding of colon carcinoma in a patient referred to FDG PET/CT for lung cancer.

3. Initial Staging of Colorectal Cancer

The preoperative staging with imaging modalities is usually limited because most patients will benefit from colectomy to prevent intestinal obstruction and bleeding. The extent of the disease

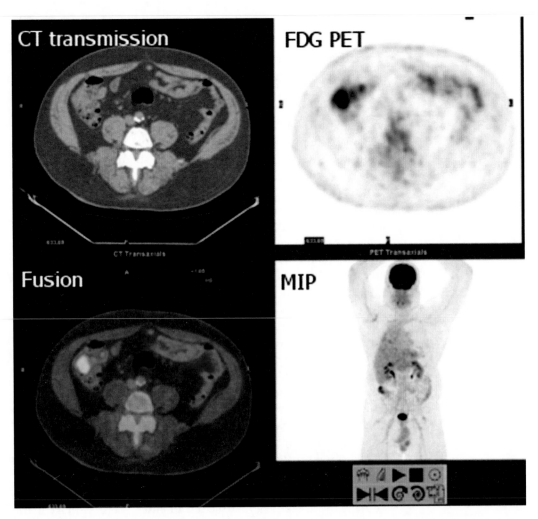

Fig. 1. A 58-year-old male with a history of stage IIIA nonsmall cell lung carcinoma treated with right pneumectomy 2 years earlier presented for evaluation of suspected recurrence. Maximum intensity projection (MIP) FDG PET image demonstrates moderate diffuse FDG uptake in the right chest consistent with the history of pneumectomy and mediastinal shift as well as a focus of markedly abnormal FDG uptake in the right upper quadrant inferior to the tip of the liver. PET/CT transaxial slices: the slice through that area demonstrates that the FDG uptake corresponds to the wall of the colon suspicious for malignancy. Follow-up: colonoscopy revealed an incidental 3 cm adenocarcinoma of the colon.

can be evaluated during surgery with excision of pericolonic and mesenteric lymph nodes along with peritoneal exploration. The performance of FDG PET preoperatively may be helpful if the detection of distant metastases will cancel surgery in patients with increased surgical risk. It may also be helpful as a baseline evaluation prior to chemotherapy and/or radiation therapy in patients with advanced stage disease as illustrated in Fig. 2.

Several studies have reported on the role of FDG PET in the initial preoperative staging of patients with colorectal carcinoma. The most recent study compared CT and FDG PET in 104 patients (12). In 14 patients, surgery was contraindicated by FDG-PET owing to the extent of disease, only 6/14 were suspected by CT. FDG-PET revealed four synchronous

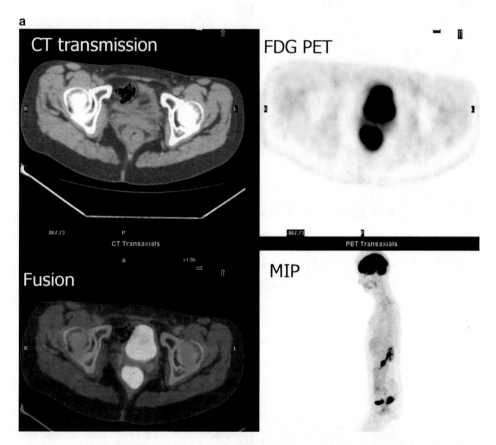

Fig. 2. A 47-year-old female with recently diagnosed rectal carcinoma was referred for initial staging with FDG PET/CT imaging (**a** and **b**). She underwent chemoradiation therapy but stopped chemotherapy prematurely due to side effects. She was referred for restaging with FDG PET/CT 6 weeks after the last treatment (**c**). MIP (**a** and **b**): the FDG PET lateral MIP image demonstrates a large area of intense focal FDG uptake behind the bladder consistent with the known primary (**a**). In addition, the FDG PET anterior MIP image demonstrates a focus of FDG uptake in the right lower quadrant (**b**). (**a**) The transaxial PET/CT slice through the lower pelvis demonstrates FDG uptake corresponding to a 4.6-cm rectal mass consistent with the primary carcinoma. (**b**) The transaxial PET/CT slice through the focus of FDG uptake in the right lower quadrant demonstrates FDG uptake in a 1.5-cm right iliac lymph node consistent with a metastasis. MIP (**c**) The FDG PET MIP image demonstrates normal distribution of FDG. (**c**) The transaxial PET/CT slice through the rectum demonstrates FDG uptake in the residual mass on the left rectal wall that has decreased in size from 4.6 to 1.8 cm. These changes represent a good response to therapy. The residual FDG uptake is consistent with a small volume of residual tumor and probably associated with inflammatory radiation changes. Follow-up: the patient refused additional therapy or surgery.

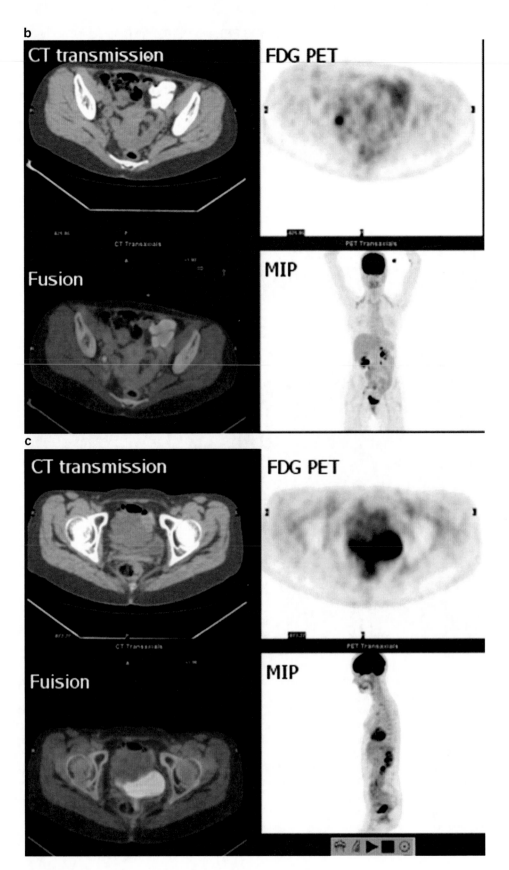

Fig. 2. (continued)

tumors. For N staging, both procedures showed a relatively high specificity but a low diagnostic accuracy (PET 56%, CT 60%) and sensitivity (PET 21%, CT 25%). For M assessment, diagnostic accuracy was 92% for FDG-PET and 87% for CT. FDG-PET results led to modification of the therapy approach in 50% of patients with unresectable disease. FDG-PET detected unsuspected disease in 19%, changed the stage in 13% and modified the surgical approach in 11%. These results confirmed results from previous studies (13, 14), and one of them also reported that FDG PET changed the treatment modality in 8% of patients and the extent of surgery in 13% (15). False-positive findings include abscesses, fistulas, diverticulitis, and occasionally adenomas.

The preoperative T-staging of rectal tumors can be performed with endorectal ultrasonography, hydro-CT, and endorectal MRI. All methods seem to be equivalent and are limited because peritumoral inflammation cannot be distinguished from infiltration by tumor (16).

4. Detection of Recurrent or Metastatic Colorectal Carcinoma

The 2005 recommendations from the American Society of Clinical Oncology for colorectal cancer surveillance following colectomy are the following (17): (1) history and physical examination every 3–6 months for the first 3 years, every 6 months during years 4 and 5, and subsequently at the discretion of the physician; (2) carcinoembryonic antigen (CEA) serum levels every 3 months postoperatively for at least 3 years after diagnosis; (3) annual computed tomography (CT) of the chest and abdomen for 3 years after primary therapy for patients who are at higher risk of recurrence and who could be candidates for curative-intent surgery, and pelvic CT scan for rectal cancer surveillance; and (4) colonoscopy at 3 years after operative treatment, and, if results are normal, every 5 years thereafter.

Most colon cancers are detected early and are treated surgically with curative intent. A recent retrospective review of 1,838 patients who underwent curative resection of nonmetastatic colorectal cancer was conducted. There were 994 patients with colon cancer and 844 patients with rectal cancer with a minimum follow-up of 3 years. The overall recurrence rate was 16.4% and the local recurrence rate, with or without systemic metastases, was 8.5% (18).

For patients who present with isolated liver metastases, hepatic resection is the only curative therapy but has the potential for significant morbidity and mortality (19). The poor prognosis of extrahepatic metastases is believed to be a contraindication to hepatic resection (20). Therefore, accurate noninvasive detection of inoperable disease with imaging modalities plays a pivotal role in selecting patients who would benefit from surgery.

5. Conventional Modalities for Detecting and Staging Recurrence

Elevated circulating levels of CEA occur in approximately two-thirds of patients with colorectal carcinoma. Serial measurements of serum CEA level are used to monitor these patients for recurrence with a sensitivity of 59% and specificity of 84%. Imaging is necessary to localize the site of recurrence (21). CT has been the conventional imaging modality used to localize recurrence. However, metastases to the peritoneum, mesentery, and lymph nodes are commonly missed on CT, and the differentiation of postsurgical changes from local tumor recurrence is often equivocal. The performance of CT for specific indications is addressed in more detail by comparison to PET in the section below. In patients undergoing exploration for recurrent colorectal cancer, the presence of adhesions or the limitations of surgical exposure (transverse upper abdominal incision for liver resection) often preclude a detailed intraoperative staging.

6. Detection and Staging Recurrent Colorectal Carcinoma with FDG PET Imaging

A number of studies have demonstrated the role of FDG PET as a functional imaging modality for detecting recurrent or metastatic colorectal carcinoma (22–43). Overall, the sensitivity of FDG PET imaging is in the 90% range and the specificity greater than 70%, both superior to CT. A meta-analysis of 11 clinical reports and 577 patients in 2000 determined that the sensitivity and specificity of FDG PET for detecting recurrent colorectal cancer were 97% and 76%, respectively (44). A comprehensive review of the PET literature (2,244 patient studies) in 2001 reported a weighted average for FDG PET sensitivity and specificity of 94% and 87%, respectively, compared to 79% and 73% for CT (45).

However, false-negative FDG PET findings have been reported with mucinous adenocarcinoma. Whiteford et al. (46) reported that the sensitivity of FDG PET imaging for detection of mucinous adenocarcinoma ($n = 16$) is significantly lower than for nonmucinous adenocarcinoma ($n = 93$), 58% and 92%, respectively ($p = 0.005$). The low sensitivity of FDG PET for detection of mucinous adenocarcinoma is most likely related to the relative hypocellularity of these tumors. Similar findings (41% sensitivity) were reported in a subsequent series of 22 patients (47).

Several studies have compared FDG PET and CT for differentiation of scar versus local recurrence (23, 24, 27–29, 33). CT was equivocal in most cases and the accuracy of FDG PET imaging was over 90%. In the largest study (76 patients) (29), the accuracy of FDG PET and CT were 95% and 65%, respectively.

Other studies have compared the accuracy of FDG PET and CT for detection of hepatic metastases (29, 30, 32, 33, 35). A 2002 meta-analysis was performed to compare the performance of noninvasive imaging methods (US, CT, MRI and FDG PET) in a mixed population of patients with colorectal, gastric, and esophageal cancers. At an equivalent specificity of 85%, FDG PET had the highest sensitivity of 90% compared to 76% for MRI, 72% for CT and 55% for US for detection of hepatic metastases on a patient-based analysis (48). A subsequent meta-analysis in 2005, including MRI with Gadolinium and superparamagnetic iron oxide particle (SPIO) enhancement, came to similar conclusions on a patient-based analysis (49). For a lesion-based analysis, FDG PET had the highest sensitivity of 76% compared to 66% for unenhanced MRI and 64% for CT. Both Gadolinium- and SPIO-enhanced MRI were superior to nonenhanced MRI, and SPIO MRI was the most sensitive technique with a sensitivity of 90% for detection of lesions greater than 1 cm, compared to 76% for FDG PET. In patients with colorectal cancer, FDG PET sensitivity for detection of hepatic metastases was compared to that of multiphase CT using intraoperative ultrasound as the reference standard for lesions of different sizes (50). The overall sensitivity was similar for PET (71%) and CT (72%). Both PET and CT missed approximately 30% of smaller lesions, resulting in a change of management in 7% of patients. There is one study comparing mangafodipir trisodium-enhanced hepatic MRI with FDG PET for detection of hepatic metastases in patients with colorectal and pancreatic cancer (51). Based on a per-patient analysis, MRI and FDG PET showed sensitivities of 97% and 93%, positive predictive values of 100% and 90%, and accuracies of 97% and 85%, respectively. On a per-lesion analysis, MRI and FDG PET showed sensitivities of 81% and 67%, positive predictive values of 90% and 81%, and accuracies of 76% and 64%, respectively. FDG PET provided additional information about extrahepatic disease and was useful in initial staging. However, significantly more and smaller (subcentimeter) hepatic metastases were detected with MRI than with FDG PET.

Flanagan et al. (34) described the use of FDG PET in 22 patients with unexplained elevation of serum CEA levels after resection of colorectal carcinoma accompanied by no abnormal findings on conventional work-up, including CT. Sensitivity and specificity of FDG PET for tumor recurrence were 100% and 71%, respectively. Valk et al. (35) reported sensitivity of 93% and specificity of 92% in a similar group of 18 patients. In both studies, PET correctly demonstrated tumor in two-thirds of patients with rising serum CEA levels and negative CT scans.

Valk et al. (35) compared the sensitivity and specificity of FDG PET and CT for specific anatomic locations and found that FDG PET was more sensitive than CT in all locations except the lung, where the two modalities were equivalent. The largest difference between PET and CT was found in the abdomen, pelvis, and retroperitoneum, where over one-third of PET-positive lesions were negative by CT. PET was also more specific than CT at all sites except the retroperitoneum, but the differences were smaller than the differences in sensitivity. Other investigators have found that FDG PET is especially useful for detecting retroperitoneal and pulmonary metastases (31, 32). In addition, by the nature of being a whole-body technique, FDG PET imaging permits identification of distant metastatic disease in the chest, abdomen, or pelvis which might not be in the field of view of routine CT staging examinations. Figure 3 illustrates the usefulness of PET/CT to detect metastastases in a patient with suspected recurrence.

7. FDG Imaging to Monitor Therapy

7.1. Systemic Chemotherapy

FDG PET is useful for monitoring the response to treatment in patients with advanced-stage colorectal carcinoma who have a typically poor prognosis. Systemic chemotherapy with 5-fluorouracil has demonstrated effective palliation and improved survival (52), although response rates are only 10–20% in patients with advanced disease. In a study of 18 patients with hepatic metastases, Findlay et al. (53) reported that responders could be discriminated from nonresponders after 4–5 weeks of chemotherapy with 5-fluorouracil by measuring FDG uptake before and during therapy. More recently, newer chemotherapeutic agents, particularly irinitecan and oxiplatin, have been shown to improve survival in combination with 5-fluorouracil-based therapies.

In a series of patients evaluated for resection of hepatic metastases, Akhurst et al. (54) compared detection of hepatic metastases in patients who underwent preoperative adjuvant chemotherapy with 5-fluorouracil within 3 months of resection versus those who did not receive adjuvant chemotherapy. In patients who underwent chemotherapy, the SUV was lower (average 4.5 vs. 6.6), the hexokinase activity was lower (14.4 vs. 23.4), and 37% of the lesions were not detected compared to 23% in patients who were not administered chemotherapy. The lower sensitivity of FDG PET in patient who underwent chemotherapy has been confirmed in multiple subsequent studies ranging from 49 to 62% compared to 65–92% for CT (55–57). The detection rate of FDG PET was especially low for small lesions, less than 20% for lesions smaller than 2 cm. The authors concluded that

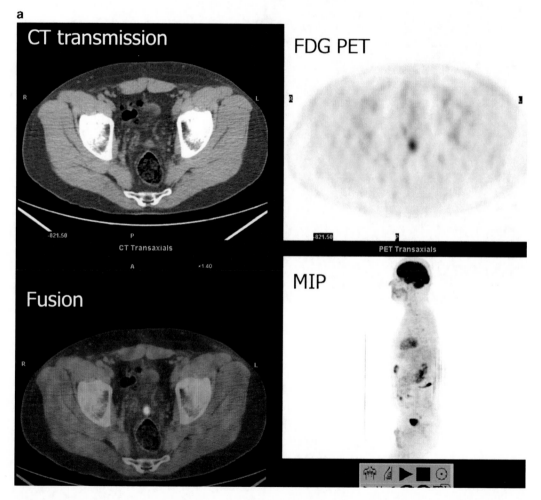

Fig. 3. A 49-year-old male with a history of colon carcinoma resected 2 years earlier presented for evaluation of suspected recurrence using FDG PET/CT imaging. Maximum intensity projection (MIP) FDG PET image demonstrates a focus of abnormal FDG uptake posterior and superior to the bladder (a) and multiple foci in the abdomen (b), the largest one on the midline at the level of the kidneys. (a) PET/CT transaxial slices: the slice through the pelvis demonstrates that the FDG uptake corresponds to a 1-cm nodule in the prerectal fat consistent with a metastasis. (b) PET/CT transaxial slices: the slice through the abdomen demonstrates that the FDG uptake corresponds a 3 cm densely calcified mass along the peritoneal surface of the anterior abdominal wall consistent with a calcified metastasis. Follow-up: biopsy of both lesions was diagnostic of metastases.

b

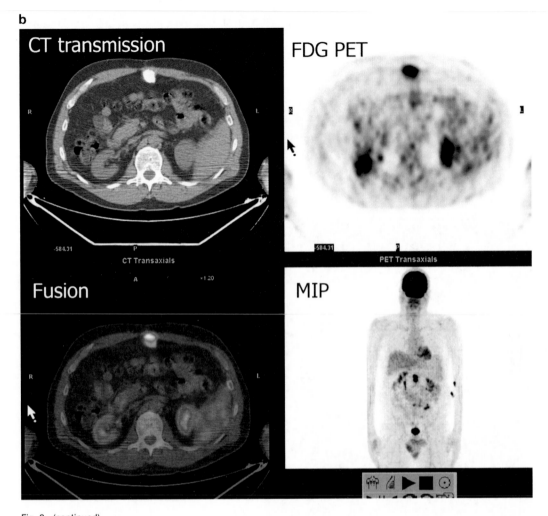

Fig. 3. (continued)

both PET and CT have a lower sensitivity for detection of hepatic metastases after chemotherapy, especially for small lesions, and CT is slightly more sensitive than PET. In addition, when there is normalization of FDG uptake in hepatic metastases after chemotherapy, complete histopathological response is seen in only 15% of lesions (58). Therefore, curative resection should not be deferred based on FDG PET.

7.2. Radiation Therapy   For patients with rectal carcinoma, systemic chemotherapy with 5-fluorouracil in combination with radiotherapy has also been shown to improve survival. In these patients, radiation-induced inflammation and necrosis makes it difficult to differentiate post-radiation changes from residual tumor using ultrasound, CT and MRI (59). A preliminary study on six patients demonstrated that

FDG uptake decreased in the primary tumor during radiation therapy, whereas the size did not change on CT (60). Another study of 44 patients demonstrated that FDG PET imaging can differentiate local recurrence from scarring after radiation therapy (61). However, increased FDG uptake immediately following radiation treatment may be due to inflammatory changes and is not always associated with residual tumor. The time course of postirradiation FDG activity has not been studied systematically; it is, however, generally accepted that FDG activity present 6 months after completion of radiation therapy most likely represents tumor recurrence. A case-controlled study of 60 FDG PET studies performed 6 months following external beam radiation therapy for rectal cancer found a sensitivity of 84% and specificity of 88% for detection of local pelvic recurrence (62). In a study of 15 patients with locally advanced rectal carcinoma, Guillem et al. (63) demonstrated that FDG PET imaging performed before and 4–5 weeks after completion of preoperative radiation and 5-fluorouracil-based chemotherapy had the potential to assess the pathological response. Subsequently, the same authors demonstrated that FDG PET imaging could predict long-term outcome after a median follow-up of 42 months (64). The mean percent decrease in SUVmax was 69% for patients free from recurrence and 37% for patients with recurrence.

7.3. Regional Therapy for Hepatic Metastases

Hepatic metastases can be treated by applying regional therapy to the liver. A variety of procedures to administer regional therapy to hepatic metastases have been investigated, including chemotherapy administered through the hepatic artery using infusion pumps, selective chemoembolization, cryoablation and alcohol ablation, radiofrequency ablation, and ^{90}Y-microspheres radioembolization (65–68).

Regional therapy to the liver by chemoembolization can be monitored using FDG PET imaging as shown by Vitola et al. (69) and Torizuka et al. (70). FDG uptake decreases in responding lesions and the presence of residual uptake in some lesions can help in guiding further regional therapy.

Radiofrequency ablation (RFA) and ^{90}Y-microspheres radioembolization are becoming the interventional techniques of choice for patients with unresectable hepatic metastases. Radiofrequency ablation is indicated for patients with a limited number of hepatic metastases measuring less than 5 cm in size. It is usually performed percutaneously under ultrasound or CT guidance. The probe tip delivers current and energy that destroy the liver tissue as it reaches 55°C. Median survival has been shown to improve with radiofrequency ablation of colorectal hepatic metastases compared to historical data (71). CT and MRI are limited in the evaluation of residual tumor because of contrast enhancement at the periphery of the ablative necrosis for up to 3 months post-RFA due to hyperemia and tissue regeneration (72). Langenhoff et al. (73) prospectively monitored 23 patients with liver metastases following RFA and cryoablation. Three weeks after therapy, 51/56 metastases became FDG negative, and there was no recurrence during 16 months follow-up; among the 5/56 lesions with persistent FDG uptake, 4/5 recurred. Data in smaller series of patients supports their findings (74, 75). Donckier et al. (76) followed 17 patients with 28 hepatic metastases at 1 week and 1 month post-RFA. FDG PET detected residual tumor in 4/28 lesions while CT imaging was negative. There were no recurrences in the 24/28 lesions negative by FDG PET after 11 months follow-up. In another study, the sensitivity for detection of residual tumor was 65% for PET/CT and 45% for CT (77). However, other studies have reported FDG uptake in the inflammatory rim making the interpretation difficult (77, 78). Antoch et al. (79) studied minipigs who underwent RFA of nontumorous liver. There was no FDG uptake within 90 min after completion of the procedure and no tissue regeneration was seen on histology, but there was a rim of enhancement on morphological imaging. This suggests that FDG imaging should be performed immediately after the procedure rather than several weeks later.

Intra-arterial hepatic radioembolization with ^{90}Y-microspheres is also an option for treatment of unresectable hepatic metastases and hepatocellular carcinoma. As most of the perfusion to the hepatic tumors comes from the hepatic artery, the labeled spheres administered intra-arterially and measuring approximately 30 μm in diameter are trapped in the capillaries. [90]Y has a half-life of 64 h and emits beta particles with an average range of 2.5 mm maximizing tumor damage. Prior to the procedure, the vascular anatomy to the liver must be assessed to avoid radioembolization in vessels perfusing other organs. Hepatopulmonary shunting can be evaluated on a separate day with ^{99m}Tc-macroaggregated albumin (MAA) scintigraphy; a lung/liver shunt fraction higher than 20% is usually a contraindication to treatment to avoid radiation pneumonitis. Wong et al. (80) have compared FDG PET imaging, CT or MRI and serum levels of CEA for monitoring the therapeutic response of hepatic metastases to ^{90}Y-glass microspheres 3 months after therapy. They found a significant difference between the FDG PET changes and the changes on CT or MRI; the changes in FDG uptake correlated better with the changes in serum levels of CEA. This was confirmed in a subsequent study by the same investigators using quantitative analysis (81). In summary, preliminary data suggest that FDG PET imaging may be able to effectively monitor the efficacy of regional therapy to hepatic metastases but these data need to be confirmed in larger series of patients.

8. Surveillance

The surveillance strategies after curative treatment of colorectal cancer were summarized in 2004 and did not include FDG PET imaging at that time (82).

A single study has reported that regular FDG PET monitoring in the follow-up of colorectal cancer patients may permit the earlier detection of recurrence, and influence therapy strategies (83). One hundred and thirty patients who had undergone curative therapy were randomized to undergo either conventional or FDG PET procedures during follow-up. Recurrence was diagnosed in 46 patients (25 in the FDG PET group, and 21 in the conventional group). PET revealed unexpected malignancies in three additional patients. There were three false-positive cases of FDG PET that led to no beneficial procedures and two false-negative cases of peritoneal carcinomatosis. Recurrences were detected earlier in the PET group (12.1 vs. 15.4 months) and were more frequently cured by surgery (ten vs. two patients).

9. Impact of FDG PET Imaging on Patient Management

In a meta-analysis of the literature performed in 2000, FDG PET imaging changed the management in 29% (102/349) of patients (44). A comprehensive review of the PET literature in 2001 reported a weighted average change of management related to FDG PET findings in 32% of 915 patients (45).

The greater sensitivity of PET compared to CT in the diagnosis and staging of recurrent tumor results from two factors: early detection of abnormal tumor metabolism, before changes have become apparent by anatomic imaging, and the whole body nature of PET imaging, which permits diagnosis of tumor when it occurs in unusual and unexpected sites. FDG PET imaging allows detection of unsuspected metastases in 13–36% of patients and has a clinical impact in 14–65% (28, 29, 31–35, 37, 41–43, 84, 85). In the study of Delbeke et al. (32), surgical management was altered by PET in 28% of patients, in one-third by initiating surgery and in two-thirds by avoiding surgery. In a survey-based study of 60 referring oncologists, surgeons, and generalists, FDG PET performed at initial staging had a major impact on the management of colorectal cancer patients and contributed to a change in clinical stage in 42% (80% upstaged and 20% downstaged) and a change in the clinical management in over 60%. As a result of the PET findings, physicians avoided major surgery in 41% of patients for whom surgery was the intended treatment (86). In a prospective study of 51 patients evaluated for resection of hepatic metastases, clinical management decisions based on conventional diagnostic methods were changed in 20% of patients based on the findings on FDG PET imaging, especially by detecting unsuspected extrahepatic disease (85). In a 2005 meta-analysis analyzing the performance of FDG PET in patients with hepatic metastases, the specificity of FDG PET (96%) was higher than CT (84%) for detection of hepatic metastases, the sensitivity of PET (91%) was higher than CT (61%) for detection of extrahepatic metastases, and PET changed the management of 31% of patients (range 20–58%) (87). PET changes the management and also improves prognostic stratification in patients with recurrent colorectal cancer (88).Two groups of symptomatic patients were studied: (1) patients with a residual structural lesion suggestive of recurrent tumor and (2) patients with pulmonary or hepatic metastases considered to be potentially resectable. Data were similar in both groups. PET detected additional sites of disease in 48 and 44% of patients. A change in planned management was documented in 66 and 49%. These management plans were implemented in 96% of patients. Follow-up data showed progressive disease in 60 and 66% of patients with additional lesions detected by PET, compared with conventional imaging, and in 36 and 39% of patients with no additional lesions detected by PET.

Although survival is not an endpoint for a diagnostic test, Strasberg et al. (84) have estimated the survival of patients who underwent FDG PET imaging in their preoperative evaluation for resection of hepatic metastases. The Kaplan–Meier test estimate of the overall survival at 3 years was 77% and the lower confidence limit was 60%. These percentages are higher than those in previously published series that ranged from 30 to 64%. In the patients undergoing FDG PET imaging prior to hepatic resection, the 3-year disease-free survival rate was 40%, again higher than that usually reported (25%).

The same group of investigators recently reported the 5-year survival after resection of metastasis from colorectal carcinoma (89). They established the 5-year survival of patients with conventional diagnostic imaging from the literature, by pooling the data of 19 studies with a total of 6,090 patients. The 5-year survival rate was 30% and appeared not to have changed over time. These results were compared to their group of 100 patients with hepatic metastases, who were preoperatively staged for resection with curative intent with the addition of FDG PET imaging. The 5-year survival rate improved to 58%, indicating that they were able to define a subgroup after conventional imaging that has a better prognosis. The main contribution was in detecting occult extrahepatic disease, leading to a reduction of futile surgeries.

10. Clinical Impact of Integrated PET/ CT Imaging

Concurrent PET/CT imaging with an integrated system may be especially important in the abdomen and pelvis. PET images alone may be difficult to interpret owing to the absence of anatomical landmarks (other than the kidneys and bladder), the presence of nonspecific uptake in the stomach, small bowel and colon, and urinary excretion of FDG. Concurrent PET/CT imaging is helpful for differentiating focal retention of urine in the ureter, for example, versus an FDG-avid lymph node.

A study of 45 patients with colorectal cancer referred for FDG PET imaging using an integrated PET/CT system concluded that PET/CT imaging increases the accuracy of interpretation and certainty of location of the lesions. In their study, (1) the frequency of equivocal and probable lesion characterization was reduced by 50% with PET/CT compared to PET alone, (2) the number of definite locations was increased by 25%, and (3) the overall correct staging increased from 78 to 89% (90).

A study of 204 patients (34 with gastrointestinal tumors) performed at Rambam Medical Center (91) using an integrated PET/CT system concluded that the diagnostic accuracy of PET is improved in approximately 50% of patients. In that study, PET/CT fusion images improved characterization of equivocal lesions as definitely benign in 10% of sites and definitely malignant in 5% of sites. It precisely defined the anatomic location of malignant FDG uptake in 6% and led to retrospective lesion detection on PET or CT in 8%. The results of PET/CT images had an impact on the management of 14% (28/204) of patients, 7/28 patients with a change of management had colorectal cancer representing 20% (7/34) of patients with gastrointestinal tumors. The changes in management in the seven patients with colorectal cancer included guiding colonoscopy and biopsy for a local recurrence ($n=2$), guiding biopsy to a metastatic supraclavicular lymph node ($n=1$), guiding surgery to localized metastatic lymph nodes ($n=3$), and referral to chemotherapy ($n=2$).

Similar conclusions were found in a study of 173 patients performed at Vanderbilt University, 24 of which had colorectal carcinoma (92).

Selzner et al. (93) have compared contrast-enhanced CT and nonenhanced PET/CT in 76 patients referred for restaging prior to resection of hepatic metastases. For detection of hepatic metastases, contrast-enhanced CT and nonenhanced PET/CT had similar sensitivities of 95% and 91%, respectively. However, for evaluation of patients with a prior hepatic resection, the PET/CT had a superior specificity of 100% compared to 50% for contrast-enhanced CT. For local recurrence, PET/CT had a superior sensitivity of 93% compared to 53% for contrast-enhanced CT. Similar conclusions were reached for extrahepatic metastases with a sensitivity of 89% for PET/CT compared to 64% for contrast-enhanced CT. There was an impact of PET/CT on the management of 21% of patients. False-negative PET/CT studies were seen for small lesions (less than 5 mm) and in some patients who underwent chemotherapy in the month prior to PET/CT.

The performance of PET/contrasted CT has also been compared to PET/low-dose CT (94, 95). PET/low-dose CT was superior to contrasted CT (without PET) in 50% of patients due to detection of additional metastases and changed therapy in 10% of patients. PET/contrasted CT was superior to PET/low-dose CT in 72% of patients mainly due to correct segmental localization of hepatic metastases, changing management in 42% (23/54) of patients. For nodal staging of patients with rectal cancer, the accuracy of PET/contrasted CT was slightly superior to PET/low-dose CT (79% compared to 70%), but the difference was not statistically significant.

CT transmission images should be carefully reviewed for detection of malignant lesions that may not be FDG-avid such as mucinous tumors or renal cell carcinomas, for example, as well other incidental findings relevant to patient care. An analysis of 250 patients demonstrated that these findings are uncommon (3% of patients) but could be important enough to warrant alterations in clinical management (96).

Concurrent PET/CT fusion images have the potential to provide better maps than CT alone to modulate field and dose of radiation therapy, also in patients with colorectal carcinoma (97, 98).

11. Limitations of FDG Imaging

Tumor detectability depends on both the size of the lesion and the degree of uptake, as well as surrounding background uptake and intrinsic resolution of the imaging system. False-negative lesions can be due to partial volume averaging, leading to underestimation of the uptake in small lesions (less than twice the resolution of the imaging system) or in necrotic or mucinous lesions, falsely classifying these lesions as benign instead of malignant. Elevated blood glucose levels decrease the sensitivity for detection of metastases also in patients with colorectal carcinoma (99). The SUV of hepatic metastases averaged 9.4 when patients were fasting (mean serum glucose 92 mg/dl) and 4.3 after i.v. glucose infusion of 4 mg/kg/min in the same patients (mean serum glucose 158 mg/dl). After glucose infusion, 6/20 metastases were not detectable and 10/20 were not well seen.

False-positive findings are due to physiologic variations of FDG distribution and FDG-avidity of inflammatory lesions. In view of the known high uptake of FDG by activated macrophages, neutrophils, fibroblasts, and granulation tissue, it is not surprising that inflamed tissue demonstrates FDG activity. Mild to moderate FDG activity seen early after radiation therapy, along recent incisions, infected incisions, biopsy sites, drainage tubing, and catheters, as well as colostomy sites can lead to errors in interpretation if the history is not known. Postradiation therapy uptake may persist for several months. Comparison with baseline FDG images and knowledge of the radiation port are helpful. Some inflammatory lesions, especially granulomatous ones, may be markedly FDG-avid and can be mistaken for malignancies; this includes inflammatory bowel disease, tuberculosis, sarcoidosis, histoplasmosis, and aspergillosis among others (100).

12. Cost and Reimbursement Issues

Including FDG PET in the evaluation of patients with recurrent colorectal carcinoma has been shown to be cost-effective in a study using clinical evaluation of effectiveness with modeling of costs and in studies using decision-tree sensitivity analysis (35, 101, 102). In both type of studies, all costs calculations were based on Medicare reimbursement rates and a $1,800 cost for a PET scan.

In a management algorithm where recurrence at more than one site was treated as nonresectable, Valk et al. (35) evaluated cost savings in 78 patients undergoing preoperative staging of recurrent colorectal carcinoma. This study was limited to preoperative patients, and demonstrated potential savings of $3,003 per patient resulting from diagnosis of nonresectable tumor by PET.

In 1997, Gambhir et al. (101) used a quantitative decision-tree model combined with sensitivity analysis to evaluate cost issues if all patients presenting with recurrent colorectal cancer undergo FDG PET imaging. The conventional strategy for detection of recurrence and determination of resectability using CEA levels and CT was compared to the conventional strategy plus PET for all patients presenting with suspected recurrence. The assumptions included prevalence of resectable disease of 3%, sensitivity and specificity of 65% and 45%, respectively for CT, and 90% and 85% for PET. The conventional strategy plus PET showed an incremental saving of $220 per patient without a loss of life expectancy.

Park et al. (101) used the decision-tree sensitivity analysis to evaluate the cost of adding FDG PET imaging in the evaluation of patients referred for suspected recurrence based on elevated CEA levels and candidates for hepatic resection. The CT plus PET strategy was higher in mean cost by $429 per patient, but resulted in an increase in the mean life expectancy of 9.5 days per patient.

In July 2001, the Center for Medical Services (CMS) approved and implemented reimbursement by Medicare for six types of malignant tumors including colorectal carcinoma. This coverage is for diagnosis, staging, and restaging, but not for monitoring therapy.

13. Guidelines and Recommendations for the use of ¹⁸F-FDG PET and PET/CT in Colorectal Carcinoma

The National Comprehensive Cancer Network (NCCN) has incorporated FDG PET and PET/CT in the evaluation and management algorithm of a variety of malignancies including colorectal cancer (103). The use of FDG PET (PET/CT where available) is recommended in the following clinical scenarios: (1) initial staging if initial conventional studies are equivocal for metastatic disease; (2) rising CEA levels or suspicious symptoms unless conventional imaging is diagnostic; (3) restaging if curative resection is considered. FDG PET is not indicated: (1) for restaging after nonsurgical treatment of metastatic disease; and (2) for posttreatment surveillance.

A multidisciplinary panel of experts reviewed meta-analyses and systematic reviews published in the FDG PET literature before March 2006 and made recommendations for the use of FDG PET in oncology (104): (1) the panel found little evidence to support the use of FDG PET for the diagnosis of colorectal carcinoma; (2) FDG PET should be used routinely in addition to conventional imaging in the preoperative diagnostic workup of patients with potentially resectable hepatic metastases from colorectal cancer; (3) FDG PET should routinely be obtained after the conventional workup, especially if CEA levels are elevated and the results of the conventional workup are negative. PET can also be used to differentiate between local relapse and postsurgical scars.

14. Potential New PET Tracers for Clinical Use

Besides evaluation of glucose metabolism with FDG, PET can assess various other biologic parameters such as perfusion, metabolism of other compounds, hypoxia, and receptor expression.

Some of these radiopharmaceuticals are labeled with positron emitters that have a short half-life, such as ^{15}O ($T1/2 = 2$ min), ^{13}N ($T1/2 = 10$ min), and ^{11}C ($T1/2 = 20$ min). The short half-life of these radioisotopes prevents any timely distribution of the radiopharmaceuticals labeled with them, so their use is restricted to institutions having a cyclotron and associated laboratories on-site. Some tracers labeled with ^{18}F, such as ^{18}F-fluoride and ^{18}F-fluorothymidine (FLT) are being investigated for clinical use.

^{18}F-fluoride was first described as a skeletal imaging agent in the 1960s but then was replaced by the ^{99m}Tc-labeled diphosphonate radiopharmaceuticals (105). With the widespread applications of FDG PET in oncology, PET imaging systems are becoming more widely available, and there is a renewed interest in ^{18}F-fluoride. Although the mechanism of uptake for ^{18}F-fluoride is similar to that for other bone-imaging radiopharmaceuticals (106), the spatial resolution of the PET technology is superior to that of both planar and SPECT imaging using the ^{99m}Tc-radiopharmaceuticals. Because of the better spatial resolution and routine acquisition of tomographic images, ^{18}F-fluoride PET imaging offers potential advantages over bone scintigraphy in detecting metastases. Although skeletal metastases are not common in colorectal cancer, ^{18}F-fluoride may have a role in the future if skeletal metastases are suspected clinically.

The rate of DNA synthesis can be assessed using ^{11}C-thymidine or FLT. Thymidine is a DNA precursor and allows direct assessment of tumor proliferation. Shields et al. (107) have developed and evaluated ^{18}FLT for clinical use because of its ^{18}F labeling. A report of 17 patients with colorectal cancer comparing FDG and FLT demonstrated that all primary tumors were visualized with both tracers, but FDG uptake was on average twofold higher with FDG compared to FLT (108) and therefore more easily seen. Pulmonary and peritoneal metastases were identified with both tracers, but the sensitivity of FLT for hepatic metastases was only 34% compared to 97% for FDG due to the high physiologic hepatic background activity seen with FLT. Therefore, the authors concluded that it was unlikely that FLT would play an important role in the evaluation of patients with colorectal carcinoma.

15. Summary

Evaluation of patients with known or suspected recurrent colorectal carcinoma is now an accepted and reimbursed indication for FDG PET imaging. PET and CT are complimentary, and therefore integrated PET/CT imaging should be performed where available. The most common indication is for diagnosis and staging of recurrence, and for preoperative staging (N and M) of known recurrence that is considered to be resectable. FDG PET/CT imaging is valuable for differentiation of posttreatment changes from recurrent tumor, differentiation of benign from malignant lesions (indeterminate lymph nodes, hepatic, and pulmonary lesions), and evaluation of patients with rising tumor markers in the absence of a known source. Addition of FDG PET/CT to the evaluation of these patients reduces overall treatment costs by accurately identifying patients who will and will not benefit from surgical procedures.

Although initial staging at the time of diagnosis is often performed during colectomy, FDG PET/CT imaging is now commonly performed preoperatively. It is particularly useful if surgery can be avoided when FDG PET demonstrates metastases. Screening for recurrence in patients at high risk has also been advocated. FDG PET imaging seems promising for monitoring patient response to therapy but larger studies are necessary.

The diagnostic implications of integrated PET/CT imaging include improved detection of lesions on both the CT and FDG PET images, better differentiation of physiologic from pathologic foci of metabolism, and better localization of the pathologic foci. This new powerful technology provides more accurate interpretation of both CT and FDG PET images and therefore more optimal patient care. PET/CT fusion images impact clinical management by guiding further procedures (biopsy, surgery, and radiation therapy), excluding the need for additional procedures, and changing both inter- and intramodality therapy.

References

1. Cancer facts and figures, 2008.
2. Smith RA, Cokkinides V, Eyre HJ. American Cancer Society Guidelines for the early detection of cancer, 2004. CA Cancer J Clin 2004;54:41–52.
3. McFarland EG, Levin B, Lieberman DA, Pickhardt PJ, Johnson CD, Glick SN, Brooks D, Smith RA. Revised colorectal screening guidelines: joint effort of the American Cancer Society, U.S. Multisociety Task Force on Colorectal Cancer, and American College of Radiology. Radiology. 2008 Sep;248(3): 717–720.
4. Yasuda S, Fujii H, Nakahara T, Nishumi N, Takahashi W, Ide M, Shohtsu A. 18F-FDG PET detection of colonic adenomas. J Nucl Med 2001;42:989–992.
5. Agress H and Cooper BZ. Detection of clinically unexpected malignant and premalignant tumors with whole-body FDG PET: histopathologic comparison. Radiology 2004;230 (2): 417–422.
6. Kamel EM, Thumshirn M, Truninger K, et al. Significance of incidental 18F-FDG accumulations in the gastrointestinal tract in PET/CT: Correlation with endoscopic and histopathological results. J Nucl Med 2004;45:1804–1810.
7. Gutman F, Alberini JL, Wartski M et al. Incidental colonic focal lesions detected by FDG PET/CT. Am J Roentgenol 2005;185 (2):495–500.
8. Israel O, Yefremov N, Bar-Shalom R, Kagana O, Frenkel A, Keidar Z, Fischer D. PET/CT detection of unexpected gastrointestinal foci of 18F-FDG uptake: incidence, localization patterns, and clinical significance. J Nucl Med. 2005 May;46(5):758–762.
9. Van Kouwen MC, Nagengast FM, Jansen JB, Oyen WJ, Drenth JP. 2-(18F)-fluoro-2-deoxy-D-glucose positron emission tomography detects clinical relevant adenomas of the colon: a prospective study. J Clin Oncol 2005;23 (16): 3713–3717.

10. Friedland S, Soetikno R, Carlisle M, Taur A, Kaltenbach T, Segall G. 18-Fluorodeoxyglucose positron emission tomography has limited sensitivity for colonic adenomas and early stage colon cancer. Gastrointest Endosc 2005;61 (3):305–400.

11. Tatlidil R, Jadvar H, Bading JR, Conti PS. Incidental colonic fluorodeoxyglucose uptake: correlation with colonoscopic and histopathologic findings. Radiology 2002;224(3):783–787.

12. Llamas-Elvira JM, Rodríguez-Fernández A, Gutiérrez-Sáinz J, Gomez-Rio M, Bellon-Guardia M, Ramos-Font C, Rebollo-Aguirre AC, Cabello-García D, Ferrón-Orihuela A. Fluorine-18 fluorodeoxyglucose PET in the preoperative staging of colorectal cancer. Eur J Nucl Med Mol Imaging. 2007 Jun; 34(6):859–867.

13. Abdel-Nabi H, Doerr RJ, Lamonica DM, Cronin VR, Galantowicz PJ, Carbone GM, Spaulding MB. Staging of primary colorectal carcinomas with fluorine-18 fluorodeoxyglucose whole-body PET: Correlation with histopathologic and CT findings. Radiology 1998;206:755–760.

14. Mukai M, Sadahiro S, Yasuda S, Ishida H, Tokunaga N, Tajima T, Makuuchi H. Preoperative evaluation by whole-body 18F-fluorodeoxyglucose positron emission tomography in patients with primary colorectal cancer. Oncol Reports 2000;7:85–87.

15. Kantorova I, Lipska L, Belohlavek O, et al. Routine 18F-FDG PET preoperative staging of colorectal cancer: Comparison with conventional staging and its impact on treatment decision making. J Nucl Med 2003;44:1784–1788.

16. Dinter DJ, Hofheinz RD, Hartel M, Kaehler GF, Neff W, Diehl SJ. Preoperative staging of rectal tumors: comparison of endorectal ultrasound, hydro-CT, and high-resolution endorectal MRI. Onkologie. 2008 May; 31(5):230–235.

17. Desch CE, Benson AB 3rd, Somerfield MR, Flynn PJ, Krause C, Loprinzi CL, Minsky BD, Pfister DG, Virgo KS, Petrelli NJ; American Society of Clinical Oncology. Colorectal cancer surveillance: 2005 update of an American Society of Clinical Oncology practice guideline. J Clin Oncol. 2005;23(33):8512–8519.

18. Yun HR, Lee LJ, Park JH, Cho YK, Cho YB, Lee WY, Kim HC, Chun HK, Yun SH. Local recurrence after curative resection in patients with colon and rectal cancers. Int J Colorectal Dis. 2008 Aug 8. [Epub ahead of print]

19. Helling TS, Blondeau B. Anatomic segmental resection compared to major hepatectomy in the treatment of liver neoplasms. HPB (Oxford). 2005;7(3):222–225. Links

20. Hughes KS, Simon R, Songhorabodi S, et al. Resection of liver for colorectal carcinoma metastases: a multi-institutional study of indications for resection. Surgery. 1988;103: 278–288.

21. Moertel CG, Fleming TR, McDonald JS, Haller DJ, Laurie JA, Tangen CA. An evaluation of the carcinoembryonic antigen (CEA) test for monitoring patients with resected colon cancer. JAMA. 1993;270:943–947.

22. Yonekura Y, Benua RS, Brill AB, et al. Increased accumulation of 2-deoxy-2[^{18}F]fluoro-D- glucose in liver metastases from colon carcinoma. J Nucl Med 1982;23:1133–1137.

23. Strauss LG, Clorius JH, Schlag P, et al. Recurrence of colorectal tumors: PET evaluation. Radiology 1989;170:329–332.

24. Ito K, Kato T, Tadokoro M, et al. Recurrent rectal cancer and scar: differentiation with PET and MR imaging. Radiology 1992;182:549–552.

25. Kim EE, Chung SK, Haynie TP, et al. Differentiation of residual or recurrent tumors from post-treatment changes with F-18 FDG-PET. Radiographics. 1992;12:269–279.

26. Gupta NC, Falk PM, Frank AL, Thorson AM, Firck MP, Bowman B. Pre-operative staging of colorectal carcinoma using positron emission tomography. Nebr Med J 1993;78:30–35.

27. Falk PM, Gupta NC, Thorson AG, et al. Positron emission tomography for preoperative staging of colorectal carcinoma. Dis Colon Rectum 1994;37:153–156.

28. Beets G, Penninckx F, Schiepers C, et al. Clinical value of whole-body positron emission tomography with [18F]fluorodeoxyglucose in recurrent colorectal cancer. Br J Surg. 1994;81:1666–1670.

29. Schiepers C, Penninckx F, De Vadder N, et al. Contribution of PET in the diagnosis of recurrent colorectal cancer: comparison with conventional imaging. Eur J Surg Oncol 1995;21:517–522.

30. Vitola JV, Delbeke D, Sandler MP, et al. Positron emission tomography to stage metastatic colorectal carcinoma to the liver. Am J Surg 1996;171:21–26.

31. Lai DT, Fulham M, Stephen MS, et al. The role of whole-body positron emission tomography with [18F]fluorodeoxyglucose in identifying operable colorectal cancer. Arch Surg. 1996;131:703–707.

32. Delbeke D, Vitola J, Sandler MP, et al. Staging recurrent metastatic colorectal carcinoma with PET. J Nucl Med 1997;38: 1196–1201.

33. Ogunbiyi OA, Flanagan FL, Dehdashti F, et al. Detection of recurrent and metastatic

colorectal cancer: comparison of positron emission tomography and computed tomography. Ann Surg Oncol 1997; 4:613–620.

34. Flanagan FL, Dehdashti F, Ogunbiyi OA, Siegel BA. Utility of FDG PET for investigating unexplained plasma CEA elevation in patients with colorectal cancer. Ann Surg 1998;227(3):319–323.

35. Valk PE, Abella-Columna E, Haseman MK, et al. Whole-body PET imaging with F-18-fluorodeoxyglucose in management of recurrent colorectal cancer. Arch Surg 1999;134:503–511.

36. Ruhlmann J, Schomburg A, Bender H, et al. Fluorodeoxyglucose whole-body positron emission tomography in colorectal cancer patients studied in routine daily practice. Dis Colon Rectum 1997;40:1195–1204.

37. Flamen P, Stroobants S, Van Cutsem E, Dupont P, Bormans G, De Vadder N, Penninckx F, Van Hoe L, Mortelmans L. Additional value of whole-body positron emission tomography withfluorine-18-2-fluoro-2-deoxy-D-glucose in recurrent colorectal cancer. J Clin Oncol. 1999 Mar; 17(3):894–901.

38. Akhurst T, Larson SM. Positron emission tomography imaging of colorectal cancer. Semin Oncol. 1999;26(5):577–583.

39. Vogel SB, Drane WE, Ros PR, Kerns SR, Bland KI. Prediction of surgical resectability in patients with hepatic colorectal metastases. Ann Surg 1994;219:508–516.

40. Imbriaco M, Akhurst T, Hilton S, Yeung HW, Macapinlac HA, Mazumdar M, Pace L, Kemeny N, Erdi Y, Cohen A, Fong Y, Guillem J, Larson SM. Whole-Body FDG-PET in patients with Recurrent Colorectal Carcinoma. A comparative Study with CT. Clin Pos Imag 2000;3(3):107–114.

41. Imdahl A, Reinhardt MJ, Nitzsche EU, Mix M, Dingeldey A, Einert A, Baier P, Farthmann EH. Impact of 18F-FDG-positron emission tomography for decision making in colorectal cancer recurrences. Arch Surg. 2000;385(2):129–134.

42. Staib L, Schirrmeister H, Reske SN, Beger HG. Is (18)F-fluorodeoxyglucose positron emission tomography in recurrent colorectal cancer a contribution to surgical decision making? Am J Surg. 2000;180(1):1–5.

43. Kalff VV, Hicks R, Ware R. F-18 FDG PET for suspected or confirmed recurrence of colon cancer. A prospective study of impact and outcome. Clin Pos Imag 2000;3:183.

44. Huebner RH, Park KC, Shepherd JE, Schwimmer J, Czernin J, Phelphs M,

Gambhir SS. A meta-analysis of the literature for whole-body FDG PET detection of colorectal cancer. J Nucl Med 2000;41: 1177–1189.

45. Gambhir SS, Czernin J, Schimmer J, Silverman DHS, Coleman RE, Phelps ME. A tabulated review of the literature. J Nucl Med 2001;42 (suppl):9S–12S.

46. Whiteford MH, Whiteford HM, Yee LF, Ogunbiyi OA, Dehdashti F, Siegel BA, Birnbaum EH, Fleshman JW, Kodner IJ, Read TE. Usefulness of FDG-PET scan in the assessment of suspected metastatic or recurrent adenocarcinoma of the colon and rectum. Dis Colon Rectum. 2000;43(6):759–67; discussion 767–770.

47. Berger KL, Nicholson SA, Dehadashti F, Siegel BA. FDG PET evaluation of mucinous neoplasms: correlation of FDG uptake with histopathologic features. Am J Roentgenol 2000;174(4):1005–1008.

48. Kinkel K, Lu Y, Both M, Warren RS, Thoeni RF. Detection of hepatic metastases from cancers of the gastrointestinal tract by using noninvasive imaging methods (US, CT, MR imaging, PET): a meta-analysis. Radiology 2002;224(3):748–756.

49. Bipat S, van Leeuwen MS, Comans EF, Pijl ME, Bossuyt PM, Zwinderman AH, Stoker J. Colorectal liver metastases: CT, MR imaging, and PET for diagnosis--meta-analysis. Radiology. 2005 Oct;237(1):123–131.

50. Wiering B, Ruers TJ, Krabbe PF, Dekker HM, Oyen WJ. Comparison of multiphase CT, FDG-PET and intra-operative ultrasound in patients with colorectal liver metastases selected for surgery. Ann Surg Oncol. 2007 Feb;14(2):818–826.

51. Sahani DV, Kalva SP, Fischman AJ, Kadavigere R, Blake M, Hahn PF, Saini S. Detection of liver metastases from adenocarcinoma of the colon and pancreas: comparison of mangafodipir trisodium-enhanced liver MRI and whole-body FDG PET. AJR Am J Roentgenol. 2005 Jul;185(1):239–246.

52. Venook A: Critical evaluation of current treatments in metastatic colorectal cancer. Oncologist 2005;10:250–261.

53. Findlay M, Young H, Cunningham D, et al. Noninvasive monitoring of tumor metabolism using fluorodeoxyglucose and positron emission tomography in colorectal cancer liver metastases: correlation with tumor response to fluorouracil. J Clin Oncol. 1996;14:700–708.

54. Akhurst T, Kates TJ, Mazumdar M, Yeung H, Riedel ER, Burt BM, Blumgart L, Jarnagin W, Larson SM, Fong Y. Recent

chemotherapy reduces the sensitivity of [18F]fluorodeoxyglucose positron emission tomography in the detection of colorectal metastases. J Clin Oncol. 2005 Dec 1;23(34):8713–8716.

55. Takahashi S, Kuroki Y, Nasu K, Nawano S, Konishi M, Nakagohri T, Gotohda N, Saito N, Kinoshita T. Positron emission tomography with F-18 fluorodeoxyglucose in evaluating colorectal hepatic metastasis down-staged by chemotherapy. Anticancer Res. 2006 Nov-Dec;26(6):4705–4711.

56. Carnaghi C, Tronconi MC, Rimassa L, Tondulli L, Zuradelli M, Rodari M, Doci R, Luttmann F, Torzilli G, Rubello D, Al-Nahhas A, Santoro A, Chiti A.Utility of 18F-FDG PET and contrast-enhanced CT scan in the assessment of residual liver metastasis from colorectal cancer following adjuvant chemotherapy. Nucl Med Rev Cent East Eur. 2007;10(1):12–15.

57. Lubezky N, Metser U, Geva R, Nakache R, Shmueli E, Klausner JM, Even-Sapir E, Figer A, Ben-Haim M. The role and limitations of 18-fluoro-2-deoxy-D-glucose positron emission tomography (FDG-PET) scan and computerized tomography (CT) in restaging patients with hepatic colorectal metastases following neoadjuvant chemotherapy: comparison with operative and pathological findings. J Gastrointest Surg. 2007 Apr; 11(4):472–8.

58. Tan MC, Linehan DC, Hawkins WG, Siegel BA, Strasberg SM. Chemotherapy-induced normalization of FDG uptake by colorectal liver metastases does not usually indicate complete pathologic response. J Gastrointest Surg. 2007;11(9):1112–9.

59. Kahn H, Alexander A, Ratinic J et al. Preoperative staging of irradiated rectal cancers using digital rectal examination, computed tomography, endorectal ultrasound, and magnetic resonance imaging does not accurately predict T0, N0 pathology. Dis Colon Rectum 1997;40:140–144.

60. Strauss LG, Clorius JH, Schlag P, et al. Recurrence of colorectal tumors: PET evaluation. Radiology 1989;170:329–332.

61. Haberkorn U, Strauss LG, Dimitrakopoulou A, Engenhart R, Oberdorfer F, Ostertag H, Romahn J, van Kaick G. PET studies of fluorodeoxyglucose metabolism in patients with recurrent colorectal tumors receiving radiotherapy. J Nucl Med. 1991;31:1485–1490.

62. Moore HG, Akhurst T, Larson SM, Minsky BD, Mazumdar M, Guillem JG. A case controlled study of 18-fluorodeoxyglucose positron emission tomography in the detection of pelvic recurrence in previously irradiated rectal cancer patients. J Am Coll Surg 2003;197(1):22–28.

63. Guillem J, Calle J, Akhurst T, et al. Prospective assessment of primary rectal cancer response to preoperative radiation and chemotherapy using 18-Fluorodeoxyglucose positron emission tomography. Dis Colon Rectum. 2000;43:18–24.

64. Guillem JG, Moore HG, Akhurst T et al. Sequential preoperative fluorodeoxyglucose-P positron emission tomography assessment of response to preoperative chemoradiation: A means for determining longterm outcomes of rectal cancer. J Am Coll Surg 2004;199: 1–7.

65. Liu LX, Zhang WH, Jiang HC. Current treatment for liver metastases from colorectal cancer. World J Gastroenterol 2003;9(2): 193–200.

66. Ruers T, Bleichrodt RP. Treatment of liver metastases, an update on the possibilities and results. Eur J Cancer 2002;38(7): 1023–1033.

67. Gray B, Van Hazel G, Hope M, Burton M, Moroz P, Anderson J, Gebsk V. Randomized trial of Sir-spheres plus chemotherapy vs chemotherapy alone for treating patients with liver metastases from primary large bowel cancer. Ann Oncol 2001;12 (12):1711–1720.

68. Nijsen JF, van het Schip AD, Hennink WE, Rook DW, van Rijk PP, de Klerk JM. Advances in nuclear oncology: microspheres for internal radionuclide therapy of liver tumours. Curr Med Chem 2002;9(1):73–82.

69. Vitola JV, Delbeke D, Meranze SG, Mazer MJ, Pinson CW. Positron emission tomography with F-18-fluorodeoxyglucose to evaluate the results of hepatic chemoembolization. Cancer. 1996;78:2216–2222.

70. Torizuka T, Tamaki N, Inokuma T, Magata Y, Yonekura Y, Tanaka A, Yamaoka Y, Yamamoto K, Konoishi J. Value of fluorine-18-FDG PET to monitor hepatocellular carcinoma after interventional therapy. J Nucl Med. 1994;35(12):1965–1969.

71. Solbiati L, Livraghi T, Golberg SN et al. Percutaneous radiofrequency ablation of hepatic metastases from colorectal cancer: long-term results in 117 patients. Radiology 2001;221:159–166.

72. Linamond P, Zimmerman P, Raman SS et al. Interpretation of CT and MRI after radiofrequency ablation of hepatic malignancies. Am J Roentgenol 2003;181:1635–1640.

73. Langenhoff BS, Oyen WJ, Jager GJ, Strijk SP, Wobbes T, Corstens FH, Ruers TJ. Efficacy of fluorine-18-deoxyglucose positron emission tomography in detecting

tumor recurrence after local ablative therapy for liver metastases: A prospective study. J Clin Oncol 2002;20:4453–4458.

74. Anderson GS, Brinkmann F, Soulen MC, Alavi A, Zhuang H. FDG positron emission tomography in the surveillance of hepatic tumors treated with radiofrequency ablation. Clin Nucl Med 2003;28:192–197.

75. Ludwig V, Hopper OW, Martin WH, Kikkawa R, Delbeke D. FDG-PET surveillance of hepatic metastases from prostate cancer following radiofrequency ablation-Case report.. Americ Surg 2003; 69:593–598.

76. Donckier V, Van Laetham JL, Goldman S et al. Fluorodeoxyglucose positron emission tomography as a tool for early recognition of incomplete tumor destruction after radiofrequency ablation for liver metastases. J Surg Oncol 2003;84:215–223.

77. Veit P, Antoch G, Stergar H et al. Detection of residual tumor after radiofrequency ablation of liver metastasis with dual-modality PET/CT: Initial results. Eur Radiol 2006;16:80–87.

78. Barker DW, Zagoria RJ, Morton KA et al. Evaluation of liver metastases after radiofrequency ablation: Utility of FDG PET and PET/CT. Am J Roentgenol 2005;184:1096–1102.

79. Antoch G, Vogt FM, Veit P et al. Qassessment of liver tissue after radiofrequency ablation: Findings with different imaging procedures. J Nucl Med 2005;46:520–525.

80. Wong CY, Salem R, Raman S, Gates VL, Dworkin HJ. Evaluating 90Y-glass microsphere treatment response of unresectable colorectal liver metastases by [18F]FDG PET: a comparison with CT or MRI. Eur J Nucl Med Mol Imag 2002;29:815–820.

81. Wong CY, Salem R, Qing F et al. Metabolic response after intra-arterial 90Y-glass microsphere treatment for colorectal metastases: Comparison of quantitative and visual analyses by 18F-FDG PET. J Nucl Med 2004; 45:1892–1897.

82. Pfister DG, Benson AB 3rd, Somerfield MR. Clinical practice. Surveillance strategies after curative treatment of colorectal cancer. N Engl J Med. 2004 Jun 3;350(23):2375–2382.

83. Sobhani I, Tiret E, Lebtahi R, Aparicio T, Itti E, Montravers F, Vaylet C, Rougier P, André T, Gornet JM, Cherqui D, Delbaldo C, Panis Y, Talbot JN, Meignan M, Le Guludec D. Early detection of recurrence by 18FDG-PET in the follow-up of patients with colorectal cancer. Br J Cancer. 2008 Mar 11;98(5):875–880.

84. Strasberg SM, Dehdashti F, Siegel BA, Drebin JA, Linehan D. Survival of patients evaluated by FDG PET before hepatic resection for metastatic colorectal carcinoma: A prospective database study. Ann Surg 2001;233:320–321.

85. Ruers TJ, Langenhoff BS, Neeleman N, Jger GJ, Strijk S, Wobbes T, Corstens FH, Oyen WJ. Value of positron emission tomography with [F-18] fluorodeoxyglucose in patients with colorectal liver metastases: A prospective study. J Clin Oncol 2002;20 (2):388–395.

86. Meta J, Seltzer M, Schiepers C, Silverman DH, Ariannejad M, Gambhir SS, Phelps ME, Valk P, Czernin J. Impact of ^{18}F-FDG PET on managing patients with colorectal cancer: The referring physician's perspective. J Nucl Med 2001;42:586–590.

87. Wiering B, Krabbe PF, Jager GJ, Oyen WJ, Ruers TJ. The impact of fluor-18-deoxyglucose-positron emission tomography in the management of colorectal liver metastases. Cancer. 2005 Dec 15;104(12):2658–2670.

88. Scott AM, Gunawardana DH, Kelley B, Stuckey JG, Byrne AJ, Ramshaw JE, Fulham MJ.PET Changes Management and Improves Prognostic Stratification in Patients with Recurrent Colorectal Cancer: Results of a Multicenter Prospective Study. J Nucl Med. 2008 Aug 14. [Epub ahead of print]

89. Fernandez FG, Drebin JA, Linehan DC, Dehdashti F, Siegel BA, Strasberg SM. Five-year survival after resection of hepatic metastases from colorectal cancer in patients screened by positron emission tomography with F-18 fluorodeoxyglucose (FDG-PET). Ann Surg 2004;240(3):438–447; discussion 447–450.

90. Cohade C, Osman M, Leal J, Wahl RL. Direct comparison of FDG PET and PET-CT imaging in colorectal carcinoma. J Nucl Med 2003;44:1797–1803.

91. Bar-Shalom R, Yefremov N, Guralnik L, et al. Clinical performance of PET/CT in the evaluation of cancer: Additional value for diagnostic imaging and patient management. J Nucl Med 2003;44:1200–1209.

92. Roman CD, Martin WH, Delbeke D. Incremental value of fusion imaging with integrated PET-CT in oncology. Clin Nucl Med 2005;30(5):470–477.

93. Selzner M, Hany TF, Wildbrett P et al. Does the novel PET/CT imaging modality impact on the treatment of patients with metastatic colorectal cancer of the liver? Ann Surg 2004;240:1027–1034.

94. Soyka JD, Veit-Haibach P, Strobel K, Breitenstein S, Tschopp A, Mende KA, Lago MP, Hany TF. Staging pathways in recurrent

colorectal carcinoma: is contrast-enhanced 18F-FDG PET/CT the diagnostic tool of choice? J Nucl Med. 2008 Mar;49(3): 354–361.

95. Tateishi U, Maeda T, Morimoto T, Miyake M, Arai Y, Kim EE. Non-enhanced CT versus contrast-enhanced CT in integrated PET/CT studies for nodal staging of rectal cancer. Eur J Nucl Med Mol Imaging. 2007 Oct;34(10):1627–1634.

96. Osman MM, Cohade C, Fishman E, Wahl RL. Clinically significant incidental findings on non-contrast CT portion of PET-CT studies: Frequency in 250 patients. J Nucl Med 2005;46:1252–1355.

97. Dizendorf E, Ciernik IF, Baumert B, et al. Impact of integrated PETCT scanning on external beam radiation treatment planning. J Nucl Med 2002;43:33P.

98. Ciernik IF, Dizendorf E, Baumert BG, Reiner B, Burger C, Davis JB, Lutolf UM, Steinert HC, Von Schulthess GK. Radiation treatment planning with integrated positron emission and computed tomography (PET/CT): A feasibility study. Int J Radiat Oncol Biol Phys 2003;57(3):853–863.

99. Crippa F et al. Tumori 1997;83 (4):748–752.

100. Kubota R, Yamada S, Kubota K, Ishiwata K, Tamahashi N, Ido T. Intratumoral distribution of fluorine-18-fluorodeoxyglucose in vivo: high accumulation in macrophages and granulocytes studied by microautoradiography. J Nucl Med. 1992;33:1972–1980.

101. Gambhir SS, Valk P, Shepherd J, Hoh C, Allen M, Phelps ME. Cost effective analysis modeling of the role of FDG-PET in the management of patients with recurrent colorectal cancer. J Nucl Med. 1997;38:90P.

102. Park KC, Schwimmer J, Sheperd JE, Phelps ME, Czernin JR, Schiepers C, Gambhir SS. Decision analysis for the cost-effective management of recurrent colorectal cancer. Ann Surg 2001;233:310–319.

103. Podoloff DA, Advani RH, Allred C, Benson AB, Brown E, Burstein HJ, Carlson RW, Coleman RE, Czuczman MS, Delbeke D, Edge SB, Ettinger DS, Grannis FW, Hillner BE, Hoffman JM, Keil K, Komaki R, Larson SM, Mankoff DA, Rozenzweig KE, Skibber JM, Yahalom J, Yu JM, Zelenetz AD. NCCN Task Force Report: Positron Emission Tomography (PET/Computed tomography (CT) scanning in cancer. J Natl Compr Canc Netw 2007;May;5 Suppl 1: S1–S22.

104. James W Fletcher, Benjamin Djulbegovic, Heloisa P. Soares, Barry A. Siegel, Val J. Lowe, Gary H. Lyman, Edward Coleman, Richard Wahl, John Christopher Paschold, Norbert Avril, Lawrence H. Einhorn W. Warren Suh, David Samson, Dominique Delbeke, Mark Gorman, Anthony F. Shields. Recommendations for the Use of FDG (fluorine-18, (2-[18F]Fluoro-2-deoxy-D-glucose) Positron Emission Tomography in Oncology. J Nucl Med 2008;49:480–508.

105. Blau M, Nagler W, Bender MA. A new isotope for bone scanning. J Nucl Med 1962;3:332–334.

106. Bang S, Baug CA. Topographical distribution of fluoride in iliac bone of a fluoride-treated osteoporotic patient. J Bone Miner Res 1990;5:S87–S89.

107. Shields AF, Grierson JR, Dohmen BM, et al. Imaging proliferation in vivo with [F-18] FLT and positron emission tomography. Nat Med 1998;4:1334–1336.

108. Francis DL, Visvikis D, Costa DC, et al. Potential impact of [(18)F]3'-deoxy-3'-fluorothymidine versus [(18)F]fluoro-2-deoxy-D-glucose in positron emission tomography for colorectal cancer. Eur J Nucl Med Mol Imaging. 2003 Jul;30(7):988–94.

Chapter 7

Functional Imaging of Neuroendocrine Tumors

Sofie Van Binnebeek, Wolfram Karges, and Felix M. Mottaghy

Abstract

Neuroendocrine tumors (NET) have several distinct pathophysiological features that can be addressed by specific radiolabeled probes. An overview on the different radiopharmaceuticals that have been developed for positron emission tomography (PET) of NET are presented. The focus is on fluordeoxyglucose (F-18 FDG), biogenic amine precursors, somatostatin analogs, and hormone syntheses markers. Due to the highly specific tracers lacking any clear anatomical landmarking, the advantages of integrated functional and morphological imaging systems such as PET-CT are obvious. Based on the up to now published literature and one's own experience, it is concluded that amine precursors (e.g. fluor-dihydroxyphenylalanin and hydroxytryptophane) should be employed in most gastroenteropancreatic NET, whereas F-18 FDG should be preserved for more aggressive less-differentiated NETs. Hormone syntheses markers have up to now only been used in few centers and their broad clinical value remains uncertain.

The different available somatostatin analogs are the most promising tracers, since they can improve dosimetry in cases where peptide receptor radiotherapies are planned. Of specific interest are the somatostatin analogs addressing several subtypes of the somatostatin receptor (e.g. DOTANOC) that allow detecting also subtypes not expressing the "classically" addressed subtype 2 and 5.

Since NET have a high variety of different features, the individual diagnostic approach using PET or integrated PET-CT should be tailored, depending on the histological classification and the differentiation of the tumor.

Key words: Positron emission tomography, Neuroendocrine tumors, Fluoro-deoxy-glucose, L-DOPA, 5-Hydroxytryptophan, F-Dopamine, C-Hydroxyephedrin, Metomidate, Somatostatin analogs, DOTATOC

1. Introduction

Neuroendocrine tumors (NET) are a heterogeneous group of neoplasias, ranging from well-differentiated and slowly growing tumors, which are the most common, to less frequent, the poorly differentiated and malignant neoplasms with an aggressive behavior (1).

Neuroendocrine cells contain secretory granules and have the capacity to produce biogenic amines and polypeptides (2).

Malik E. Juweid and Otto S. Hoekstra (eds.), *Positron Emission Tomography*, Methods in Molecular Biology, vol. 727,
DOI 10.1007/978-1-61779-062-1_7, © Springer Science+Business Media, LLC 2011

Due to their capacity to take up and decarboxylate amine precursors, neuroendocrine cells were classified as amine precursor uptake and decarboxylation (APUD) cells (3). NETs may express hormonal activity similar to the endocrine cell from which they originated. Functional NETs are characterized by a clinical or biochemical hormone excess, while nonfunctional NETs are devoid of clinically apparent hormonal activities, despite immunohistological detection of hormone expression in the tumor. The clinical presentation may be diverse, which is reflected in the imaging workup.

NETs have also the capacity to express several different peptide receptors in high quantities (4). The most investigated peptide receptors are the somatostatin receptors (SSR). SSR are heptahelical G-protein-coupled glycoprotein trans-membrane receptors (5). Up to now five SSR subtypes have been identified (6).

Important factors affecting the choice of method and combination of imaging modalities are the type of primary tumor, the presence or absence of hormone activity (functionality), the presence of SSR, and the extent of the disease. After the initial diagnostic workup and tumor staging, the imaging requirements may differ in patients considered for surgical resection and medical therapy, respectively.

The classification of NET based on their anatomic origin (7) was abandoned lately (8) and replaced by a classification that mainly takes into account the tumor differentiation and the proliferation rate. According to the WHO classification of NET, three classes are distinguished: type 1a is well-differentiated NET (Ki <2%), type 1b well-differentiated neuroendocrine carcinomas (Ki 2–10%), and type 2 poorly differentiated neuroendocrine carcinomas.

Despite the small size of the NET and carcinomas, compared to most other tumors, they can have a large clinical effect due to the release of hormones or biogene amines. Therefore, conventional anatomic imaging often fails to visualize the primary tumor or its metastases and most importantly cannot depict their specific endocrine features.

Their ability to take up and accumulate amine precursors, produce amines and peptides, and express several peptide receptors forms the basis for functional and molecular imaging of NETs. Over the past decade, probes have been developed for these tumors (9). The focus of this paper is on positron emission tomography (PET) probes.

During the last few years, PET using F-18-labeled deoxyglucose (F-18 fluordeoxyglucose (FDG)) has evolved as a powerful imaging modality in oncology. The recent introduction of PET-CT, i.e. a PET camera with a CT scanner in the same gantry, has led to several advantages over a stand-alone PET camera.

There are at least four different radiopharmaceutical classes that address the different metabolic pathways or molecular properties of these tumors:

- The glucose derivate F-18-FDG)

- The biogene amine precursors (such as [C-11]-hydroxytryptophane (HTP), [C-11]- or [F-18]-dihydroxyphenylalanine (DOPA) or [F-18]-fluorodopamine (dopamine))

- Synthesis, storage, and hormone-releasing analogs and inhibitors (e.g. [C-11]-hydroxyephedrine (HE) or the enzyme inhibiting substrate [C-11]-metomidate)

- The peptide receptor ligands: [Ga-68] labeled somatostatin analogs (10)

2. F-18 Fluordeoxyglucose

F-18 FDG is the most common tumor imaging agent in PET. It is taken up via a glucose transporter (Glut-1) and phosphorylated (11). Due to the presence of the fluorine atom in the C-2 position, this phosphate derivative does not undergo further glycolysis but is metabolically trapped in the cell. Generally, malignant tumors have an increased accumulation of fluor-deoxy-glucose or F-18 FDG compared to most normal tissues. F-18 FDG PET may therefore be used to distinguish malignant from benign tumors. Other applications are tumor staging, diagnosis of recurrent disease, monitoring of therapy, and detection of an occult tumor in case of metastases from an unknown primary (1). Several studies have investigated its usefulness in different NETs (7–9). Most pheochromocytomas accumulate F-18 FDG. However, uptake is found in a greater percentage of malignant than benign pheochromocytomas. In a comparative study on 21 consecutive patients, it was concluded that F-18 FDG PET is especially useful in defining the distribution of those pheochromocytomas that fail to accumulate metaiodobenzylguanidine (MIBG). In one study, F-18 FDG PET was directly compared to somatostatin receptor scintigraphy (SRS). In the few patients that were studied, PET imaging of GEP-NETs revealed increased glucose metabolism only in less-differentiated GEP tumors with high proliferative activity and metastasizing medullary thyroid carcinomas (MTC) associated with rapidly increasing CEA levels. The authors conclude that additional F-18 FDG PET should be performed only if SRS is negative, and that it might be reasonable to include it as a diagnostic tool in those patients with poorly differentiated NETs (12, 13).

Another group found comparable results (14). This capacity of F-18 FDG PET is also proven with poorly differentiated or aggressive pancreatic NETs, which could not be visualized on In-111 scintigraphy, still described as the first line nuclear medicine imaging technique (15).

In a comparative study, it was concluded that F-18 FDG PET seemed to be useful to identify those NETs characterized by rapid growth or aggressive behavior. The authors speculate that F-18 FDG uptake by the tumor may be related to a worse prognosis. Furthermore F-18 FDG PET contributed to better staging of advanced disease.

In a series of carcinoid tumors ($n = 17$) SRS and F-18 FDG PET findings were correlated to Ki-67 expression (16). Since most tumors were typical carcinoids with low Ki-67 expression, no correlation was found between the histological features and the tracer's uptake. The authors concluded that F-18 FDG PET should be reserved to patients with negative results on SRS (16).

In a multicenter study on MTC, conventional radiological and nuclear medicine diagnostic procedures were compared to F-18 FDG PET (17). In the studied patients, F-18 FDG PET showed the highest lesion detection probability for MTC tissue with a high sensitivity and specificity, and therefore it was concluded that F-18 FDG PET is a useful method in the staging and follow-up of MTC (17). Another group presented comparable results in a unicenter trial (18).

Recent studies confirm the superiority of the F-18 FDG PET-CT in detecting metastatic deposits in recurrent MTC patients. Furthermore, in some patients with a limited loco-regional metastatic spread the F-18 FDG PET-CT findings were useful to accurately plan surgery (19). In the study by Ong, there seemed to be a correlation between the detection rate of metastatic MTC and the calcitonin levels after thyroidectomy: more determined, a higher chance of disease detection in the presence of higher calcitonin levels. In practice, F-18 FDG PET can be used in a clinically meaningful manner in patients with calcitonin levels of more than 1.000 pg/mL (sensitivity 78%), but its utility appears limited if the calcitonin level is below 500 pg/mL (20). These promising results in detecting MTC lesions with F-18 FDG are also observed in a study by Rufini et al. However, as F-18 FDG only seemed useful in patients with very high calcitonin levels and high progression rate, F-18 FDG in MTC seems limited in its use, as it depends on lesion size and to some extent, on the grade of differentiation and biologic aggressiveness of the tumor (21).

In conclusion, F-18 FDG seems to be reasonable in fast growing NET with histopathologically detected high Ki-67 values that show a poor differentiation (Fig. 1a). In most well-differentiated tumors and carcinomas peptide, receptor ligands or MIBG scintigraphy seems to be superior.

F-18 FDG

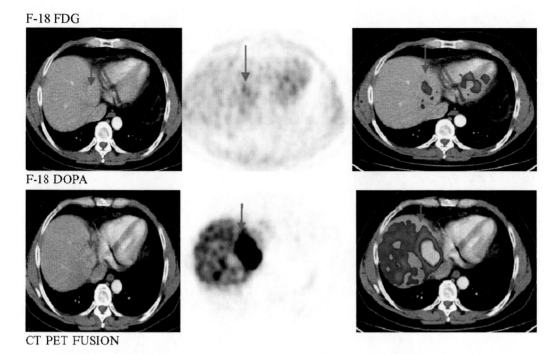

F-18 DOPA

CT PET FUSION

Fig. 1. Well-differentiated neuroendocrine tumor of the duodenum with suspicion of a hepatic metastasis visualized with F-18 FDG and F-18 DOPA. It is shown that almost no F-18 FDG taken up by well-differentiated tumors, F-18 DOPA, on the other hand gives an excellent visualization of the tumor localization.

3. Amine Precursors

NETs are characterized by the capacity for APUD. Thus, amine precursors such as 5-hydroxy-L-tryptophan (5-HTP) and L-dihydroxyphenylalanine (L-DOPA) may be taken up into the tumor cells where they are decarboxylated by the action of the enzyme aromatic amino acid decarboxylase (AADC). This reaction converts the precursors into their corresponding amines, dopamine and serotonin. These are stored in secretory granules within the cytoplasm and released from the cell by exocytosis in response to stimuli. By the action of the enzyme monoamine oxidase, 5-HTP is further metabolized and excreted into the urine as 5-hydroxyindoleacetic acid (U-HIAA) (1).

Of all the NETs, especially NETs of the jejunum and ileum produce 5-HT, whereas in other NETs (bronchial carcinoids and endocrine pancreatic tumors), 5-HT production is rare; therefore, 5-HIAA is rarely increased. Still, production of 5-HTP can also occur in these groups; therefore, immunohistochemical staining for 5-HT maybe positive (22).

3.1. l-Dihydroxy-phenylalanine-PET

Based on this concept of amine metabolism, C-11-labeled and F-18-labeled L-dihydroxyphenylalanine (C-11-L-DOPA, F-18-L-DOPA) have been used in a number of studies to visualize NETs (Figs. 2 and 3).

In 17 patients with histologically confirmed gastrointestinal NETs (23), F-18-L-DOPA-PET was performed and the results were compared with those of F-18 FDG PET, SRS and morphological

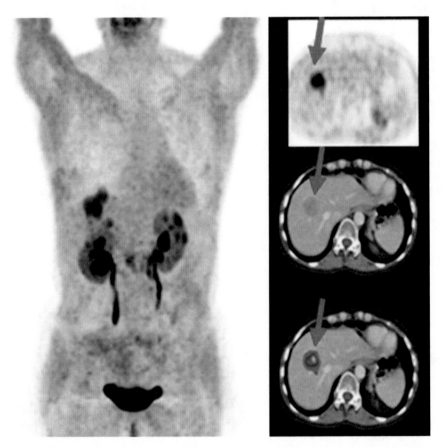

Fig. 2. Maximum intensity projection (MIP) and transaxial PET, CT and fused F-18 DOPA PET-CT images of liver metastases in a patient with status after resection of a well-differentiated pancreatic head neuroendocrine carcinoma.

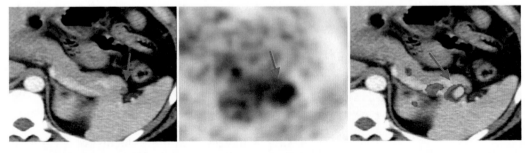

Fig. 3. Small insulinoma (*red arrows*) in the pancreas tail with intense F-18 DOPA uptake, not depicted on the CT alone (transaxial slices of the F-18 DOPA PET, CT and the fused PET-CT images).

imaging (CT and/or MRI) (23). A higher sensitivity was found for morphological imaging (73%) than for F-18-L-DOPA-PET (65%), SRS (57%) and F-18 FDG PET (29%), but F-18DOPA enabled best the localization of primary tumors and lymph node staging.

In another study (24) on 23 patients with histologically confirmed NETs, F-18-L-DOPA-PET was compared to SRS, with morphological imaging (CT, MRI, US) as the reference. When applying a region-based assessment F-18-L-DOPA-PET performed better than SRS because it was the most sensitive for bone metastases (even better than CT), mediastinal tumors, and pancreatic lesions, almost equally sensitive in detecting metastases in the liver and in lymph nodes, and equally poor sensitive in visualizing lung involvement.

F-18-L-DOPA-PET, compared with F-18 FDG PET, SRS and conventional diagnostic imaging procedures, has also been investigated for visualization of medullary thyroid cancer with elevated calcitonin levels (14). On a lesion-by-lesion basis, the sensitivity was 63% for F-18-DOPA-PET, 44% for F-18 FDG PET, 52% for SRS, and 81% for morphological imaging (CT/MRI). The highest specificity, on the other hand, was obtained with F-18-DOPA. Moreover, the data indicate that no single procedure provides adequate diagnostic certainty. Thus, F-18-DOPA provides a more specific diagnosis of primary tumor and local recurrence and improves the lymph node staging. DOPA PET was also superior to F-18 FDG PET, SRS, and conventional diagnostic imaging procedures in gastrointestinal carcinoid tumors (23).

F-18-L-DOPA-PET was further on compared to I-123-MIBG scintigraphy in 14 patients suspected of having pheochromocytoma, utilizing MRI as the reference. F-18-L-DOPA-PET was highly sensitive and specific for detection of pheochromocytomas and superior to MIBG scintigraphy (25). The same was shown for glomus tumors (26). Although F-18-DOPA has been used thus far almost exclusively for brain examinations, it also enables whole-body examinations for NET such as carcinoid tumors. However, similar to C-11-DOPA uptake, there is a considerable variability in tracer uptake. This variability is explained with the heterogeneous nature of the neuroendocrine gastrointestinal tumors, which present considerable differences in biologic, histologic, and clinical characteristics (23).

3.2. 5-Hydroxy-L-tryptophan-PET

The promising findings of a higher tumor uptake of C-11-5-HTP than of C-11-L-DOPA in EPTs initiated a study in 18 consecutive patients with histopathologically verified NETs in whom C-11-D-HTP-PET was compared with CT. It was found that all 18 patients had increased uptake of C-11-5-HTP in tumor tissue. In patients with liver metastases or lymph node metastases, every incident of metastases was detected (27). Tumor involvement of abdominal lymph nodes was much easier to visualize with PET than with CT, and especially the high liver metastases-to-normal liver background SUV ratio contributed to the better tumor visibility with PET.

A drawback in the image interpretation at PET was the sometimes very high radioactivity concentration in the urinary collecting system. In some patients, this considerably deteriorated the image quality with a risk of disguising tumor lesions at the level of the kidney pelvises (28).

These problems, related to high urinary concentrations of C-11, could be reduced by administration of carbidopa before C-11-HIAA treatment (29). Carbidopa blocks the AADC enzyme and slows down the decarboxylation of C-11-5-HTP, its conversion to C-11-5-hydroxytryptamine, and the ensuing formation of C-11-HIAA, so that a decrease in C-11-concentration follows. Also, the tumor tracer uptake increased by these pretreatments. Consequently, the administration of carbidopa is now a standard procedure in all patients examined with C-11-5-HTP-PET.

In a study of Orlefors et al., an unselected number of patients with histopathologically characterized NETs, both different primary tumors and metastases, were examined with PET in comparison with SRS and CT. As tracer the C-11-labeled 5-HT precursor 5-HTP was used (22). The greatest number of lesions was visualized with C-11-5-HTP-PET. In 95% of the patients, PET could visualize positive lesions, and in 58% of cases, could visualize more lesions than SRS and CT.

PET could also contribute substantially in visualization of the primary tumors. These tumors are often small, and therefore, can be difficult to detect. In this sense, the high tumor-to-background ratio and spatial resolution of PET compared with CT were of great importance. For very tiny lesions, the approach is rather endoscopic.

In a subgroup of 13 patients with mid-gut carcinoids, C-11-5-HTP-PET had a higher detection rate for abdominal lymph node, liver, mediastinal lymph node, and bone metastases than SRS and CT imaging. In addition to better diagnostic value, PET also achieved better spatial resolution and a higher tumor to background ratio than SRS; this is important for preoperative assessment. Also of great significance was the fact that liver lesions as small as 5 mm were hardly detectable by abdominal sonography, or CT were readily imaged by C-11-5-HTP-PET, owing to the good resolution of the camera. PET did not visualize nonfunctioning or poorly differentiated NETs and neither tumor with a high proliferation index (>40%). In common for these three cases is a low peptide hormone production and therefore, almost normal biochemical markers. This might indicate that the amine precursor uptake system is not as well expressed in these tumors, resulting in a low uptake of the radiolabeled amine precursor 5-HTP and thereby a poor tumor imaging. In these cases and also in occasional lesions such as necrotic tumors, F-18 FDG PET is a better choice for tumor visualization.

A recent study by Koopmans et al. (30) established once more F-18-DOPA PET-CT as the optimal imaging method for Carcinoid tumors and C-11-5-HTP PET-CT for islet cell tumors.

In combination with conventional radiology, SRS probably is sufficient as workup in a majority of patients with NETs, but as this study indicates, C-11-5-HTP-PET contributes in the majority of cases, especially with regard to small tumor lesions (0.5–1.5 cm) and in the detection of the nature of the lesion. This new and fairly expensive technology is probably most beneficial in selected patients such as those with biochemical evidence of an endocrine tumor or tumor recurrence but with negative imaging workup, as well as to find possible metastases in patients where the aim is curative surgery. Another situation where C-11-5-HTP-PET can contribute is when considering liver transplantation in a patient with solely liver metastases of a NET. In this case, it is crucial to exclude extra hepatic tumor sites before introducing potent immunosuppressive treatment (22).

3.3. F-18-Fluorodopamin

Dopamine is a better substrate for the norepinephrine transporter than most other amines, including norepinephrine. Thus, a labeled analog of dopamine should be useful as a scintigraphic imaging agent. 6-F-18-Fluorodopamine, a sympathoneuronal imaging agent, is a positron-emitting analog of dopamine and a good substrate for both the plasma membrane and intracellular vesicular transporters in catecholamine-synthesizing cells (31).

The ability of NETs to accumulate and decarboxylate 5-hydroxytryptamine (5-HTP) and L-3,4-dihydroxyphenylalanine (L-DOPA) is well known; it led to the original APUD concept of Pearse (2). Increased activity of L-DOPA decarboxylase was found to be a hallmark of NETs.

In a study of Ilias et al. (31), 16 patients with metastatic PHEO were examined with CT/MRI, F-18-DA PET and I-131-MIBG. All patients were positive with F-18-DA, whereas I-131-MIBG was negative in 7 of the 16 patients. CT and MRI are already proven to have a sensitivity that approaches 98.3% and more for the detection of adrenal PHEO, but in extra-adrenal, metastatic, or recurrent PHEO this result decreases to 90.9% or lower. The specificity in both imaging methods is approximately 50% and thus rather limited. I-131-MIBG, on the contrary, has an excellent specificity but the sensitivity is imperfect (see below). I-123-MIBG has a sensitivity around 90%, which is much higher, because of a higher administered dose and better imaging characteristics than I-131-MIBG, but this tracer is only available in a few academic medical centers.

In patients with PHEO, like in all NETs, it is important to localize the primary tumor but also possible metastatic lesions.

Without metastases, a PHEO can be considered for surgical treatment. Alternatively, if a metastatic PHEO is present, it is crucial to detect as many lesions as possible to optimize treatment; sometimes, surgery is still an option, unless the disease is widespread.

In this study, F-18-DA is an excellent and highly specific agent for localization of adrenal and extra-adrenal PHEO, including metastatic lesions. Other advantages are a lower radiation dose, no particular adverse effect on the thyroid, immediate scanning after injection, and better spatial resolution of the images. The images are superior in terms of spatial resolution compared with the planar images, obtained by I-131-MIBG.

A recent study by the same group confirms the superiority of dopamine PET as imaging modality with regard to MIBG scintigraphy and somatostatin receptor analogs-PET in patients with metastatic pheochromocytoma. Morphological imaging methods had the same sensitivity, but the specificity was higher in dopamine PET (32). As investigated by Kaji et al. (33), F-18-DA PET combined with CT or MRI is the most effective method for the proper localization of von Hippel–Lindau-related adrenal pheochromocytoma. Dopamine PET was found to be a superior imaging modality with regard to MIBG scintigraphy in patients with metastatic pheochromocytoma, most of the visualized lesions were also seen on CT or MRI, but the specificity was higher in dopamine PET (31).

Taken together, biogene amine precursors are superior to F-18 FDG, unless the tumor is afunctional, poorly differentiated, rapidly growing, or necrotic. They address a neuroendocrine specific pathophysiology and seem to be superior to conventional imaging methods and peptide receptor ligands. Peptide receptor ligands, however, still defend their place as the functional imaging method of choice for NETs due to their availability and capacity to reflect the expression of SSR, which forms the basis for therapy with nonradioactive and β-emitting-labeled somatostatin analogs (peptide receptor radionuclide therapy). It might be reasonable to include amine precursor PET (Fig. 1c, d). However, a direct and technically fair comparison between somatostatin analogs and DOPA-, HPT-, dopamine-PET does not exist up-to-date.

4. Analogs and Inhibitors

4.1. Hydroxyephedrin

Carbon-11-HE is the first available positron-emitting probe of the sympathetic nervous system suitable for administration in men. HE is more polar than MIBG and bears closer structural similarity to norepinephrine. Biodistribution studies in experimental animals and man have shown selective uptake in organs with rich sympathetic innervations, including the heart and adrenal medulla.

When HE is labeled with C-11, its distribution can be mapped with PET. PET offers improved imaging technology over conventional single photon techniques: the use of agents labeled with short-lived radionuclides allows administration of larger tracer doses, resulting in images of higher count density and superior quality; and the three-dimensional reconstruction more precisely depicts the spatial relationship of areas of uptake to the location of nearby organs. It was assumed that C-11-HE would rapidly (within minutes post-injection, vs. MIBG that accumulates within days after injection) concentrate in pheochromocytomas and, that, using PET to detect focal accumulations of HE, both the anatomic site and the functional nature of adrenergic tumors could be portrayed in high quality images within minutes after injection. Some negative aspects of C-11-HE are the complexity of its synthesis and its short half-life which requires on-site production for each patient (34).

So far, mainly the specific hormonal synthesis of adrenocortical tumors as well as pheochromocytomas was addressed. HE concentrates in adrenergic nerve terminals and therefore, besides its application in cardiac nuclear imaging, was evaluated in pheochromocytomas (34). HE has a high sensitivity and specificity in pheochromocytoma (35). This finding was confirmed by another study that demonstrated a higher sensitivity and specificity with regard to MIBG scintigraphy (36).

4.2. Metomidate

Incidentalomas, accidentally detected masses at the site of the adrenals, are frequently revealed by CT or MRI. Most often, the incidentalomas are benign adrenal cortical adenomas without clinical or biochemical manifestations of hormone excess. Some incidentalomas that represent pheochromocytoma, metastasis to the adrenal, or are of other nonadrenal origin.

Presently available imaging methods are seldom capable of diagnosing the origin and potential malignancy of the lesion. Therefore, the need to develop methods to discriminate adenomas form other lesions, such as pheochromocytomas, metastasis, cysts, and lipomas was high. These methods could also be used to visualize metastases from adrenocortical carcinoma.

Etomidate, an imidazole-based ethyl ester, has been used as an anesthesia-induction agent, but has also been documented as a potent inhibitor of 11β-hydroxylase, a key enzyme in the synthesis of cortisol and aldosterone within the adrenal cortex. Metomidate, the corresponding methyl ester, has similar properties. As proven in previous studies (37), C-11-etomidate and C-11-metomidate have very high uptake in adrenal cortex and adrenal cortical tumors, but very low uptake in other organs, except the liver.

The enzyme inhibiting radiotracer C-11-metomidate, selected because of better synthetic characteristics, was first tested in nonhuman primates (37) and later validated in patients with adrenocortical tumors (38). It was shown that this tracer has the potential to differentially characterize adrenal masses with the ability to discriminate lesions of adrenal cortical origin from non-cortical lesions (38, 39). C-11-metomidate is an indicator of 11β-hydroxylase tissue content and high expression of this enzyme is the basis for visualization by C-11-metomidate PET. Because high uptake was also observed in adrenocortical adenomas, which are hormonally silent, it is apparent that the enzyme expression is not the factor governing the lack of hormone synthesis. This is advantageous concerning the application, because silent adenomas constitute the largest group of incidentalomas and these are the ones that often fail to be correctly diagnosed by blood analyses.

A recent comparative study by Henning et al. (40) between CT/MRI and C-11-metomidate in the detection of adrenal masses shows that CT and MRI already are accurate methods to detect adrenal masses, but C-11-Metomidate PET has maximal sensitivity and specificity and therefore can be used for better characterization of adrenal masses.

Both tracers, C-11-metomidate and C-11-etomidate, are highly selective and are potentially promising approaches for adrenal tumors, and however, have been introduced in only few PET centers up to now. The potential role of PET and C-11-metomidate in clinical practice must also be judged in relation to other available diagnostic methods. CT and MRI are the basis for the detection of an adrenal mass, but their major drawback is a lack of specificity. NP-59 (I-131-labeled 6-beta-iodomethyl-19-norcholesterol) SPECT has a high specificity and a 90–95% accuracy for the identification of adrenalocortical lesions, but the images are obtained as late as 4–7 days after tracer injection. Another drawback is that glucocorticoids must be given for a few days before and after tracer administration to suppress the normal adrenal uptake. PET with F-18 FDG has high accuracy to detect metastases from other primary tumors in the adrenal cortex, but had only low uptake in adrenocortical masses (38).

5. Peptide Receptor Ligands

A variety of different peptide receptors are expressed by NETs. Several (e.g. bombesin/gastrin releasing peptide receptors (GRPR) (41) have been observed by imaging approaches, however, at the moment the only clinically relevant PET tracer target is the somatostatin receptor. These SSR were the first ones to be addressed by in vivo targeting of human cancers (42). Besides the diagnostic impact of the in vivo receptor scintigraphy for the localization of tumors and their metastases, there is also a serious therapeutic impact of radiolabeled somatostatin analogs (43). The standard procedure has been planar and single-photon emission tomography (SPECT) imaging using indium-111 octreotide. Limiting problems with this method consisted of the relatively low spatial resolution of the gamma camera and the improvable affinity for SSR. In order to improve the in vivo molecular imaging of SSR-positive tumors, several radiolabeled somatostatin analogs (e.g. DOTANOC or DOTATOC) for PET imaging have been introduced (Fig. 4). Labeling has been performed with the positron emitters C-11, F-18, Cu-64, and Ga-68.

Currently, the metallic positron emitter Ga-68 is of great interest because of its suitable radiophysical properties: its positron yield is high, its half-life is 68 min and matches the pharmacokinetics of many peptides and other small molecules owing to a fast blood clearance, quick diffusion, and target localization.

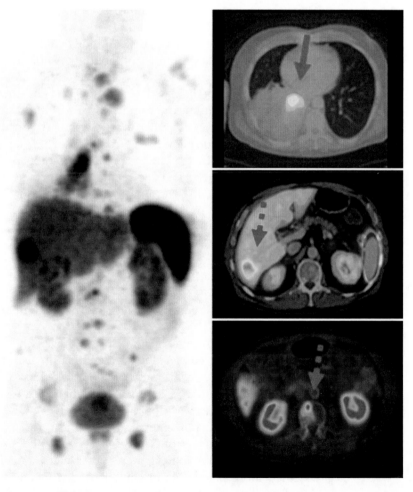

Fig. 4. MIP of a Ga-68 DOTATOC PET in a patient with a metastasized bronchial carcinoid. The transaxial fusion PET-CT shows the primary tumor, a liver and bone metastases (red arrows).

Peptide-chelators, based on somatostatin analogs were investigated and compared; and it was shown that DOTA, coupled to the octapeptide, e.g. (Tyr[3])octreotide or (Nal[3])octreotide, had about a fivefold increased affinity to the somatostatin receptor subtype 2 (SSR2) (44).

DOTATOC and DOTANOC have a different structural formula, with DOTATOC equals DOTA-Tyr[3]-octreotide and DOTANOC is DOTA-1-Nal[3]-octreotide. Ga-68-DOTANOC has a larger affinity spectrum for SSR, more determined it binds SSR2, SSR3, and SSR5 with high affinity, whereas Ga-68-DOTATOC is only a ligand of SSR2 and SSR5.

However, most clinical applications have used Ga-68-labeled DOTATOC (45–48). In a study by Hofmann et al. (46), the production of Ga-68-DOTATOC, the biokinetics in tumor and nontumor tissue and its clinical performance in detecting SSR-positive tumors and metastases were addressed. Because of a half-life of 68 min, the time window for Ga-68 imaging is short, which could be used to investigate early tumor to nontumor ratios compared with conventional imaging using In-111-octreotide scintigraphy. Many former experiences with antibody and peptide imaging have shown that sufficient lesion contrast is not always achieved within such short periods. Two factors contribute to the early tumor contrast obtained with Ga-68-DOTATOC: the rapid accumulation of activity in the tumors (80% within 30 min) and the rapid renal clearance together with low activity concentrations in tissues without expression of SST-receptors. The pharmacokinetics of Ga-68-DOTATOC is so far unique for radiopeptides, even in comparison with DOTATOC containing other metal ions. This combination of a high tumor to nontumor contrast, within a period of 30–40 min postinjection, and the superior imaging characteristics of PET, allowed the detection of very small lesions, which may become of decisive importance when SSR-PET is used in clinical routine, e.g. for staging and therapy decisions.

The same results were obtained in a comparison study by Kowalski et al. (47), with Ga-68-DOTATOC and In-111-DTPAOC-SPECT for the detection of small neuroendocrine lesions.

Therefore, also the imaging of SSR even in small meningiomas by Ga-68-DOTATOC, as described in a study by Henze et al. (48) was very promising. This SSR-PET-tracer offered excellent imaging properties and a very high tumor-to-background ratio in comparison with In-111-DTPAOC.

A study by Buchmann et al. (49) confirms these findings, and some other advantages of Ga-68-DOTATOC PET in comparison with In-111-DTPA-SPECT were observed. Ga-68-DOTATOC seemed more practicable in clinical routine and was superior in guiding the clinical management. Another asset of Ga-68-DOTATOC is the higher affinity of Ga-68 versus In-111 towards the receptors, and therefore lower unspecific radiation exposure, the possibility of quantifying findings, including the use of data for monitoring of therapy response. Finally, Ga-68 is a generator nuclide and easily accessible. Future studies will have to investigate the value of Ga-68-DOTATOC PET in comparison to In-111-DTPAOC SPECT for the selection of patients eligible for radionuclide DOTATOC treatment and for the prediction of outcome.

The use of Ga-68-DOTANOC was also investigated in two recent studies. Fanti et al. (50) performed a study of Ga-68-DOTA-NOC PET to evaluate the role of this somatostatin receptor analog in NET of uncommon presentation. Since its mechanism is receptor-based, it provides a good visualization of well-differentiated NET and data on the receptor status. The synthesis of Ga-68-DOTA-peptides is very easy as Gallium-68 can be easily eluted from a commercially available generator and used for labeling of DOTA-peptides. In this study the results were good in all, even uncommon, tumors, confirming that Ga-68-DOTA-peptides may have a relevant role for studying all NETs. In particular, the evaluation of patients with paraganglioma was very promising. But it was also observed that Ga-68-DOTA-NOC showed increased uptake in the presence of inflammatory tissue, usually with a mild degree of uptake; so like other PET radiopharmaceuticals, Ga-68-DOTA-NOC is not an absolute oncologic tracer (50).

In a following comparative study (51) two tracers, F18-DOPA and Ga-68-DOTA-NOC, have been investigated because they present different mechanisms of action and are therefore able to detect different aspects of tumor biology. While F18-DOPA uptake by NET cells is directly related to a specific tumor cell metabolism (see above for details), binding to somatostatin surface cell receptors, Ga-68-labeled peptides are an indirect measure of tumor cells differentiation. Ga-68-DOTANOC was found to be more accurate than F-18-DOPA for the detection of NET primary tumor and metastatic sites of the disease. Radioactive somatostatin gives also information on tumor cell receptors status which is crucial in planning any targeted radionuclide therapy.

It is also, in addition, necessary to mention that in our own experience the sensitivity of the integrated DOTATOC PET-CT outperforms that of DOTATOC PET due to two factors (Fig. 1d): first, the additional anatomical information allows to disentangle also very small lesions that might be overseen with PET alone and second, the improved attenuation correction improves the intrinsic resolution.

6. Conclusion

The lack of anatomic landmarks on PET images, especially using highly specific tracers such as biogene amines, somatostatin analogs or hormone synthesis markers makes a consistent fusion to cross-sectional anatomic data extremely useful. In several F-18 FDG PET studies, it was shown that addition of CT to PET improves specificity foremost, but also sensitivity, and the addition of PET to CT adds sensitivity and specificity in tumor imaging (52, 53). PET-CT is more accurate than either of its individual components and therefore has been one of the fastest growing diagnostic devices (54). So far, no prospective trials on PET-CT in NET have been published (55). The broad spectrum of NET requires tailoring the individual diagnostic approach using PET or the integrated PET-CT, depending on the histological classification and the differentiation of the tumor.

References

1. Sundin, A., Garske, U., Örlefors, H. (2007) Nuclear imaging of neuroendocrine tumors *Best Pract Res Clin Endocrinol Metab* **21**, 69–85.

2. Pearse, A.G. (1968). Common cytochemical and ultrastructural characteristics of cells producing polypeptide hormones (the APUD series) and their relevance to thyroid and ultimobranchial C cells and calcitonin *Proc R Soc Lond B Biol Sci* **170(18)**, 71–80.

3. Pearse, A.G. (1980). The APUD concept and hormone production *Clin Endocrinol Metab* **9(2)**, 211–22.

4. Reubi, J.C. (2003). Peptide receptors as molecular targets for cancer diagnosisand therapy *Endocr Rev* **24(4)**, 389–427.

5. Patel, R.C., Kumar, U., Lamb, D.C., et al. (2002) Ligand binding to somatostatin receptors induces receptor-specific oligomer formation in live cells *Proc Natl Acad Sci U S A* **99(5)**, 3294–9.

6. Patel, Y.C., Greenwood, M.T., Panetta, R., Demchyshyn, L., Niznik, H., Srikant, C.B. (1995) The somatostatin receptor family *Life Sci* **57(13)**, 1249–65.

7. Williams, E.D., Sandler, M. (1963) The classification of carcinoid tumors *Lancet* **1**, 238–9.

8. Solcia, E., Klöppel, G., Sobin, L. (2000) Histological typing of endocrine tumors, 2nd edition. Berlin, Heidelberg Springer Verlag.

9. Pacak, K., Eisenhofer, G., Goldstein, D.S. (2004) Functional imaging of endocrine tumors: role of positron emission tomography *Endocr Rev* **25(4)**, 568–80.

10. Lamberts, S.W., Bakker, W.H., Reubi, J.C., Krenning, E.P. (1990) Somatostatin-receptor imaging in the localization of endocrine tumors *N Engl J Med* **323(18)**, 1246–9.

11. Brown, R.S., Wahl, R.L. (1993) Overexpression of Glut-1 glucose transporter in human breast cancer. An immunohistochemical study *Cancer* **72(10)**, 2979–85.

12. Adams, S., Baum, R.P., Hertel, A., Schumm-Drager, P.M., Usadel, K.H., Hor, G. (1998) Metabolic (PET) and receptor (SPET) imaging of well- and less well-differentiated tumors: comparison with the expression of the Ki-67 antigen *Nucl Med Commun* **19(7)**, 641–7.

13. Adams, S., Baum, R., Rink, T., Schumm-Drager, P.M., Usadel, K.H., Hor, G. (1998) Limited value of fluorine-18 fluorodeoxyglucose positron emission tomography for the imaging of neuroendocrine tumors *Eur J Nucl Med* **25(1)**, 79–83.

14. Hoegerle, S., Altehoefer, C., Ghanem, N., Brink, I., Moser, E., Nitzsche, E. (2001) 18F-DOPA positron emission tomography for tumor detection in patients with medullary thyroid carcinoma and elevated calcitonin levels *Eur J Nucl Med* **28(1)**, 64–71.

15. Kok, J., Lin, M., Wong, V., et al. (2008) (18F) FDG PET-CT in pancreatic neuroendocrine tumors associated with von Hippel Lindau Syndrome *Clin Endocrinol* **70(4)**, 657–9.

16. Belhocine, T., Foidart, J., Rigo, P., et al. (2002) Fluorodeoxyglucose positron emission tomography and somatostatin receptor scintigraphy for diagnosing and staging carcinoid tumors: correlations with the pathological indexes p53 and Ki-67 *Nucl Med Commun* **23**, 727–34.

17. Diehl, M., Risse, J.H., Brandt-Mainz, K., et al. (2001) Fluorine-18 fluorodeoxyglucose positron emission tomography in medullary thyroid cancer: results of a multicentre study *Eur J Nucl Med* **28:(11)**, 1671–6.

18. Szakall, S., Jr., Esik, O., et al. (2002) 18F-FDG PET detection of lymph node metastases in medullary thyroid carcinoma *J Nucl Med* **43(1)**, 66–71.

19. Rubello, D., Rampin, I., Nanni, C., et al. (2008) The role of ^{18}F-FDG PET-CT in detecting metastatic deposits of recurrent medullary thyroid carcinoma: A prospective study *Eur J Surg Oncol* **34**, 581–6.

20. Ong, S.C., Schröder, H., Patel, S.G., et al. (2007) Diagnostic accuracy of ^{18}F-FDG PET in restaging patients with medullary thyroid carcinoma and elevated calcitonin levels *J Nucl Med* **48**, 501–7.

21. Rufini, V., Treglia, G., Perotty, G., et al. (2008) Role of PET in medullary thyroid carcinoma *Minerva Endocrinol* **33**, 67–73.

22. Orlefors, H., Sundin, A., Garske, U., et al. (2005) Whole-body (11)C-5-hydroxytryptophan positron emission tomography as a universal imaging technique for neuroendocrine tumors: comparison with somatostatin receptor scintigraphy and computed tomography *J Clin Endocrinol Metab* **90(6)**, 3392–400.

23. Hoegerle, S., Altehoefer, C., Ghanem, N., et al. (2001) Whole-body ^{18}F dopa PET for detection of gastrointestinal carcinoid tumors *Radiology* **220(2)**, 373–80.

24. Becherer, A., Szabo, M., Karanikas, G., et al. (2004) Imaging of advanced neuroendocrine tumors with (18)F-DOPA PET *J Nucl Med* **45**, 1161–7.

25. Hoegerle, S., Nitzsche, E., Altehoefer, C., et al. (2002) Pheochromocytomas: detection with ^{18}F DOPA whole body PET – initial results *Radiology* **222(2)**, 507–12.

26. Hoegerle, S., Ghanem, N., Altehoefer, C., et al. (2003) ^{18}F-DOPA positron emission tomography for the detection of glomus tumors *Eur J Nucl Med Mol Imaging* **30(5)**, 689–94.

27. Örlefors, H., Sundin, A., Ahlström, H., et al. (1998) Positron emission tomography with 5-hydroxytryptophan in neuroendocrine tumors *J Clin Oncol* **16**, 2534–42.

28. Sundin, A., Eriksson, B., Bergström, M., et al. (2004) PET in the diagnosis of neuroendocrine tumors *Ann NY Acad Sci* **1014**, 246–57.

29. Orlefors, H., Sundin, A., Lu, L., et al. (2006) Carbidopa pretreatment improves image interpretation and visualization of carcinoid tumors with ^{11}C-5-hydroxytryptophan positron emission tomography *Eur J Nucl Med Mol Imaging* **33(1)**, 60–5.

30. Koopmans, K., Neels, O., Kema, I., et al. (2008) Improved staging of patients with carcinoid and islet cell tumors with ^{18}F-dihydroxy-Phenyl-alanine and ^{11}C-5-Hydroxy-Tryptophan positron emission tomography *J Clin Oncol* **26**, 1489–1495.

31. Ilias, I., Yu, J., Carrasquillo, J.A., et al. (2003) Superiority of 6-[^{18}F]-fluorodopamine positron emission tomography versus [^{131}I]-metaiodobenzylguanidine scintigraphy in the localization of metastatic pheochromocytoma *J Clin Endocrinol Metab* **88(9)**, 4083–7.

32. Ilias, I., Chen, C.C., Carrasquillo, J.A., et al. (2008) Comparison of 6-18F-fluorodopamine PET with ^{123}I-metaiodobenzylguanidine and ^{111}In-pentreotide scintigraphy in localization of nonmetastatic and metastatic pheochromocytoma. *J Nucl Med* **49(10)**, 1613–9.

33. Kaji, P., Carrasquillo, J.A., Linehan, M.W., et al. (2007) The role of 6-(^{18}F)fluorodopamine positron emission tomography in the localization of adrenal pheochromocytoma associated with von Hippel-Lindau syndrome *Eur J Endocrinol* **156**, 483–7.

34. Shulkin, B.L., Wieland, D.M., Schwaiger, M., et al. (1992) PET scanning with hydroxyephedrine: an approach to the localization of pheochromocytoma *J Nucl Med* **33(6)**, 1125–31.

35. Trampal, C., Engler, H., Juhlin, C., Bergstrom, M., Langstrom, B. (2004) Pheochromocytomas: detection with ^{11}C hydroxyephedrine PET *Radiology* **230(2)**, 423–8.

36. Mann, G.N., Link, J.M., Pham, P., et al. (2006) [^{11}C]metahydroxyephedrine and [^{18}F] fluorodeoxyglucose positron emission tomography improve clinical decision making in suspected pheochromocytoma *Ann Surg Oncol* **13(2)**, 187–97.

37. Bergstrom, M., Bonasera, T.A., Lu, L., et al. (1998) In vitro and in vivo primate evaluation of carbon-11-etomidate and carbon-11-metomidate as potential tracers for PET imaging of the adrenal cortex and its tumors *J Nucl Med* **39(6)**, 982–9.

38. Bergstrom, M., Juhlin, C., Bonasera, T.A., et al. (2000) PET imaging of adrenal cortical tumors with the 11beta-hydroxylase tracer ^{11}C-metomidate *J Nucl Med* **41(2)**, 275–82.

39. Hennings, J., Lindhe, O., Bergstrom, M., Langstrom, B., Sundin, A., Hellman, P. (2006) [^{11}C]metomidate positron emission tomography of adrenocortical tumors in correlation with histopathological findings *J Clin Endocrinol Metab* **91(4)**, 1410–4.

40. Hennings, J., Hellman, P., Ahlström, H., et al. (2007) Computed tomography, magnetic resonance imaging and ^{11}C-metomidate positron emission tomography for evaluation of adrenal incidentalomas *Eur J Radiol* **69(2)**, 314–23.

41. Oliveira, P.G., Brenol, C.K., Edelweiss, M. et al. (2008) Effect of an antagonist of the bombesin/gastrin releasing peptide receptor

on complete Freund's adjuvant-induced arthritis in rats *Peptides* **29(10)**, 1726–31.

42. Krenning, E.P., Bakker, W.H., Breeman, W.A., et al. (1989) Localization of endocrine-related tumors with radioiodinated analogue of somatostatin *Lancet* **1(8632)**, 242–4.

43. Valkema, R., Pauwels, S., Kvols, L.K., et al. (2006) Survival and response after peptide receptor radionuclide therapy with [^{90}Y-DOTA0,Tyr3]octreotide in patients with advanced gastroenteropancreatic neuroendocrine tumors *Semin Nucl Med* **36(2)**, 147–56.

44. Antunes, P., Ginj, M., Zhang, H., et al. (2007) Are radiogallium-labelled DOTA- conjugated somatostatin analogues superior to those labeled with other radiometals *Eur J Nucl Med Mol Imaging* **34(7)**, 982–93.

45. Henze, M., Schuhmacher, J., Hipp, P., et al. (2001) PET imaging of somatostatin receptors using [^{68}Ga]DOTA-D-Phe1-Tyr3-octreotide: first results in patients with meningiomas *J Nucl Med* **42(7)**, 1053–6.

46. Hofmann, M., Maecke, H., Borner, R., et al. (2001) Biokinetics and imaging with the somatostatin receptor PET radioligand (68) Ga-DOTATOC: preliminary data *Eur J Nucl Med* **28(12)**, 1751–7.

47. Kowalski, J., Henze, M., Schuhmacher, J., Macke, H.R., Hofmann, M., Haberkorn, U. (2003) Evaluation of positron emission tomography imaging using [^{68}Ga]-DOTA-D Phe(1)-Tyr(3)-Octreotide in comparison to [^{111}In]-DTPAOC SPECT. First results in patients with neuroendocrine tumors *Mol Imaging Biol* **5(1)**, 42–8.

48. Henze, M., Dimitrakopoulou-Strauss, A., Milker-Zabel, S., et al. (2005) Characterization of ^{68}Ga-DOTA-D-Phe1-Tyr3-octreotide kinetics in patients with meningiomas *J Nucl Med* **46(5)**, 763–9.

49. Buchmann, I., Henze, M., Engelbrecht, S., et al. (2007) Comparison of ^{68}Ga-DOTATOC PET and ^{111}In-DTPAOC (Octreoscan) SPECT in patients with neuroendocrine tumors *Eur J Nucl Med Mol Imaging* **34(10)**, 1617–26.

50. Fanti, S., Ambrosini, V., Tomassetti, P., et al. (2008) Evaluation of unusual neuroendocrine tumors by means of ^{68}Ga-DOTA-NOC PET *Biomed Pharmacother* **62**, 667–71.

51. Ambrosini, V., Tomassetti, P., Castellucci, P., et al. (2008) Comparison between ^{68}Ga-DOTA-NOC and 18F-DOPA PET for the detection of gastro-entero-pancreatic and lung neuro-endocrine tumors *Eur J Nucl Med Mol Imaging* **35**, 1431–8.

52. Von Schulthess, G.K., Steinert, H.C., Hany, T.F. (2006) Integrated PET-CT: current applications and future directions. *Radiology* **238(2)**, 405–22.

53. Mottaghy, F.M., Sunderkotter, C., Schubert, R., et al. (2007) Direct comparison of [^{18}F]FDG PET-CT with PET alone and with side-by-side PET and CT in patients with malignant melanoma *Eur J Nucl Med Mol Imaging* **34(9)**, 1355–64.

54. Beyer, T., Townsend, D.W., Brun, T., et al. (2000) A combined PET-CT scanner for clinical oncology *J Nucl Med* **41(8)**, 1369–79.

55. Mottaghy, F.M., Reske, S.N. (2006) Functional imaging of neuroendocrine tumors with PET *Pituitary* **9(3)**, 237–42.

Chapter 8

Melanoma

Esther Bastiaannet, Harald J. Hoekstra, and Otto S. Hoekstra

Abstract

This chapter discusses the value of FDG-PET and combined FDG-PET/CT in staging and follow-up of melanoma patients. For melanoma patients, the presence or absence of regional lymph node metastases is one of the most important prognostic factors; the recent development of sentinel lymph node biopsy offers a highly sensitive staging method. FDG-PET has shown a limited sensitivity to detect microscopic lymph node metastases in this selected group of patients with stages I and II melanoma. However, for the detection of distant metastases, FDG-PET is frequently used. Although there is no consensus, some surgeons pursue surgical excision of metastatic disease if only one or a few sites of disease are apparent. Precise identification of the location and number of metastatic lesions could therefore be important for surgical planning. Even though patients with metastatic melanoma generally have a poor prognosis (5-year survival 3–16%), there is still a need for accurate staging. Firstly, to identify those patients who may benefit from a surgical procedure, while avoiding these potentially harmful surgical procedures for patients with multiple distant metastases. Secondly, accurate staging is important to improve the efficiency of clinical trials, and thirdly, to provide patients with detailed information about their prognosis. Taking the published literature together, and reasoning that FDG-PET/CT is the current standard in PET imaging, there may be a case for the combined PET/CT in the setting of metastatic melanoma. However, further research is needed as the benefit of the combined FDG-PET/CT vs. FDG-PET alone seems to be less than reported for other tumor entities, which may be due to the high avidity of melanoma for FDG, so that many of the metastases are detected with FDG-PET and the additional CT does not increase the sensitivity.

Key words: FDG-PET, FDG-PET/CT, Melanoma, Melanoma metastases, Staging

1. Introduction

The incidence of melanoma, which causes a large proportion of all deaths related to skin cancer, has increased dramatically in Caucasian populations in all parts of the world. It is one of the tumors with the most rapidly increasing incidence among all malignancies. Particularly among whites in areas of high sun exposure, the incidence has steadily increased in the last decades (1). For the United States, it is estimated that 1 in 82 women and

Malik E. Juweid and Otto S. Hoekstra (eds.), *Positron Emission Tomography*, Methods in Molecular Biology, vol. 727,
DOI 10.1007/978-1-61779-062-1_8, © Springer Science+Business Media, LLC 2011

1 in 58 men will develop melanoma during their lifetime (2). This accounts for more than 55,000 new cases per year and approximately 7,600 deaths; it is also the most common cancer among women of 20–29 years of age (2–4). In the European Community, the incidence is 17,000/year and annually 5,000 patients die of melanoma (5). Predictions of melanoma incidence show an increase of 99% in the total number of melanoma patients by the year 2015 in the Netherlands, with the largest increase for males (6). World-wide, the incidence of melanoma is highest in Australia and New Zealand. There is strong evidence that increased exposure to the ultraviolet solar radiation is the main cause of the rising incidence, with severe sunburn in early life correlating best with melanoma risk (7–9). The ultraviolet radiation promotes malignant change in the skin by (1) direct mutagenic effects on DNA, (2) promoting reactive oxygen species of melanin that cause the DNA damage and suppress apoptosis, (3) reducing the cutaneous immune defense, and (4) stimulating the cellular constituents of the skin to produce growth factors (7, 10). Other risk factors for the development of melanoma include familial melanoma (HR 3-70), multiple atypical naevi (HR 11), freckling (HR 2.5), skin type I (HR 1.7), and history of severe sunburn (HR 2.5) (7). Consequently, efforts to reduce the incidence of melanoma have focused on identifying and screening people at high risk and on promoting sun protection (11).

The most important factor for successful management of melanoma is early diagnosis, allowing treatment to be undertaken at a stage when cure is still achievable (7). Wide local excision with proper resection margins according to the thickness of the lesion remains the treatment for localized melanoma (stages I and II). Sentinel lymph node biopsy (SLNB), as a staging procedure, can be considered for patients with melanoma thicker than 1 mm (11). The additional benefit of complete lymph node dissection (CLND) and the survival benefits of the SLNB are still under study, but an interim analysis showed a survival benefit (12–14). Patients with lymph node metastases (stage III), synchronous or metachronous, are candidates for a lymph node dissection if no distant metastases are present. For patients with distant metastases (stage IV), no trials of any specific drug or a combination of drugs have shown a convincing survival benefit (11, 15). However, surgical resection, which can be performed if there are only a few resectable distant metastases, seems to have a survival benefit: a 5-year survival of 40% can be achieved by metastasectomy (16). Probably as a result of increased awareness, melanoma is diagnosed at an earlier stage of disease. Nevertheless, some patients still present or recur with lymph node or distant metastases. The 10-year survival rates for stage I are 79–88%, for stage II 32–64%, for stage III 15–63%, and for stage IV 3–16% depending on the number and site of distant metastases (1).

Prognostic factors for recurrence and survival are Breslow thickness of the primary melanoma, ulceration, mitotic index, gender, localization, and nodal status (17, 18). Besides, in patients with lymph node metastases, the number and size of metastatic nodes and extranodal growth are of prognostic importance (17, 19, 20).

Melanomas are typically F-18 FDG-avid; and together with the erratic pattern of spread, high-risk patients are good candidates to screen with F-18 FDG-PET(–CT) for distant metastases. Several studies have suggested that F-18 FDG-PET is more sensitive and specific for the detection of melanoma metastases than conventional diagnostic tests (21–23). Even though whole-body PET does not provide the same anatomical detail as CT or MRI, it can easily cover the entire body and target-background contrasts are usually high, to allow for relatively easy identification of suspected sites. Furthermore, semiquantitative measurement of glucose metabolism (by calculating standard uptake values) might have prognostic relevance to predict disease-specific survival (24). Disadvantages of PET include its limited ability to detect brain metastases and lesions 5 mm, its limited availability, and its high cost compared to CT (25–28).

This chapter discusses the value of F-18 FDG-PET and combined F-18 FDG-PET–CT in staging and follow-up of melanoma patients. The additional value of F-18 FDG-PET above the conventional staging modalities as well as the limitations of F-18 FDG-PET is discussed. Finally, we propose a guideline for the use of F-18 FDG-PET in clinical practice for melanoma patients.

2. F-18 FDG-PET Acquisition and Criteria

The typical scan trajectory for most oncology F-18 FDG-PET or PET–CT studies comprises skull base to mid femur. Since melanoma may metastasize to virtually any organ, it is one of the indications to perform a true whole-body F-18 FDG-PET scan (scan from the skull vertex to the feet). However, this requires extending the scan by an additional six to seven bed positions at 3–5 min per position, nearly doubling the emission scanning time (although nowadays 1–2 min per position with a higher dose of F-18 FDG is also performed) (29). With the use of PET–CT, the additional radiation exposure by the CT scan is not negligible, particularly in patients for whom the scan is performed for surveillance purposes (29). Niederkohr et al. assessed the additional benefit of scanning the lower extremities and skull in PET–CT evaluation of metastatic melanoma in 173 patients (29). Unanticipated metastatic melanoma in the lower extremities outside the routine imaging field of view were identified in eight scans (2.7% of all scans) and two scans (0.7% of all scans) identified unanticipated metastatic lesions in the brain or scalp on PET–CT (29). The authors suggest that three categories of patients should have a true whole body scan: (1) primary melanoma in the head or neck region or at the lower extremities; (2) known or suspected metastases in the head or neck region, or lower extremities; and (3) clinical suspicion of aggressive or widespread disease (29). In another study of 153 patients with suspected or recurrent melanoma (30), the authors recommend a true whole-body scan for patients with previous melanoma manifestations to the legs.

Definitions of PET positivity are variable in the literature and often, criteria are not specified. In the studies where PET positivity criteria are mentioned, different criteria prevail, usually a definition where PET positivity is "any tracer uptake exceeding normal uptake." Standardization of these criteria, and extending them with criteria of combined PET and CT interpretations would facilitate metaanalysis, and this should be part of further research.

3. F-18 FDG-PET in the Staging of Melanoma

A retrospective review of 257 melanoma patients in three university centers in the Netherlands showed that most scans were requested for staging, and mainly to detect distant metastases in stage III patients (31). At initial presentation, most patients with melanoma have disease confined to the skin, and extensive staging procedures are inappropriate because of the extremely low detection rate of distant metastases (32). As is the case with all diagnostic tests, high rates of false positivity are to be expected in settings with low prevalence.

3.1. F-18 FDG-PET to Detect Regional Lymph Node Metastases

The presence or absence of regional lymph node metastases is an important prognostic factor for patients with melanoma and the recent development of SLNB offers a highly sensitive staging method. F-18 FDG-PET has shown a limited sensitivity to detect microscopic lymph node metastases in this selected group of patients with stages I and II melanoma (33, 34). The average sensitivity of F-18 FDG-PET for subclinical nodal disease in stages I and II melanoma was 14–17%, whereas sentinel node biopsy reached 86–94% sensitivity (34–36). Recent studies in 2006 and 2007 confirmed that PET has no place in the initial work-up of patients without any clinical evidence of regional lymph node metastases (37, 38). The low yield in nodal staging is readily explained since sizes of tumor deposits are within nonenlarged, i.e., clinically normal lymph nodes are too small to be identified with F-18 FDG-PET (30 μm) (34, 39). Therefore, SLNB remains the technique of choice for initial nodal staging in patients without clinically apparent lymph node metastases. Not surprisingly, the accuracy of F-18 FDG-PET to detect lymph node metastases is higher in patients with clinically suspicious or palpable lymph nodes: Blessing et al. reported a sensitivity of 74% at a specificity of 93% in such patients (40). However, the clinical relevance of these findings in lymph node stations is limited since biopsies are usually quite effective to solve the clinical problem (41).

Crippa et al. (42) studied the relation between size and sensitivity: sensitivity was only 23% for lymph nodes less than 5 mm, but increased to 83 and 100% for lymph nodes with a size of 6–10 mm and greater than 10 mm, respectively. Even though performance of PET is partly related to scanner performance and image reconstruction algorithms, these clinical data are in line with the predictions based upon histomorphometric analysis and in vitro PET data as shown by Mijnhout et al. (43).

3.2. F-18 FDG-PET to Detect Distant Metastases

Although there is no consensus, some surgeons pursue surgical excision of metastatic disease if only one or a few sites of disease are apparent (16, 23). Precise identification of the location and number of metastatic lesions could therefore be important for surgical planning. As mentioned before, the "not guideline-driven" clinical indication for F-18 FDG-PET is to detect distant metastases in high-risk melanoma patients. There is an apparent paradox that even though patients with metastatic melanoma generally have a poor prognosis (5-year survival 3–16%), there still is a need for accurate staging. Firstly, to identify those patients who may benefit from a surgical procedure, while avoiding these potentially harmful surgical procedures for patients with multiple distant metastases (41). Patients with lymph node metastases (without distant metastases) can benefit from a lymph node dissection, while patients in whom distant metastases are found could benefit from other individualized treatment including surgery, immunotherapy, and chemotherapy. Secondly, accurate staging is important to improve the efficiency of clinical trials, for example, patients with a limited number of distant metastases. Thirdly, to provide patients with detailed information about their prognosis (41).

Several studies found F-18 FDG-PET to be highly sensitive to detect distant metastases. In a systematic review and metaanalysis of all literature before July 1999, Mijnhout and co-authors found a pooled sensitivity of 79% (95% CI 66–93%) and a specificity of 86% (95% CI 78–95%) for the detection of melanoma metastases (lymph nodes and distant) in all stages of disease (44). Schwimmer et al. found a range of overall sensitivity and specificity of 92% (95% CI 88.4–95.8) and 90% (95% CI 83.3–96.1), respectively, for the detection of *recurrent* melanoma reported in literature from 1980 to 1999 (45). Finally, the review of Prichard (literature between 1980 and 2000) found ranges of sensitivity from 74 to 100% and specificity from 67 to 100% in the detection of distant metastases (46). However, one of the problems in determining accuracy is the definition of the reference test; e.g., the appropriate time of follow-up in the case of a negative scan and the gold standard to confirm metastases if pathological confirmation is not possible. Two studies assessed the accuracy of F-18 FDG-PET to detect distant metastases in exclusively stage III patients, where F-18 FDG-PET seems to have the most value. The largest study of 251 patients with palpable lymph node metastases found that 27.1% of the patients were upstaged to stage IV as a result of the F-18 FDG-PET scan (47). F-18 FDG-PET scan was significantly better for identifying bone and subcutaneous metastases than CT (Fig 1). Overall, F-18 FDG-PET

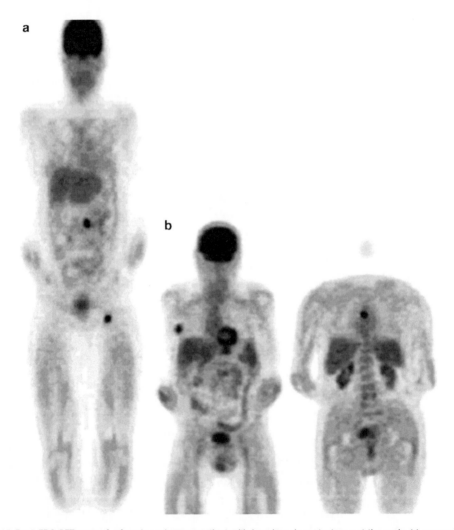

Fig. 1. (a) F-18 FDG-PET scan of a female melanoma patient with lymph node metastases at the groin 11 years after the primary melanoma at the leg (Breslow thickness 1.3 mm). The abdominal lesion turned out to be an adenoma. (b) F-18 FDG-PET scan of a male patient with lymph node metastases at the axilla 1 year after the primary melanoma at the trunk (Breslow 5.0 mm). F-18 FDG-PET depicted a midthoracic bone metastasis not seen at CT. The metastasis was confirmed with MRI.

depicted more metastases than CT ($p = 0.017$), and in 34 patients (13.5%) F-18 FDG-PET had an additional value in the management of these patients above spiral CT. Tyler et al. examined 95 patients with clinically evident lymph node and/or in-transit metastases. F-18 FDG-PET changed the management of 15% (95% CI 9.5–23.1) of the patients, as compared to 19.1% (95% CI 14.7–24.4) in the study of Bastiaannet et al. (47). Both studies found a high sensitivity (87.3 and 86.1%) and positive predictive value (78.6 and 85.0%) for the detection of distant metastases in stage III patients; however, direct comparison is difficult as one analysis was patient-based (48).

Taken the published literature together and reasoning that F-18 FDG-PET–CT is the current standard in PET imaging, there may be a case for the combined PET–CT in the setting of metastatic melanoma. Reinhardt et al. recently reported a significant increase in sensitivity and accuracy with F-18 FDG-PET–CT for M-stage assessment of 250 melanoma patients (all stages) in comparison to F-18 FDG-PET alone and CT alone, although not better than PET alone for N-stage assessment (49). In a retrospective study, Lagaru et al. also concluded that the best performance of the combined F-18 FDG-PET–CT scanner was in patients with advanced stage of disease; overall, the addition of CT increases the specificity of PET–CT over PET alone, and added diagnostic data for small lesions, such as small pulmonary metastases (50). However, it has been shown that CT can also miss small lesions in liver and lung (47, 51). Finally, Mottaghy et al. performed a retrospective study of 127 scans in patients with all stages of melanoma: PET alone, side-by-side PET and CT, and integrated PET–CT were independently and separately interpreted (28). With histological proof or follow-up as gold standard, PET, side-by-side PET and CT, and PET–CT had a sensitivity of 86, 89, and 91%, at similar specificity (94%), no difference in PPV (96%) and a NPV of 80, 83, and 87%, respectively (lesion-based). The benefit seems less than reported for other tumor entities, which may be due to the high avidity of melanoma for F-18 FDG, so that many of the metastases are detected with F-18 FDG-PET and the additional CT does not increase the sensitivity.

4. Other Modalities for Staging Melanoma in Comparison with F-18 FDG-PET(–CT)

The diagnostic accuracy of imaging tools to detect distant metastases of melanoma depends on the method of examination, the technique used, the organ, and the size of the tumor (52). Several studies compared F-18 FDG-PET with other diagnostic tools. Gulec et al. studied 49 patients with metastatic melanoma; patients first underwent conventional imaging with

CT and MRI after which a treatment plan was formulated, followed by an F-18 FDG-PET scan (53). The F-18 FDG-PET scan identified more metastatic sites in 55% of the patients and led to treatment changes in 49%; F-18 FDG-PET was more accurate to depict the extent of disease in patients with metastatic melanoma. A recent study of Brady et al. explained the clinical utility of F-18 FDG-PET if it was used in addition to standard imaging in patients with preoperative stages IIC, III, and IV melanoma (22). Imaging findings led to a change in clinical management in 36 of the 103 patients (35%); in 32 (89%) of these patients the information was accurate. However, as the authors note in the discussion, a possible bias in this study was introduced as approximately one third of the patients who were referred for resection had a CT scan before referral; so patients with unresectable metastases would not have been referred. Two studies have compared staging with F-18 FDG-PET and CT in all stages of melanoma patients; both found F-18 FDG-PET to be superior in terms of sensitivity and specificity to CT in all stages of melanoma (54, 55). In contrast to the previous publications, Krug et al. were not convinced of the diagnostic value of F-18 FDG-PET as a potential routine clinical procedure (52). They conclude that F-18 FDG-PET is inferior to CT (patient-based) for the detection of lung and liver metastases, and should therefore not be used alone to exclude metastasis. Direct comparison of F-18 FDG-PET and CT in stage III patients showed correct upstaging in 27.1% by F-18 FDG-PET and in 24.3% with CT ($p = 0.178$) (47). F-18 FDG-PET detected more metastatic sites (141 vs. 112, $p = 0.017$), significantly more bone and skin metastases. Treatment changed in 19.1%; in 79.2% as result of both scans, 16.6% exclusively F-18 FDG-PET, and 4.2% exclusively CT.

5. Change in Treatment as a Result of the F-18 FDG-PET Scan

Results of the F-18 FDG-PET scan can lead to a change in treatment, especially in stage III or IV melanoma patients. Several studies assessed this change in treatment (Table 1). Overall, in all stages of melanoma F-18 FDG-PET lead to a change in treatment in 17–48% of the patients. Three studies included stage IIC–IV patients and found a change in treatment from 34 to 49%; a single study in exclusively stage III patients found a change in treatment in 19.1% of the patients. Mijnhout et al. studied the change in treatment in patients with recurrent melanoma and found a change in 17% of the patient as a result of the F-18 FDG-PET scan.

Table 1
Change in treatment as a result of F-18 FDG-PET in melanoma patients in different stages of disease

Authors	Year	Stage	Tests before F-18 FDG-PET	N	Change in treatment (%)
Damian et al. (56)	1996	All stages	None	100	22
Stas et al. (57)	2002	All stages	Chest X-ray, liver US, blood analysis, CT. Subgroup: diagnostic modalities for distant metastases	84	26
Wong et al. (27)	2002	All stages	Different modalities	51	29
Reinhardt et al. (58)	2006	All stages	None	250	48.4
Bastiaannet et al. (31)	2006	All stages	Different modalities	257	17.1
Brady et al. (22)	2006	IIC, III and IV	CT scan	103	35
Gulec et al. (53)	2003	III or IV	CT and MRI	49	49
Harris et al. (59)	2005	92% III or IV	CT	92	34
Bastiaannet et al. (47)	2009	III	Chest X-ray	251	19.1
Mijnhout et al. (60)	2002	Recurrent disease	Different modalities	58	17

6. Unexpected Findings Other than Melanoma

F-18 FDG-PET has the potential to detect other unexpected (pre) malignant lesions besides melanoma which can lead to a change in treatment. A study with 257 melanoma patients found unexpected, clinically relevant, pathology mainly of the colon and rectum in 4.3% ($n = 11$) of the patients (21). Additionally, another study depicted 58 (3%) abnormalities (malignant or premalignant) in 1,750 F-18 FDG-PET scans (all malignancies), which were not clinically apparent and needed treatment and follow-up (61). Also, in two studies with the combined whole-body PET–CT scanner new, unexpected F-18 FDG-avid primary malignant tumors were detected in 1.2 and 1.7%, respectively, of the patients with known malignancies (62, 63).

7. Response Assessment with F-18 FDG-PET

There is very little literature concerning the value of F-18 FDG-PET in the evaluation of response to treatment in patients with melanoma. Mercier studied three patients who underwent F-18

FDG-PET before and 1 month after isolated limb perfusion (64). A reduction in the number of visualized limb lesions was seen, but also a diffusely enhanced uptake throughout the perfused limb, probably as a result of posttreatment inflammation. Hofman et al. performed a pilot study (seven patients) to evaluate the value of F-18 FDG-PET–CT to assess the early response to chemotherapy in metastatic melanoma (65). The study showed the potential use of F-18 FDG-PET and F-18 FDG-PET–CT to assess the response to chemotherapy in patients with distant metastases; as distant metastases were accurately depicted by PET. According to the authors, metabolic imaging may improve the palliation of patients receiving chemotherapy for metastatic melanoma by identifying patients unlikely to respond and thereby avoiding ineffective further chemotherapy (65). The largest study so far with 41 patients treated for melanoma metastases, showed PET–CT was suitable for response assessment in patients with proven melanoma metastases (66). In all patients, therapy response was assessed using visual criteria and change of DeltaSUV(max) or total lesion glycolysis; correlations between these and S-100 were both excellent showing that the PET–CT findings did correlate with response. A study that evaluates the effect of treatment with bevacizumab with PET is currently conducted in the Netherlands. However, other and larger prospective studies need to be performed.

8. F-18 FDG-PET in the Follow-up of Melanoma Patients

There is no universally accepted consensus advocating the routine use of F-18 FDG-PET in the follow-up of melanoma (67, 68). Most recurrences are actually detected by the patient and the most essential component of surveillance to detect recurrences or new primary melanoma is the history and physical examination (69, 70). A recent study assessed the methods to detect recurrent disease after SLNB (71). Of the 1,062 patients, 198 had a recurrence: established by symptoms and self-detection in 109 patients (55%), physician detection in 89 (45%), nearly half of which by a scheduled radiographic test (chest X-ray 16%, CT 29%, PET 1%). A Finnish study explained the impact of F-18 FDG-PET to detect clinically silent metastases in the follow-up of patients with high-risk melanoma (67). F-18 FDG-PET was performed (together with CT and physical examination) in 30 asymptomatic patients (stages IIB–IIIC) and was able to detect six of the seven recurrences. The authors conclude that F-18 FDG-PET could be a valuable modality in the follow-up of high-risk melanoma to diagnose recurrences and to select patients who are suitable for metastasectomy. However, at this moment, there is no place for F-18 FDG-PET in the follow-up of melanoma patients outside a clinical study.

9. On the Role of F-18 FDG Quantification

The standardized uptake value (SUV), which represents the F-18 FDG accumulation in the tumor or metastasis, could be a useful index in different cancers. It could be used to predict the prognosis, as metabolic activity correlates with tumor proliferation; and tumor proliferation is related to the clinical behavior (72, 73). Several studies in different tumors (breast, head and neck, pancreatic cancer, lung cancer) have shown that a high F-18 FDG uptake was associated with a lower disease-free survival (DFS) or overall survival (OS) (74–76). However, there are also studies published where the SUV value had no significant association with survival (77, 78). As far as the authors know, only one study has been published in patients with cutaneous melanoma (24). This retrospective study included 38 stage III melanoma patients and showed that DFS was prolonged in melanoma patients with a low SUVmean in the lymph nodes ($p=0.009$) compared to patients with a high SUVmean. There are many factors that may influence the F-18 FDG uptake: glucose and insulin levels, patient size, and the interval between F-18 FDG injection and image acquisition (79). SUV estimates suffer from poor reproducibility between centers because of the lack of standardization in acquisition and processing protocols in the past (79). This makes the SUV cutoff value only applicable in the center where the study was performed, while multicenter trials need standardization of acquisition, reconstruction, and data analysis. Recently, standardization of scanner calibration, acquisition, and analysis protocols was achieved for different institutes in the Netherlands (see Chap. 18) (79). Hopefully, this standardization will also be performed in other countries, so SUV values will be easily compared.

As a result of the current methodological heterogeneity, there is no consensus on the optimal SUV threshold to distinguish between malignant or benign tissues, and no cut-off value has been established to define subgroups of different prognosis (80). Additional prospective studies need to be performed to determine these values. The SUV value could be used, in addition to the number of positive nodes, tumor size, and extranodal growth, to decide for adjuvant radiotherapy. However, to be a practical prognostic factor in routine practice, a single SUV threshold allowing distinguishing between long and short survival patients remains to be validated and agreed upon (81).

10. Limitations and Pitfalls

There are several limitations and pitfalls with the use of F-18 FDG-PET in melanoma patients; first, due to physiological uptake of F-18 FDG in the brain, cerebral metastases are difficult to detect. Besides, F-18 FDG-PET has a low ability to detect pulmonary metastases, which has been attributed to lowering of target–nontarget contrast due to blurring by respiratory movement, partial volume effects (function of scanner quality, biological contrast and image reconstruction techniques), scatter from other organs in basal lung fields, and different levels of background activity in normal lung tissue (82). However, a recent study also showed that lung metastases detected with F-18 FDG-PET were not detected with CT (47). The review of Prichard et al. showed a high sensitivity of F-18 FDG-PET to detect metastases in the mediastinum, abdomen, and lymph nodes (abdominal and peripheral) (46). Besides, sensitivity of F-18 FDG-PET to detect lung metastases was 70% with a specificity of 100% (46). Ghanem et al. compared MRI and F-18 FDG-PET to detect liver metastases in 35 patients; sensitivity was higher for MRI (100%) compared to F-18 FDG-PET (47%). However, sensitivity was higher (71%) if only lesions >1 cm were assessed (83). A recent study comparing F-18 FDG-PET and CT discussed that in retrospect several of the bone metastases were seen in a second reading of the CT, suggesting that the bone structures were not routinely evaluated (enough) with CT (47).

It is unlikely that a generalizable, quantitatively correct added value of F-18 FDG-PET will become available in this setting. Total body CT generates huge amounts of data (300–400 images) to be reviewed with several windows settings. Moreover, the erratic spreading pattern of melanoma requires scrutinous survey of all tissues. This may just be too much for what a human brain can consistently manage. In our experience, reviewing the CT after PET usually identifies the anatomical substrate for the PET findings at CT in normal-sized structures or retrospectively abnormal ones. This is the strength of combined PET–CT as a "one stop-shop" procedure in these patients, together usually providing the basis for management decisions.

11. Recommendation for Use of F-18 FDG-PET(–CT) in Melanoma

Most studies assess the sensitivity and specificity of F-18 FDG-PET which is level 2 in the proposed hierarchical model of efficacy for diagnostic tests (84, 85). To justify F-18 FDG-PET in the clinical practice, the technique should also be valuable in diagnostic work-up (level 3) and have a beneficial effect on the patients' management plan (level 4). This is true for stage III and IV melanoma patients. Next, level 5 studies should measure or compute the effect of the information on patient outcomes, which has not been performed for melanoma patients. Finally, at level 6, costs and benefits of a diagnostic imaging technology for society in general can be examined. It is unlikely that such data will be provided within the next few years, if at all.

Since there are currently no standardized or universally agreed guidelines regarding the stage-specific use of imaging modalities available for clinicians caring for patients with melanoma (69), we provide a proposal for such guideline of F-18 FDG-PET(–CT) in melanoma patients (Fig 2). In stages I and II, and SNB-positive patients, F-18 FDG-PET has no additional value. However, for patients with palpable, proven lymph node metastases with no suspicion for lung metastases on chest X-ray, F-18 FDG-PET(–CT) does have additional value vs. CT alone in terms of treatment

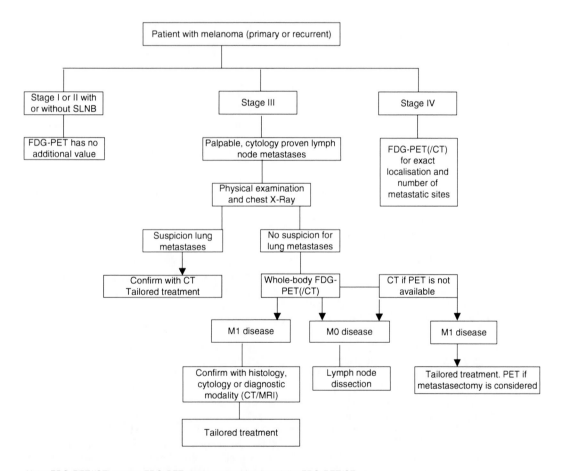

Note: FDG-PET(/CT) means FDG-PET single or combined modality FDG-PET/CT

Fig. 2. Proposed guideline for the use of F-18 FDG-PET(–CT) in melanoma patients for the different stages of disease.

planning (47). Also, for stage IV melanoma patients F-18 FDG-PET may be of importance to localize the distant metastases if surgical treatment is considered. Verification of PET and CT findings remains necessary in patients to prevent that potentially beneficial surgery for localized disease is withheld.

References

1. Balch, C.M., Buzaid, A.C., Soong, S.J., et al. (2001) Final version of the American Joint Committee on Cancer staging system for cutaneous melanoma *J Clin Oncol* **19**, 3635–48.

2. Tyler, D., Seigler, H. Malignant melanoma. In: Rakel R, Bope E eds. Conn's Current Therapy. Philadelphia: W.B. Saunders, 2006:998–1003.

3. Jemal, A., Tiwari, R.C., Murray, T., et al. (2004) Cancer statistics *CA Cancer J Clin* **54**, 8–29.

4. National Cancer Institute, SEER cancer statistics review, 1975-2001. Internet Communication

5. De Braud, F., Khayat, D., Kroon, B.B., et al. (2003) Malignant melanoma *Crit Rev Oncol Hematol* **47**, 35–63.

6. De Vries, E., van de Poll-Franse, L.V., Louwman, W.J., et al. (2005) Predictions of skin cancer incidence in the Netherlands up to 2015 *Br J Dermatol* **152**, 481–8.

7. Thompson, J.F., Scolyer, R.A., Kefford, R.F. (2005) Cutaneous melanoma *Lancet* **365**, 687–701.

8. Armstrong, B.K., Kricker, A. (1994) Cutaneous melanoma *Cancer Surv* **19-20**, 219–40.

9. Tucker, M.A., Fraser, M.C., Goldstein, A.M., et al. (1993) Risk of melanoma and other cancers in melanoma-prone families *J Invest Dermatol* **100**, 350S–355S.

10. Meyskens, F.L., Jr., Farmer, P.J., Anton-Culver, H. (2004) Etiologic pathogenesis of melanoma: a unifying hypothesis for the missing attributable risk *Clin Cancer Res* **10**, 2581–3.

11. Tsao, H., Atkins, M.B., Sober, A.J. (2004) Management of cutaneous melanoma *N Engl J Med* **351**, 998–1012.

12. Morton, D.L., Cochran, A.J., Thompson, J.F., et al. (2005) Sentinel node biopsy for early-stage melanoma: accuracy and morbidity in MSLT-I, an international multicenter trial. *Ann Surg* **242**, 302–11.

13. Morton, D.L., Thompson, J.F., Cochran, A.J., et al. (2006) Sentinel-node biopsy or nodal observation in melanoma *N Engl J Med* **355**, 1307–17.

14. Morton DL, Thompson JF, Cochran AJ, Elashoff R. Sentinel node biopsy and immediate lymphadenectomy for occult metastases versus nodal observation and delayed lymphadenectomy for nodal recurrence: fourth interim analysis of MSLT-I. Ann Surg Oncol. 2010;17(Suppl.1):S22–S23.

15. Atkins, M.B., Buzaid, A.C., Houghton, A., Jr. (2003) Chemotherapy and biochemotherapy. In: Balch C, Houghton A, Sober A et al. eds. Cutaneous melanoma. St. Louis: Quality Medical Publishing; 589–604.

16. Ollila, D.W. (2006) Complete metastasectomy in patients with stage IV metastatic melanoma *Lancet Oncol* **7**, 919–24.

17. Leiter, U., Meier, F., Schittek, B., et al. (2004) The natural course of cutaneous melanoma *J Surg Oncol* **86**, 172–8.

18. Francken, A.B., Shaw, H.M., Thompson, J.F., et al. (2004) The prognostic importance of tumor mitotic rate confirmed in 1317 patients with primary cutaneous melanoma and long follow-up *Ann Surg Oncol* **11**, 426–33.

19. Reintgen, D.S., Cox, C., Slingluff, C.L., Jr. et al. (1992) Recurrent malignant melanoma: the identification of prognostic factors to predict survival *Ann Plast Surg* **28**, 45–9.

20. Soong, S.J., Harrison, R.A., McCarthy, W.H., et al. (1998) Factors affecting survival following local, regional, or distant recurrence from localized melanoma *J Surg Oncol* **67**, 228–33.

21. Bastiaannet, E., Oyen, W., Meijer, S., et al. (2006) Impact of FDG-PET on surgical management of melanoma patients *Br J Surg* **93(2)**, 243–9.

22. Brady, M.S., Akhurst, T., Spanknebel, K., et al. (2006) Utility of preoperative [(18)] F-fluorodeoxyglucose-positron emission tomography scanning in high-risk melanoma patients *Ann Surg Oncol* **13**, 525–32.

23. Rohren, E.M., Turkington, T.G., Coleman, R.E. (2004) Clinical applications of PET in oncology *Radiology* **231**, 305–32.

24. Bastiaannet, E., Hoekstra, O.S., Oyen, W.J., et al. (2006) Level of fluorodeoxyglucose uptake predicts risk for recurrence in melanoma patients presenting with lymph node metastases *Ann Surg Oncol* **13**, 919–26.

25. Buzaid, A.C., Tinoco, L., Ross, M.I., et al. (1995) Role of computed tomography in the staging of patients with local- regional metastases of melanoma *J Clin Oncol* **13**, 2104–8.

26. Karakousis, C.P., Velez, A., Driscoll, D.L., et al. (1994) Metastasectomy in malignant melanoma *Surgery* **115**, 295–302.

27. Wong, C., Silverman, D.H., Seltzer, M., et al. (2002) The impact of 2-deoxy-2[18F] fluoro-D-glucose whole body positron emission tomography for managing patients with melanoma: the referring physician's perspective *Mol Imaging Biol* **4**, 185–90.

28. Mottaghy, F.M., Sunderkotter, C., Schubert, R., et al. (2007) Direct comparison of [18F] FDG PET-CT with PET alone and with side-by-side PET and CT in patients with malignant melanoma *Eur J Nucl Med Mol Imaging* **34**, 1355–64.

29. Niederkohr, R.D., Rosenberg, J., Shabo, G., et al. (2007) Clinical value of including the head and lower extremities in 18F-FDG PET-CT imaging for patients with malignant melanoma *Nucl Med Commun* **28**, 688–95.

30. Loffler, M., Weckesser, M., Franzius, C., et al. (2003) Malignant melanoma and (18)F-FDG-PET: Should the whole body scan include the legs *Nuklearmedizin* **42**, 167–72.

31. Bastiaannet, E., Oyen, W.J., Meijer, S., et al. (2006) Impact of [18F]fluorodeoxyglucose positron emission tomography on surgical management of melanoma patients *Br J Surg* **93**, 243–9.

32. Kumar, R., Mavi, A., Bural, G., et al. (2005) Fluorodeoxyglucose-PET in the management of malignant melanoma *Radiol Clin North Am* **43**, 23–33.

33. Prichard, R.S., Hill, A.D., Skehan, S.J., et al. (2002) Positron emission tomography for staging and management of malignant melanoma *Br J Surg* **89**, 389–96.

34. Havenga, K., Cobben, D.C., Oyen, W.J., et al. (2003) Fluorodeoxyglucose-positron emission tomography and sentinel lymph node biopsy in staging primary cutaneous melanoma *Eur J Surg Oncol* **29**, 662–4.

35. Wagner, J.D., Schauwecker, D., Davidson, D., et al. (1999) Prospective study of fluorodeoxyglucose-positron emission tomography imaging of lymph node basins in melanoma patients undergoing sentinel node biopsy *J Clin Oncol* **17**, 1508–15.

36. Belhocine, T., Pierard, G., De Labrassinne, M., et al. (2002) Staging of regional nodes in AJCC stage I and II melanoma: 18FDG PET imaging versus sentinel node detection *Oncologist* **7**, 271–8.

37. Maubec, E., Lumbroso, J., Masson, F., et al. (2007) F-18 fluorodeoxy-D-glucose positron emission tomography scan in the initial evaluation of patients with a primary melanoma thicker than 4 mm *Melanoma Res* **17**, 147–54.

38. Clark, P.B., Soo, V., Kraas, J., et al. (2006) Futility of fluorodeoxyglucose F 18 positron emission tomography in initial evaluation of patients with T2 to T4 melanoma *Arch Surg* **141**, 284–8.

39. Acland, K.M., Healy, C., Calonje, E., et al. (2001) Comparison of positron emission tomography scanning and sentinel node biopsy in the detection of micrometastases of primary cutaneous malignant melanoma *J Clin Oncol* **19**, 2674–8.

40. Blessing, C., Feine, U., Geiger, L., et al. (1995) Positron emission tomography and ultrasonography. A comparative retrospective study assessing the diagnostic validity in lymph node metastases of malignant melanoma *Arch Dermatol* **131**, 1394–8.

41. Friedman, K.P., Wahl, R.L. (2004) Clinical use of positron emission tomography in the management of cutaneous melanoma *Semin Nucl Med* **34**, 242–53.

42. Crippa, F., Leutner, M., Belli, F., et al. (2000) Which kinds of lymph node metastases can FDG PET detect? A clinical study in melanoma *J Nucl Med* **41**, 1491–4.

43. Mijnhout, G.S., Hoekstra, O.S., van Lingen, A., et al. (2003) How morphometric analysis of metastatic load predicts the (un)usefulness of PET scanning: the case of lymph node staging in melanoma *J Clin Pathol* **56**, 283–6.

44. Mijnhout, G.S., Hoekstra, O.S., van Tulder, M.W., et al. (2001) Systematic review of the diagnostic accuracy of (18)F-fluorodeoxyglucose positron emission tomography in melanoma patients *Cancer* **91**, 1530–42.

45. Schwimmer, J., Essner, R., Patel, A., et al. (2000) A review of the literature for whole-body FDG PET in the management of patients with melanoma *Q J Nucl Med* **44**, 153–67.

46. Prichard, R.S. (2002) Positron emission tomography for staging and management of malignant melanoma *Br J Surg* **89**, 389–96.

47. Bastiaannet, E., Wobbes, T., Hoekstra, O.S., et al. (2009) Prospective comparison of [18F] FDG-PET and CT in patients with melanoma with palpable lymph node metastases: diagnostic accuracy and impact on treatment *J Clin Oncol* **27**(28), 4774–80.

48. Tyler, D.S., Onaitis, M., Kherani, A., et al. (2000) Positron emission tomography scanning in malignant melanoma *Cancer* **89**, 1019–25.

49. Reinhardt, M.J., Joe, A.Y., Jaeger, U., et al. (2006) Diagnostic performance of whole body dual modality 18F-FDG PET/CT imaging for N- and M-staging of malignant melanoma: experience with 250 consecutive patients *J Clin Oncol* 24:1178–87.

50. Iagaru, A., Quon, A., Johnson, D., et al. (2007) 2-Deoxy-2-[F-18]fluoro-D-glucose positron emission tomography/computed tomography in the management of melanoma *Mol Imaging Biol* 9, 50–7.

51. Senft, A., de Bree, R., Hoekstra, O.S., et al. (2008) Screening for distant metastases in head and neck cancer patients by chest CT or whole body FDG-PET: a prospective multicenter trial *Radiother Oncol* 87, 221–9.

52. Krug, B., Dietlein, M., Groth, W., et al. (2000) Fluor-18-fluorodeoxyglucose positron emission tomography (FDG-PET) in malignant melanoma. Diagnostic comparison with conventional imaging methods *Acta Radiol* 41, 446–52.

53. Gulec, S.A., Faries, M.B., Lee, C.C., et al. (2003) The role of fluorine-18 deoxyglucose positron emission tomography in the management of patients with metastatic melanoma: impact on surgical decision making *Clin Nucl Med* 28, 961–5.

54. Swetter, S.M., Carroll, L.A., Johnson, D.L., et al. (2002) Positron emission tomography is superior to computed tomography for metastatic detection in melanoma patients *Ann Surg Oncol* 9, 646–53.

55. Holder, W.D., Jr., White, R.L., Jr., Zuger, J.H., et al. (1998) Effectiveness of positron emission tomography for the detection of melanoma metastases *Ann Surg* 227, 764–9.

56. Damian, D.L., Fulham, M.J., Thompson, E., et al. (1996) Positron emission tomography in the detection and management of metastatic melanoma *Melanoma Res* 6, 325–9.

57. Stas, M., Stroobants, S., Dupont, P., et al. (2002) 18-FDG PET scan in the staging of recurrent melanoma: additional value and therapeutic impact *Melanoma Res* 12, 479–90.

58. Reinhardt, M.J., Joe, A.Y., Jaeger, U., et al. (2006) Diagnostic performance of whole body dual modality 18F-FDG PET-CT imaging for N- and M-staging of malignant melanoma: experience with 250 consecutive patients *J Clin Oncol* 24, 1178–87.

59. Harris, M.T., Berlangieri, S.U., Cebon, J.S., et al. (2005) Impact of 2-deoxy-2[F-18]fluoro-D-glucose positron emission tomography on the management of patients with advanced melanoma *Mol Imaging Biol* 7, 304–8.

60. Mijnhout, G.S. (2002) Reproducibility and clinical value of 18F-fluorodeoxyglucose positron emission tomography in recurrent melanoma *Nucl Med Commun* 23, 475–81.

61. Agress, H., Jr., Cooper, B.Z. (2004) Detection of clinically unexpected malignant and premalignant tumors with whole-body FDG PET: histopathologic comparison *Radiology* 230, 417–22.

62. Ishimori, T., Patel, P.V., Wahl, R.L. (2005) Detection of unexpected additional primary malignancies with PET-CT *J Nucl Med* 46, 752–7.

63. Even-Sapir, E., Lerman, H., Gutman, M., et al. (2006) The presentation of malignant tumours and pre-malignant lesions incidentally found on PET-CT *Eur J Nucl Med Mol Imaging* 33, 541–52.

64. Mercier, G.A., Alavi, A., Fraker, D.L.(2001) FDG positron emission tomography in isolated limb perfusion therapy in patients with locally advanced melanoma: preliminary results *Clin Nucl Med* 26, 832–6.

65. Hofman, M.S., Constantinidou, A., Acland, K., et al. (2007) Assessing response to chemotherapy in metastatic melanoma with FDG PET: early experience *Nucl Med Commun* 28, 902–6.

66. Strobel, K., Skalsky, J., Steinert, H.C., et al. (2007) S-100B and FDG-PET-CT in therapy response assessment of melanoma patients *Dermatology* 215, 192–201.

67. Koskivuo, I.O., Seppanen, M.P., Suominen, E.A., et al. (2007) Whole body positron emission tomography in follow-up of high risk melanoma *Acta Oncol* 46, 685–90.

68. Poo-Hwu, W.J., Ariyan, S., Lamb, L., et al. (1999) Follow-up recommendations for patients with American Joint Committee on Cancer Stages I-III malignant melanoma *Cancer* 86, 2252–8.

69. Choi, E.A., Gershenwald, J.E. (2007) Imaging studies in patients with melanoma *Surg Oncol Clin N Am* 16, 403–30.

70. Francken, A.B., Bastiaannet, E., Hoekstra, H.J. (2005) Follow-up in patients with localised primary cutaneous melanoma *Lancet Oncol* 6, 608–21.

71. Moore, D.K., Zhou, Q., Panageas, K.S., et al. (2008) Methods of detection of first recurrence in patients with stage I/II primary cutaneous melanoma after sentinel lymph node biopsy *Ann Surg Oncol* 15, 2206–14.

72. Oshida, M., Uno, K., Suzuki, M., et al. (1998) Predicting the prognoses of breast carcinoma patients with positron emission

tomography using 2-deoxy-2-fluoro[18F]-D-glucose *Cancer* **82**, 2227–34.

73. Oyama, N., Akino, H., Suzuki, Y., et al. (2002) Prognostic value of 2-deoxy-2-[F-18]fluoro-D-glucose positron emission tomography imaging for patients with prostate cancer *Mol Imaging Biol* **4**, 99–104.

74. Oshida, M., Uno, K., Suzuki, M., et al. (1998) Predicting the prognoses of breast carcinoma patients with positron emission tomography using 2-deoxy-2-fluoro[18F]-D-glucose *Cancer* **82**, 2227–34.

75. Minn, H., Lapela, M., Klemi, P.J., et al. (1997) Prediction of survival with fluorine-18-fluoro-deoxyglucose and PET in head and neck cancer *J Nucl Med* **38**, 1907–11.

76. Sperti, C., Pasquali, C., Chierichetti, F., et al. (2003) 18-Fluorodeoxyglucose positron emission tomography in predicting survival of patients with pancreatic carcinoma *J Gastrointest Surg* **7**, 953–9.

77. Sugawara, Y., Quint, L.E., Iannettoni, M.D., et al. (1999) Does the FDG uptake of primary non-small cell lung cancer predict prognosis? A work in progress *Clin Positron Imaging* **2**, 111–8.

78. Van Westreenen, H.L., Plukker, J.T., Cobben, D.C., et al. (2005) Prognostic value of the standardized uptake value in esophageal cancer *AJR Am J Roentgenol* **185**, 436–40.

79. Westerterp, M., Pruim, J., Oyen, W., et al. (2007) Quantification of FDG PET studies using standardised uptake values in multi-centre trials: effects of image reconstruction, resolution and ROI definition parameters *Eur J Nucl Med Mol Imaging* **34**, 392–404.

80. Allal, A.S., Dulguerov, P., Allaoua, M., et al. (2002) Standardized uptake value of 2-[(18)F]fluoro-2-deoxy-D-glucose in predicting outcome in head and neck carcinomas treated by radiotherapy with or without chemotherapy *J Clin Oncol* **20**, 1398–1404.

81. Berghmans, T., Dusart, M., Paesmans, M., et al. (2008) Primary tumor standardized uptake value (SUVmax) measured on fluoro-deoxyglucose positron emission tomography (FDG-PET) is of prognostic value for survival in non-small cell lung cancer (NSCLC): a systematic review and meta-analysis (MA) by the European Lung Cancer Working Party for the IASLC Lung Cancer Staging Project *J Thorac Oncol* **3**, 6–12.

82. Miyauchi, T., Wahl, R.L. (1996) Regional 2-[18F]fluoro-2-deoxy-D-glucose uptake varies in normal lung *Eur J Nucl Med* **23**, 517–23.

83. Ghanem, N., Altehoefer, C., Hogerle, S., et al. (2005) Detectability of liver metastases in malignant melanoma: prospective comparison of magnetic resonance imaging and positron emission tomography *Eur J Radiol* **54**, 264–70.

84. Fryback, D.G., Thornbury, J.R. (1991) The efficacy of diagnostic imaging *Med Decis Making* **11**, 88–94.

85. Thornbury, J.R. (1994) Eugene W. Caldwell lecture. Clinical efficacy of diagnostic imaging: love it or leave it *AJR Am J Roentgenol* **162**, 1–8.

Chapter 9

Breast Cancer

Johannes Czernin, Matthias R. Benz, and Martin S. Allen-Auerbach

Abstract

Diagnostic imaging modalities utilized in the care of cancer patients must fulfill several requirements: they must diagnose and characterize tumors with high accuracy, must reliably stage and restage the disease, and should allow for monitoring the effects of therapeutic interventions on the course of the disease. They should impact management by guiding treating physicians to appropriate individualized treatment strategies. There is ample evidence that positron emission tomography (PET) and PET-computed tomography (CT) imaging can meet these requirements.

This chapter discusses the role and contributions of PET and PET-CT imaging using ^{18}F-fluorodeoxyglucose in diagnosing, staging, restaging, and treatment monitoring of breast cancer. Novel molecular imaging probes and devices that have been developed and translated into early clinical research protocols are also introduced.

Key words: PET, PET-CT, Breast cancer, FDG, FLT, Treatment monitoring, Staging

1. Introduction

Breast cancer is the leading malignancy and second leading cause of cancer mortality in women. However, over the last decade, early detection and novel therapeutic approaches have led to a marked change in the outcome of breast cancer patients. Since 1990, breast cancer mortality has decreased by more than 20%, of which close to 50% can be ascribed to mammographic screening and advances in adjuvant therapy (1, 2).

While cure of more advanced disease has remained an elusive goal, this previously devastating disease is now often manageable like a more chronic disorder. Targeted treatments of breast cancer are now available that, however, only benefit selected patients (3). Moreover, several lines of nontargeted therapies are available that, if selected appropriately, can improve patient survival (4).

Malik E. Juweid and Otto S. Hoekstra (eds.), *Positron Emission Tomography*, Methods in Molecular Biology, vol. 727,
DOI 10.1007/978-1-61779-062-1_9, © Springer Science+Business Media, LLC 2011

Diagnostic imaging modalities utilized in the care of cancer patients must fulfill several requirements: they must diagnose and characterize tumors with high accuracy, must reliably stage and restage the disease, and should allow for monitoring the effects of therapeutic interventions on the course of the disease. They should impact management by guiding treating physicians to appropriate individualized treatment strategies. There is ample evidence that positron emission tomography (PET) (5, 6) and PET-computed tomography (CT) (7) imaging can meet these requirements (4).

In this chapter, we discuss the role and contributions of PET imaging using ^{18}F-fluorodeoxyglucose (F-18 FDG) in diagnosing, staging, restaging, and monitoring of breast cancer. We also describe the potential impact of novel imaging modalities such as PET-CT and dedicated PET breast imaging devices on the care of breast cancer patients. Throughout this chapter, we attempt to review the role of PET-CT imaging in the context of other available imaging modalities deployed in breast cancer care.

Since different therapeutics target a variety of cellular processes that are altered in malignant degeneration, we will also briefly discuss other emerging PET imaging approaches for phenotyping of breast cancer.

2. Diagnosing Breast Cancer

The decline in breast cancer mortality over the last decade has been ascribed to successful mammographic screening. However, cancer detection remains unsatisfactory in large sections of the population. The sensitivity of mammography decreases with increased breast density (8, 9). Its sensitivity is only marginally improved by using digital mammography, as shown in more than 3,000 patients with heterogeneously or extremely dense breasts (10). Overall, the sensitivity of mammography remains low at less than 40% in women with very dense breasts (10).

The sensitivity is also lower in women on estrogen replacement therapy (8, 11) and in those with prior surgical interventions leading to scarred breast tissue (12), but is not affected by age or ethnicity. Limited reader experience/competence together with suboptimal imaging techniques is an important additional factor that can also lower the sensitivity of the test (13). The sensitivity of mammography does not exceed 85% in any population (8).

A well-established and better recognized limitation of mammography is its low specificity. The majority of tissue samples obtained from breast biopsies performed as a consequence of mammographic findings demonstrate benign pathology. For instance, Breast Imaging Reporting and Data System (BI-RADS;

developed by the American College of Radiology) class IV findings on mammography (suspicious on mammogram), the most frequent indication for biopsy, carry a positive predictive value of only 40% for cancer. Only BI-RADS class V is near-diagnostic for breast cancer with a positive predictive value of 97% (14). The implications of these data on health care expenditures are evident and have been discussed before (15).

Mammography is nevertheless the only accepted breast cancer screening tool. In the absence of robust data, we cannot recommend other imaging approaches for breast cancer screening in the general population.

However, alternative strategies such as magnetic resonance imaging (MRI) or ultrasound are now more frequently included for breast cancer detection in populations with either "difficult to image" breasts (for instance, dense breast, very dense breast, scars, or implants) or in women at increased risk for developing breast cancer such as those with BRCA1 or BRCA2 mutations (16). In these high-risk populations, highly sensitive tests for cancer detection are justified even at the expense of low specificity and at high cost. MRI detected breast cancer with sensitivities of close to 100% in these patients (17–19). In a comparative study of more than 300 high-risk women (19), MRI detected twice as many breast cancers than ultrasound (12 vs. 24 cancers). A total of 101 false-positive findings were reported for MRI, but only 25 for ultrasound. Thus, the high sensitivity of MRI occurred at the expense of a significantly lower specificity. However, because of its low sensitivity, ultrasound is not a useful screening test in women at high risk for breast cancer.

3. Determinants of F-18 FDG Uptake in Breast Cancer

Increased glucose metabolism and hence F-18 FDG uptake is explained by the switch of cancer cells to use glucose even under normoxic conditions. This process is known as the Warburg effect (20) which appears to be the result of activation of transcription factors such as c-Myc and HIF-1a, as recently shown in 12 breast cancer cell lines (21). In general, glycolytic rates of cancer cells were correlated with HIF-1a and c-Myc expression resulting in considerable variability in glycolytic activity among 12 cell lines, as determined by tritiated deoxyglucose cell uptake assay.

Such variability in glycolytic activity is also seen on F-18 FDG PET images in breast cancer patients. Obviously, tumor size (partial volume effect) has a considerable impact on lesion detection with PET (22). In addition, tumor proliferation rates (23) (Fig. 1, b), and histological/morphological features might also determine F-18 FDG uptake. For instance, lobular breast

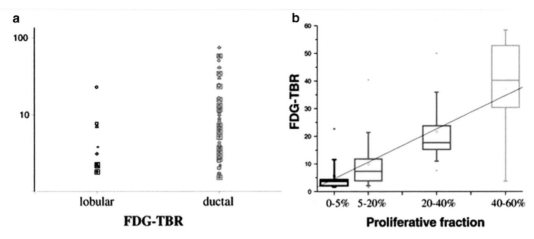

Fig. 1. (**a**) F-18 FDG tumor to background ratios (TBR) for lobular and infiltrating ductal carcinoma. Note the wide range of data. Overall, TBR are higher for ductal than for lobular cancers ($p = 0.05$); (**b**) TBR for F-18 FDG are expressed as a function of proliferative fraction based on the expression of Ki-67. The correlation between Ki-67 staining index and F-18 FDG TBR was significant ($p < 0.0001$); Reprinted with permission from Buck et al. (23).

cancers exhibit low, very low, or no discernable F-18 FDG uptake (24).

Buck et al. (23) found no correlation between F-18 FDG uptake and tumor grade, estrogen and progesterone receptor status, or axillary lymph node status. These authors also confirmed the significantly lower F-18 FDG uptake in lobular than in infiltrating ductal carcinoma (Fig. 1, a). The lack of a relationship between estrogen receptor status and F-18 FDG uptake had already been reported in a previous study by Dedashti et al. (25).

A comprehensive study to determine the reasons for the variability in F-18 FDG uptake has been undertaken by Bos et al. (26) who correlated F-18 FDG uptake in vivo with various markers expressed in tumor tissues of 55 patients. Among others, the tumors were examined for the expression of Glut-1; hexokinase I, II, and III; VEGF; and hypoxia-induced factor (HIF)-1 alpha. Tumor microvessel density and, because of their glycolytic activity, macrophage and lymphocyte content of tumors were also measured. Several significant correlations were found. Importantly, by stepwise logistic regression, a combination of mitotic activity index, Glut-1 expression, HIF-1α, and HK II predicted F-18 FDG uptake best. A different set of parameters (Glut-1, mitotic activity index, tumor cell density, and % necrosis) predicted the degree of F-18 FDG uptake in lobular cancer.

In another study (27), F-18 FDG uptake was related to histological tumor type, growth pattern, and tumor cell proliferation. The number of neoplastic cells as a fraction of all cells in tumors was also, albeit weakly, related to F-18 FDG uptake.

One study has suggested that tumor F-18 FDG uptake was directly correlated with microvascular density (28). In contrast to this observation, Avril (27) found that lower microvascular density tended to be associated with higher F-18 FDG uptake. This supports the notion that poorly perfused, and therefore, more hypoxic tumors revert to a more glycolytic phenotype. No relationship between F-18 FDG uptake and expression of GLUT1, axillary lymph node involvement, or tumor size was observed in this study.

The above studies strongly suggest that F-18 FDG uptake is correlated with tumor cell proliferation but not with hormone receptor status or tumor size. As suggested by Bos et al. (26), a set or combination of various parameters appears to determine F-18 FDG uptake. More fundamentally, multiple mechanisms including oncogenic factors such as c-Myc and HIF-1a determine the glycolytic phenotype of cancer as imaged with F-18 FDG PET.

As discussed above, F-18 FDG uptake in breast cancer varies among patients. The degree of F-18 FDG tumor uptake carries important prognostic information. Oshida et al. (28) studied 70 patients with primary breast cancer. Tumor F-18 FDG uptake was quantified using the differential uptake ratio (DAR) calculated as the tumor activity concentration (Bq/g) divided by injected dose (Bq) normalized to body weight (g). Patients with cancers exhibiting DAR >3 had a significantly worse overall and progression-free survival. In another study, a high pretreatment tumor F-18 FDG uptake was associated with a poor response to treatment (29).

4. Detection of Breast Cancer

F-18 FDG PET imaging is not proposed as a general screening test for breast cancer (30). However, several studies reported a good accuracy of F-18 FDG PET imaging for detection of breast cancer or for the characterization of breast tumors. Yet many of these investigations were hampered by a selection bias, in that frequently only patients already selected for biopsy or those with palpable breast lesions were included. Thus, populations under study were at high risk for cancer. While these studies do provide evidence that most breast cancers exhibit markedly increased F-18 FDG uptake, the accuracy of F-18 FDG PET for detecting cancer in a true screening population has not been established. Due to the high costs of PET relative to mammography and the large number of women to be enrolled, designing and conducting such a study would be extremely difficult if not impossible.

Most breast cancers have increased rates of glycolysis and can, therefore, readily be visualized on F-18 FDG PET images. Cancer

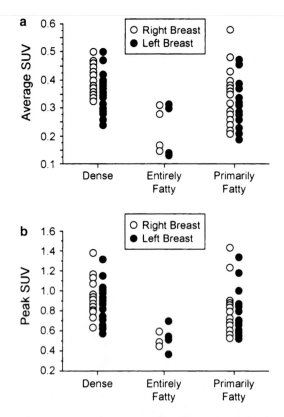

Fig. 2. Average SUV (**a**) and peak SUV (**b**) plotted for different breast-density groups. Data are presented separately for left and right breasts. Entirely fatty breasts had lowest SUVs. Reprinted with permission from Vranjesevic et al. (31).

detectability with PET is not compromised by breast density as in mammography, since F-18 FDG uptake is only marginally higher in dense breasts compared to that in fatty breasts (31, 32) (Fig. 2).

Several investigators have, by studying metabolic characteristics of primary cancers, attempted to define sensitivity and specificity of F-18 FDG PET imaging for breast cancer detection (33–42). Sensitivities ranged from 68 to 100% in these studies. However, carcinoma in situ and lobular carcinomas cannot be reliably detected, at least with conventional PET systems (23, 43).

Frequently, the specificity of F-18 FDG PET was superior to that of mammography and MRI (see Table 1). Multifocal disease was detected with a significantly higher sensitivity by F-18 FDG PET than with mammography or ultrasound as demonstrated in 117 patients (38). Moreover, accurate evaluation of postsurgical breasts, a difficult task for other imaging modalities, is feasible with F-18 FDG PET (12, 44).

Comprehensive insights into breast cancer detection with F-18 FDG PET were provided by Avril et al. (45). Their study included 144 patients who were scheduled for breast surgery (thus

Table 1
F-18 FDG PET in the detection of breast cancer – summary of the literature

Author	N	FDG-PET			Mammography		
		Sensitivity	Specificity	Accuracy	Sensitivity	Specificity	Accuracy
Bassa et al. (34)	16	100	100	100	62.5	100	64.7
Rostom et al. (35)	93	90.7	83.3	89.2			72.1[a]
Utech et al. (36)	124	100					
Noh et al. (37)	26	95.7	100	96.8	78.9	25.0	62.9
Schirrmeister et al. (38)	117	93	75	89			
Tse et al. (39)	14	80	100	85.7	80	50	71.4
Nieweg et al. (40)	19	90.9	100	94.7			
Adler et al. (41)	28	96.3	100	97.1			
Berg (53)	77	90[b]	86[b]	88[b]	92[c]	48[c]	71[c]
Avril et al. (42)	51						
Visual analysis							
Sensitive approach		83	84	–	–	–	–
Specific approach		68	97	–	–	–	–
Quantitative analysis							

PVC, partial volume corrected
[a] Mammography was performed in 86 patients
[b] Sensitivity, specificity, and accuracy of positron emission mammography (PEM)
[c] Sensitivity, specificity, and accuracy of conventional imaging (i.e., mammography and ultrasound)

the population was again at high risk for cancer). PET images were analyzed by 2 blinded readers and SUVs were calculated. Histology revealed 132 cancers in this population. In addition, 53 benign breast tumors were found. Mean tumor size was 3.1 ± 2.1 cm. Approximately 25% of all malignant tumors were lobular cancers. Two ways of visual image analyses were used. In one, only focally and markedly increased F-18 FDG uptake was considered malignant. In the other approach, diffuse and/or moderately increased focal activity was also considered malignant. Thus, the first approach was expected to result in higher specificity and the second one in a higher sensitivity. Using these criteria, the diagnostic accuracy of the specific approach was 73%, while that of the sensitive approach was 79% (with comparable confidence intervals). Of note, SUVs did not provide additional diagnostic information.

When tumors were smaller than 1 cm, the sensitivity of F-18 FDG PET was very low. For instance, no cancer smaller than

0.5 cm and only one of 8 cancers smaller than 1 cm were detected. Tumors ranging in size from 2 to 5 cm were detected with sensitivities of 80.6% (for the specific interpretation) to 92% (for the sensitive interpretation), respectively. Of note, 3 of 14 cancers larger than 5 cm did not exhibit increased FD uptake. Using the sensitive reading, only 50% of multicentric cancers were detected. Sixty-five percent of infiltrating lobular cancers and 24% of infiltrating ductal carcinomas were missed. The number of false-positive findings in this study was low.

Thus the major limitation of F-18 FDG PET imaging was the identification of small lesions. To overcome this limitation, attempts were made to improve imaging protocols and advance technology to allow for the detection of smaller lesions (46).

One approach uses prone imaging which resulted in increased sensitivity for cancer detection from 83% to 97% (47). Dual time-point imaging, whereby PET images of the breast are obtained early and late after F-18 FDG injection, has also improved the sensitivity of F-18 FDG PET. This approach is based on the notion that F-18 FDG uptake does not reach a plateau 60 min after intravenous injection but continues to increase in malignant tissue (48, 49). It needs to be seen whether these data can be confirmed in larger, well-designed clinical trials.

Recently, dedicated high-resolution breast imaging devices have been introduced that might further improve breast cancer detection with F-18 FDG PET (50, 51). One such device, the high-resolution positron-emission mammography (PEM) device obtains images by positioning the breast between two detector plates. Because of the close vicinity of the detectors to the breast tissue, the resolution of this system should be superior to that of whole body imaging systems (52) (Fig. 3). This device has been

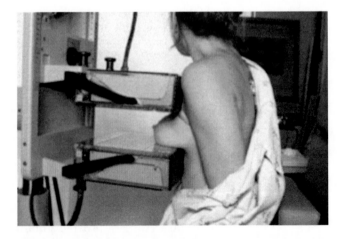

Fig. 3. Dedicated breast imaging device; note the close vicinity between breast and detectors resulting in improved sensitivity. Reprinted with permission from Tafra et al. (52).

tested prospectively in 77 women (53). Of those tested, 55% had breast cancer that was detected with a sensitivity and specificity of 90% and 86%, respectively, and positive and negative predictive values of 88%. The overall accuracy was 88%. A total of 10 of 11 carcinomas in situ were detected.

Using dedicated breast imaging devices, therefore, represents a promising approach for several reasons: first, scanners are relatively inexpensive; second, they have a small footprint and can therefore be placed in small offices; third, because of the close vicinity between detectors and breast tissue, they appear to detect cancer with improved sensitivity and accuracy. Finally, breast surveys in women at high risk for breast cancer could be offered at relatively low cost. Nevertheless, large multicenter studies are needed to define the ability of dedicated breast PET imaging devices to detect cancer.

In summary, F-18 FDG PET characterizes breast masses with a good diagnostic accuracy which is not affected by breast density. It will, therefore, find its place as an adjunct modality in women with difficult-to-image breasts, those with scarred breasts or after breast augmentation, and in women who are at high risk for primary breast cancer as well as multifocal or recurrent disease. Moreover, the glucose metabolic phenotype of primary breast cancers might have prognostic significance, and measuring F-18 FDG uptake is a prerequisite for monitoring therapeutic responses before starting neoadjuvant therapy (54).

5. Lymph Node Staging

Axillary, internal mammary, and mediastinal lymph node staging provides important prognostic information. The nodal stage of the disease also determines the best treatment approach. Sentinel node scintigraphy followed by biopsy assesses lymph node involvement with an accuracy of greater than 90% (55). The accuracy of PET for lymph node staging is, therefore, measured against this modestly invasive procedure. After initial reports of moderate-to-high accuracy of PET imaging for detecting lymph node metastases (34–36, 39, 56–60), Schirrmeister et al. reported already in 2001 that the false-negative rate of F-18 FDG PET at about 20% was too high to consider this test as a replacement for the sentinel lymph node approach.

The relatively low sensitivity of F-18 FDG PET was subsequently confirmed in a prospective multicenter trial (61) that included 360 women with initially diagnosed breast cancer. Using pathology as the gold standard, the sensitivity of PET for detecting metastatic disease in axillary nodes was only 61%, with a specificity of 80% (Table 2). Reasons for the low sensitivity included

Table 2
Axillary node staging by PET in women with newly diagnosed breast cancer (61)

	n	Sensitivity	Specificity	PPV	NPV
Visual analysis	308	61	80	62	79
Quantitative analysis (SUV-lean cut-off=2.0)	102	25	99	93	71

NPV, negative predictive value; *PPV*, positive predictive value; SUV-lean, single-pixel maximal standardized uptake value normalized to lean body mass

micro-metastases and small and few cancer-involved nodes. These data provide evidence that F-18 FDG PET cannot replace invasive axillary node staging.

Because of its ability to assign even small areas of sometimes only mildly increased F-18 FDG uptake to distinct anatomical structures, PET-CT imaging might be better equipped for axillary lymph node staging. This was investigated prospectively by Fuster et al. (62) in 60 patients with primary breast cancers measuring more than 3 cm in largest diameter. These rather large primary tumors were included to enrich the population for axillary node involvement. The performance of PET-CT for detecting axillary and extra-axillary lymph node involvement as well as distant disease was compared to that of conventional imaging including chest CT, ultrasound, and bone scan. Histology for all primary lesions, axillary nodes, and at least one site of suspected distant metastasis as well as clinical follow-up for at least 1 year served as reference standard. Lymph node involvement was diagnosed by F-18 FDG PET-CT with a sensitivity and specificity of 70 and 100%, respectively. However, distant disease was identified with a sensitivity of 100% and a specificity of 98%, which compared favorably with conventional imaging (68% and 80%, respectively). PET-CT changed the stage in 42% of the patients.

Internal mammary or mediastinal node involvement occurs in patients with advanced disease and carries a poor prognosis (63). A retrospective analysis of 73 eligible patients (64) reported a prevalence of suspected mediastinal or mediastinal involvement in 40% of the patients by F-18 FDG PET and 23% by CT. Concordant information was obtained in around 80% of the patients. The gold standard of biopsy was available in 33 patients. In these patients, the accuracy of PET for characterizing/detecting internal mammary node and mediastinal involvement was higher than that of CT ($p < 0.05$).

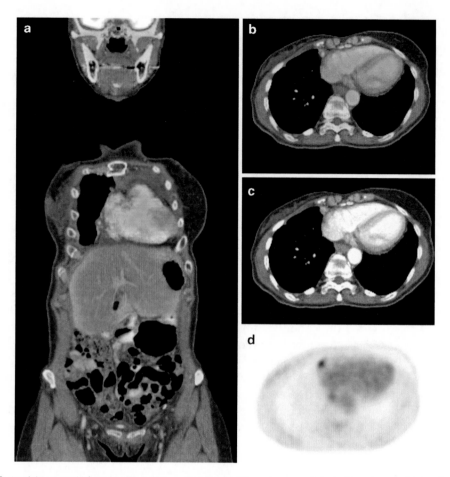

Fig. 4. Forty-eight-year-old female with a history of right-sided breast cancer. Selected fused coronal (**a**) and axial (**b**) PET-CT, as well as axial CT (**c**) and PET (**d**) slices demonstrate significant F-18 FDG uptake in a right internal mammary lymph node.

In a subsequent study, Tran et al. (65) investigated the relationship between location of the primary tumor (inner vs. outer quadrant Fig. 4), extra-axillary disease involvement, and prognosis. Patients with inner quadrant lesions had a sixfold greater frequency of isolated extra-axillary metastasis, and a threefold risk for disease progression.

These studies have significant implications: First, staging of the axilla remains the domain of the sentinel node approach but PET-CT provides the unique advantage of comprehensive whole body staging in a single diagnostic session at the time of initial staging. Second, internal mammary and mediastinal node involvement is better assessed with F-18 FDG PET than with CT. Finally, patients with inner quadrant lesions might be under-staged if axillary node involvement is not present.

6. Whole Body Staging and Restaging

The survival rate of breast cancer patients can be predicted from the extent of disease (66). The 5-year relative survival rate of patients with local limited disease approaches 80%, while prognosis remains poor at about 25% 5-year survival for women with metastatic disease.

A variety of noninvasive and invasive methods are used to determine the extent of disease prior to and after treatment. These include bone scanning, X-ray techniques, MRI, ultrasound, and tissue biopsy. Whole body staging is also important for designing the appropriate therapeutic approach. While limited disease is treated with surgery, chemotherapy, and radiation treatment, metastatic disease frequently requires palliation, and endocrine therapy with or without chemotherapy.

Rostom et al. (35) reported that all known distant metastatic lesions in 18 patients were accurately detected by F-18 FDG PET. Importantly, only the combination of ultrasound, CT, and bone scanning achieved the same accuracy.

Whether a single whole body survey using F-18 FDG PET-CT (Fig. 5) could be used to replace these multiple tests has also been investigated recently (67). In this study of 119 women with breast cancer and suspected metastatic disease, the performance of PET-CT was compared to that of chest CT, ultrasound of

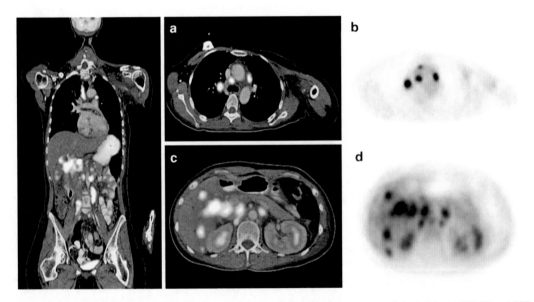

Fig. 5. Thirty-four-year-old female with a history of metastatic left-sided breast cancer. Selected fused PET-CT and PET axial slices demonstrate intense F-18 FDG uptake in mediastinal (**a**, **b**) as well as hepatic and retroperitoneal (**c**, **d**) metastases.

the abdomen, CT, and bone scanning. Of the 119 patients, 69 had newly diagnosed cancer. Sensitivity, specificity, and accuracy of PET for detection of metastases was 87%, 83%, and 86%, respectively, while the sensitivity of combined conventional imaging procedures including chest radiography, abdominal ultrasound, and bone scintigraphy was only 43%, with a corresponding specificity of 98%. CT was more sensitive than PET for detecting liver and lung metastases, while F-18 FDG PET was superior for detecting lymph node and bone metastases. The authors conclude that the combination of PET-CT imaging could obviate the need for other imaging tests for staging and restaging of breast cancer.

Similar observations were made by Fuster et al. (62) in a prospective study of 60 patients and in other retrospective studies (68–70).

An interesting approach for initial staging, termed F-18 FDG PET-CT mammography, was proposed by the group from Essen (71). Their F-18 FDG PET-CT protocol is divided into two parts. First, a standard whole PET-CT from head to thighs is performed in the supine position. This is followed by a second PET-CT scan during which the patients are imaged in the prone position using a breast positioning device (Fig. 6). Forty women with suspected breast cancer were enrolled in this study and the sensitivity for primary cancer detection was 95%. There were only two false-negative studies, both of which occurred in patients with lobular cancer.

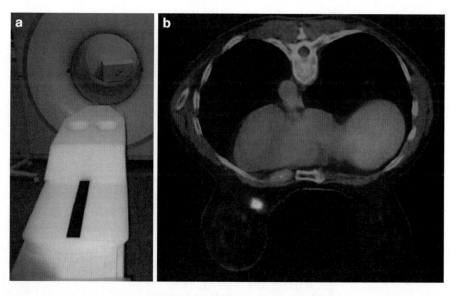

Fig. 6. (a) Positioning device for prone F-18 FDG PET-CT mammography, the Mamma Comfort Board (Additec GmbH), made from foam plastic. (b) Transverse F-18 FDG PET-CT mammogram of F-18 FDG PET-positive breast cancer lesion. Reprinted with permission from Heusner et al. (71).

PET-CT detected axillary lymph node involvement in 8/10 patients, extra-axillary lymph node metastases in 3/3 patients, and distant metastases in 10/10 patients.

The comprehensive protocol changed the management in 12.5% of the patients. While MRI was better suited to define the T-stage, PET was superior to conventional imaging for detecting distant disease.

7. PET Evaluations of the Skeletal System

The role of radionuclide bone imaging in general and F-18 FDG PET in particular for evaluating the skeletal system has been controversial. In early stage cancer, the prevalence of bone metastasis is low at 0–6% in stage I and 2–10% in stage II disease (72, 73). In another study (74), 14% of stage III patients had bone metastases.

The guideline from the British Association of Surgical Oncology suggests that in breast cancer patients who are surgical candidates, bone scanning does not yield useful information unless the patient is symptomatic. This notion was confirmed in a study by Kasem et al. (75) who reported that the number of false-positive bone scans by far exceeded that of true positive findings and that patient management was only affected in 3% of all patients at the time of presurgical staging.

F-18 FDG PET imaging is superior to conventional bone scintigraphy for detecting osteolytic metastases (Fig. 7). Conversely, blastic lesions are better detected with conventional bone scanning (76) (Fig. 8).

A retrospective review of more than 400 patients suggests that decreases in F-18 FDG uptake of bone lesions in response to treatment carry a favorable prognosis for progression-free survival (77).

Many osteolytic lesions convert to osteoblastic appearance on CT following chemotherapy. To better understand the significance of osteoblastic lesions that are positive on MDP bone scanning but negative on F-18 FDG PET, Du et al. (78) performed sequential F-18 FDG PET-CT imaging studies in 408 consecutive patients with known or suspected recurrent breast cancer. In this population with a prevalence of bone metastases of about 16%, osteolytic lesions were almost uniformly characterized by increased glycolytic activity (93.5%), while blastic lesions were less frequently F-18 FDG avid (61%). Following treatment, more than two-thirds of the osteolytic F-18 FDG-positive lesions became negative when examined by F-18 FDG PET. On the other hand, only approximately 50% of the F-18 FDG-positive blastic metastases became F-18 FDG negative. However, most

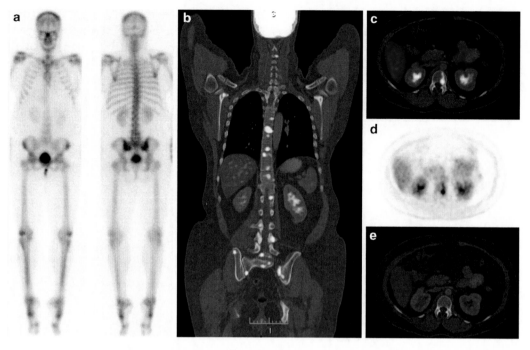

Fig. 7. Sixty-seven-year-old female with a history of right-sided breast cancer metastatic to the bone. A whole body bone scan (**a**) did not demonstrate any areas of abnormal uptake. Selected fused coronal (**b**) demonstrates significant F-18 FDG uptake in multiple lytic bone lesions throughout the skeleton in general and axial fused PET-CT (**c**), as well as in axial PET (**d**) and CT (**e**) slices in a lytic vertebral bone lesion at the level of Th12 in particular (special thanks to Klaus Oppenstaelk for providing this image).

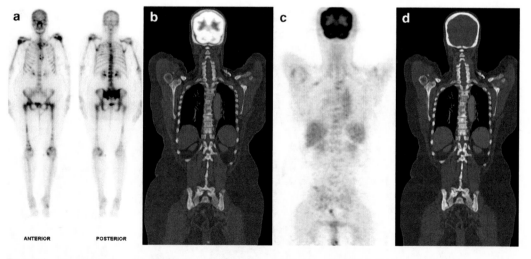

Fig. 8. Fifty-six-year-old female with a history of left-sided breast cancer metastatic to the bone. A whole body bone scan (**a**) demonstrates multiple areas of abnormal tracer uptake including the ribs, spine, pelvis, and bilateral femora. Blastic bone metastasis can be seen on the bone window of the selected coronal fused PET-CT (**b**) and CT (**d**) images. Most of the blastic bone lesions do not demonstrate any significant F-18 FDG uptake on PET (**c**).

of these lesions remained abnormal on CT, suggesting that morphological assessment cannot be used to determine therapeutic responses. By Kaplan Meier survival analysis, patients with F-18 FDG-positive lesions that converted to F-18 FDG-negative metastases had a significantly better long-term survival than patients whose lesions remained F-18 FDG positive (Fig. 9).

A different approach uses PET(-CT) with F-18 sodium fluoride for evaluating the skeletal system (Fig. 10). F-18 fluoride is a positron-emitting isotope that was first used in the clinic in the

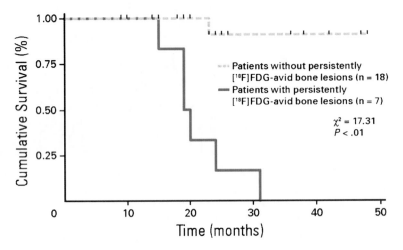

Legend:
- - - Patients without persistently [^{18}F]FDG-avid bone lesions (n = 18)
— Patients with persistently [^{18}F]FDG-avid bone lesions (n = 7)

$\chi^2 = 17.31$
$P < .01$

Fig. 9. Patient without residual F-18 FDG uptake in bone after treatment exhibits a significantly better survival than those with persistent F-18 FDG uptake. Reprinted with permission from Du et al. (78).

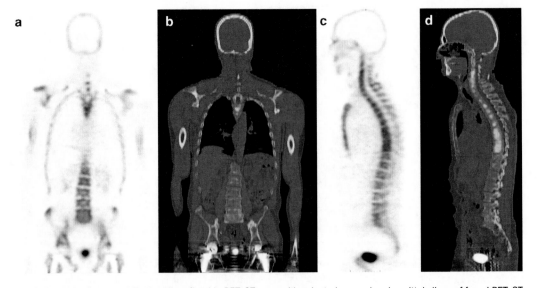

Fig. 10. Example of a normal F-18 sodium fluoride PET-CT scan with selected coronal and sagittal slices of fused PET-CT (**b**, **d**) and PET (**a**, **c**) images.

1960s (79). It binds to hydroxyapatite and its uptake is therefore increased in regions of increased osteoblastic activity. The PET-CT approach has several potential advantages: first, because of the superior spatial resolution of PET when compared with that of planar conventional bone scintigraphy, an improved sensitivity of this approach would be expected. Second, because of the addition of CT, the specificity of this approach should also be improved. Initial studies suggest that these assumptions hold true.

Schirrmeister et al. (80) compared conventional bone imaging with F-18 sodium fluoride PET for detecting bone metastases in 34 patients with breast cancer, most of whom had suspected bone involvement. CT and MRI served as reference standard. The area under curve was larger for PET than that for conventional bone imaging for both patient and lesion analysis. Clinical management was changed in 12% and adjusted in 17.6% of patients. The authors summarized the advantages of the PET approach as follows: F-18 sodium fluoride PET is more effective for revealing and excluding bone disease, and allows for monitoring of therapeutic responses, a feature not met well by conventional bone imaging.

An initial study evaluating the ability of sodium fluoride PET-CT imaging to detect/rule out bone metastases in patients with a variety of cancers reported an improved sensitivity (100% vs. 88%; $p < 0.05$) and also a trend toward improved specificity of PET-CT (56 vs. 88%) (81).

Comprehensive comparisons between conventional and PET-CT bone scintigraphy with F-18 sodium fluoride have not been performed to date but are currently being initiated.

8. Monitoring of Therapeutic Interventions and Prognostic Implications

The unique value of F-18 FDG PET imaging for assessing treatment effects early and late after the start of treatment has been demonstrated unequivocally in numerous studies. Several studies have clearly shown that anatomical imaging cannot be used to assess treatment responses reliably (83).

In breast cancer, F-18 FDG PET has been proven useful for monitoring the effects of therapeutic interventions (34, 84–87). For instance, F-18 FDG PET was used to monitor treatment responses in 22 patients with locally advanced breast cancer (88). Clinical responses were determined by MRI tumor size measurements and by histopathological evaluation of the excised tumor tissue. After the second cycle of chemotherapy, the predictive accuracy of changes in F-18 FDG uptake for histopathological response was 91% (using an SUV reduction by 55%

from baseline). Thus, treatment monitoring using F-18 FDG PET was feasible and useful in these patients. In another study that included 30 patients with locally advanced noninflammatory breast cancer, PET predicted the treatment response with a sensitivity of 90% and a specificity of 74% (89).

A complete pathological response after neoadjuvant chemotherapy is associated with favorable clinical outcome in breast cancer patients (90). It is important to identify patients who respond to treatment early after the start of therapy to avoid the toxicity associated with chemotherapy. Standard imaging approaches such as mammography, ultrasound, and MRI fail to identify early treatment responders. In contrast, a recent study strongly suggests that this can be accomplished with F-18 FDG PET. Rousseau and coworkers (91) conducted a prospective study in 64 patients with stage II or III breast cancer. The study included a baseline F-18 FDG PET scan and repeated scans after the first, second, third, and sixth cycle of chemotherapy. Pathological response was used as reference standard for the changes in F-18 FDG-SUV in response to treatment. Importantly, already after a single cycle of chemotherapy, the specificity of F-18 FDG PET for treatment response by using a reduction in SUV by 60% as threshold was 96%. However, at this time point, some responses were missed by PET. After two cycles of treatment, the sensitivity, specificity, and negative predictive value of PET were 89%, 95%, and 85%, respectively. At the same time points, neither mammography nor ultrasound predicted treatment responses with any useful accuracy. After completion of chemotherapy, F-18 FDG tumor uptake was reduced by about 50% in nonresponders, while it was reduced to background levels in responders (Fig. 11) (91). This finding has important implications. First, threshold values for response predictions with F-18 FDG PET need to be evaluated in prospective studies. Furthermore, standardized imaging protocols with simple response criteria that can be applied across institutions need to be established.

F-18 FDG PET has also been used to monitor therapeutic responses in patients with locally advanced (92) or metastatic breast cancer. In more than 50 patients with locally advanced breast cancer, tumor blood flow and various parameters of tumor F-18 FDG kinetics were quantified before and at the midpoint of neoadjuvant treatment. Progression-free and overall survival served as study endpoints. In a multivariate analysis, the baseline ratio of the metabolic rate of F-18 FDG uptake and blood flow was a predictor of relapse. Higher tumor blood flow at mid-therapy was independently associated with an elevated risk for mortality. Finally, the risk of death was higher for patients with little to no change or a proportionate increase in tumor blood flow or metabolic rates of F-18 FDG uptake. Changes in F-18 FDG SUV failed to predict patient outcome.

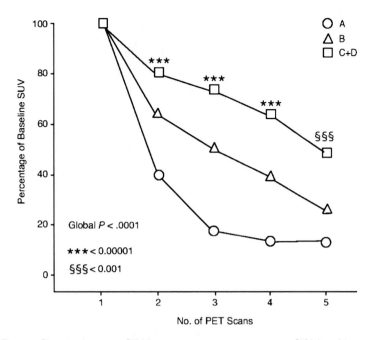

Fig. 11. Changes in tumor SUV in response to treatment tumor SUV (*y*-axis) were measured several times. Pathological tumor response served as gold standard as follows: A near-total therapeutic effect (grade A), more than 50% therapeutic effect but less than total or near-total effect (grade B), less than 50% therapeutic effect but visible effect (grade C), or no therapeutic effect (grade D). Two major regression groups, the responders (grades A and B) and nonresponders (grades C and D), were thus defined. Reprinted with permission from Rousseau et al. (91).

In another pilot study of 11 patients (93), PET imaging was performed after the first and the second cycle of chemotherapy. No significant decrease in SUV was observed in nonresponders to treatment as defined by other imaging modalities, while SUV decreased by about 50% after two cycles of chemotherapy in responders. Moreover, PET response was a strong predictor of patient survival, with responders surviving for 19 months, while nonresponders had a limited survival of only 9 months. Similar findings in patients with metastatic breast cancer were reported in 20 patients by Couturier et al. (94). In this study, F-18 FDG PET was performed after the first and the third cycle of chemotherapy. Only changes in F-18 FDG uptake after three cycles of therapy were predictive of treatment responses, as determined by long-term outcome. A large study evaluated F-18 FDG PET as a biomarker for response predictions in patients with metastatic breast cancer who underwent high-dose chemotherapy supported by autologous stem cell transplant (95). This controversial treatment approach is associated with considerable toxicity, and identification of responders early after the start of treatment is, therefore, of great clinical importance. PET findings were compared to

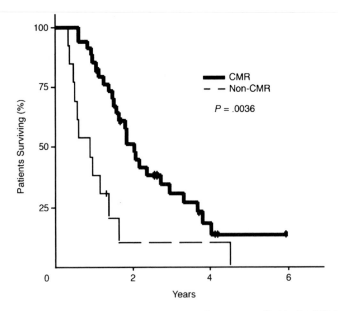

Fig. 12. Survival following high-dose chemotherapy. Data are stratified by F-18 FDG-PET result. Patients with a complete response (CMR; *solid line*) had a significantly longer survival than those with an abnormal PET scan (non-CMR; *dashed line*) after completion of high-dose chemotherapy. (p=0.0036). Reprinted with permission from Cachin et al. (95).

conventional imaging tests. PET was performed after the last cycle of chemotherapy. Patient survival served as gold standard. After the final cycle of treatment, 72% of the patients had a complete metabolic response, i.e., the PET scan was normal. The survival duration of complete metabolic responders was significantly better than that of metabolic nonresponders (24 vs. 10 months; p=0.036; Fig. 12).

9. Impact on Patient Management

Any novel imaging test for diagnosing, staging, or restaging of cancer patients should add information to other already available diagnostic tests. The degree to which F-18 FDG PET imaging adds important information or impacts patient management has been studied by several groups. In a recent retrospective study of 46 women with suspected recurrent breast cancer based on elevated tumor markers, the ability of F-18 FDG PET-CT imaging to detect disease sites was evaluated. PET-CT findings led to changes in the subsequent clinical management of 51% of these patients (initiation of chemotherapy or radiation treatment in 16 patients, treatment modification in 2 patients, and referral for biopsy in 6 with subsequent surgery in 2 patients) (69). Yap et al. used a different approach for determining the impact of PET on the management of 50 breast cancer patients (96). In their survey of referring physicians, PET changed the clinical stage in 36% (28% upstaged, 8% downstaged) and altered the clinical management in about 40% of the patients. Both reports are in line with the recently published results of the National Oncology PET registry (97). In this registry, which did not include patients with breast cancer, PET had an impact on management in about 40% of cancer patients.

10. Recent Advances in Breast Cancer Phenotyping with PET

New novel targeted and nontargeted breast cancer drugs make it increasingly important to identify patients who might benefit from these therapies. This might be feasible with a number of new PET imaging probes which target specific features of the malignant phenotype. For example, F-18 3′-deoxy-3′-fluorothymidine (FLT) (98, 99), a fluorinated thymidine analog, is transported from the plasma into tumor cells by nucleoside transporters. This imaging probe is subsequently phosphorylated by thymidine kinase 1 (TK1) to FLT-5-phoshate. The phosphorylated FLT ends up being essentially trapped in the cytoplasm of tumor cells, since FLT is not incorporated into DNA. The amount of FLT trapped inside the malignant cells thus reflects the activity of TK1, an enzyme closely involved with cellular proliferation (100).

Smyczek-Gargya et al. (101) reported that all but one primary tumor and all but one involved regional lymph node region were identified with F-18 FLT PET. The tracer uptake ratio between tumor and background was higher for F-18 FLT than that for F-18 FDG due to low soft tissue accumulation of F-18 FLT. This implies that proliferative activity of malignant tumors can be imaged with F-18 FLT PET.

F-18 FLT has also been used for monitoring treatment responses in breast cancer patients (102). One such study looked at the therapeutic responses in 13 patients with stage II–IV breast cancer. In this study, all tumors demonstrated increased F-18 FLT uptake at baseline. All six patients with complete or partial responses by CT measurement (RECIST) 60 days after the start of treatment had evidence of a significant reduction in F-18 FLT uptake as soon as 1 week after the start of treatment. Since this decrease in F-18 FLT uptake preceded any changes in tumor size, this would suggest that in breast cancer, early monitoring of therapeutic effects with F-18 FLT PET might yield useful information about the chemosensitivity of the cancer. Similar response predictions were reported by Pio et al. (103) with F-18 FLT

PET used for treatment monitoring 2 weeks after the start of chemotherapy.

Since F-18 fluoroestradiol (F-18-FES) uptake in breast cancer correlates with ER expression by tissue assays, this tracer can be used to determine *estrogen receptor expression* in primary breast cancer and metastatic disease (25, 104). With this information, predicting responses to endocrine treatments (105) might be possible. This is of particular importance since estrogen receptor expression varies among primary tumors and metastatic lesions even within individual patients (Fig. 13).

Although *angiogenesis inhibitors* have been used successfully for the treatment of breast cancers (106), response rates to these drugs alone or in combination are limited (107). Predicting responses to treatment would therefore be important. Kenny et al. (108)

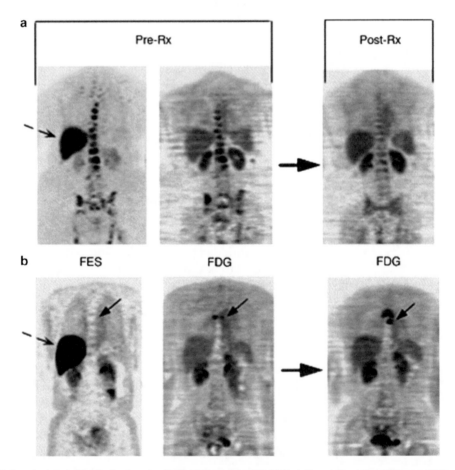

Fig. 13. Imaging examples: Pretreatment with F-18 fluoroestradiol (FES; *left*) and fluorodeoxyglucose (FDG; *middle*) scans and follow-up with F-18 FDG post-therapy (*right*) are shown. *Dashed arrows* show normal liver FES uptake. (**a**) Bone metastasis with intense F-18 FES and F-18 FDG uptake; Near-normal F-18 FDG scan at 3 months. (**b**) Bone metastasis (*solid arrow*) without F-18 FES but with F-18 FDG uptake; progressive disease at 6 months. Rx, treatment. Reprinted with permission from Linden et al. (105).

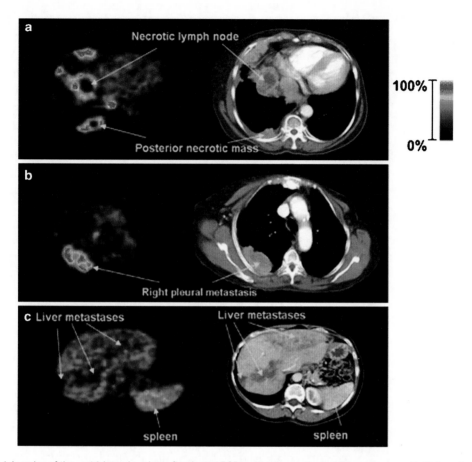

Fig. 14. Imaging of the αvβ3 integrin using a fluorinated RGD peptide in a patient with breast cancer. Multiple metastatic lesions are seen on CT images (*right*). Lesions exhibit heterogeneous uptake (**a**, **b**) and liver lesions (**c**) appear as cold defects (due to high normal background activity). Reprinted with permission from Kenny et al. (108).

recently published a phase I trial of a fluorinated RGD peptide targeting the avb3 integrin receptor (Fig. 14). Of 18 tumors detected by CT, all were visualized using this imaging probe (due to high normal background activity in the liver, tumors appeared as cold lesions in this organ). This probe showed rapid plasma clearance and stable retention in tumor tissue, and thus seems to be a promising tool for predicting and monitoring the effects of anti-angiogenic treatments.

Smith-Jones et al. (109) proposed a novel approach for measuring the pharmacodynamics of a breast cancer therapeutic agent. These authors used animal PET imaging with a microPET to study the response of breast cancer xenografts to a geldana-mycin derivative in HER2-expressing tumors. The antitumor activity of this heat shock protein-90 inhibitor results from deg-radation of HER2. Initially, HER2 expression was imaged with the gallium-68-labeled HER2 ligand (and drug) Herceptin.

Subsequently, because of a much shorter serum half-life, a gallium-68-labeled F(ab')2 fragment of Herceptin was used.

Retention of both imaging probes was correlated with HER2 expression by immunoblotting. Because gallium-68 has a short half-life of only 68 min, serial microPET imaging to measure the effects of the study drug on tumor HER2 activity was feasible. Treatment resulted in >50% reductions in tumor tracer uptake at 24 h after administration of the study drug and in concordant reductions in HER2 expression levels in excised tumor tissue by 80%. The same group (110) subsequently demonstrated that the HER2 inhibition preceded reductions in tumor glucose utilization and even more prominently reductions in tumor size.

Potential human trials could use Ga-68-F(ab')2-herceptin to identify noninvasively breast cancer patients who overexpress HER2 and are therefore more likely to respond to Herceptin treatment. In addition, HER2 expression levels of metastatic lesions that might differ from those in primary tumors could be studied, and the effects of the study drug on target expression could be measured.

Thus, in vivo phenotyping by PET imaging is emerging as a new powerful tool for predicting and monitoring therapeutic responses in breast cancer patients (111).

In summary, molecular PET imaging permits the metabolic characterization of breast cancer. Whole body F-18 FDG PET-CT imaging will continue to play an increasingly important role in diagnosing, staging, restaging, and monitoring of breast cancer patients. In addition to glucose metabolic phenotyping with F-18 FDG, processes such as tumor cell proliferation angiogenesis (112), tumor hypoxia (113), or estrogen or Her2neu receptor expression can be examined with PET. In the future, these targeted imaging approaches will enable treating physicians to individualize therapies in breast cancer patients.

References

1. Berry, D., Cronin, K., Plevritis, S., Fryback, D., Clarke, L., Zelen, M., et al. (2005) Effect of screening and adjuvant therapy on mortality from breast cancer. *N Engl J Med* **353**, 1784–92.

2. Jemal, A., Clegg, L.X., Ward, E., et al. (2004) Annual report to the nation on the status of cancer, 1975–2001, with a special feature regarding survival. *Cancer* **10(1)**, 3–27.

3. Slamon, D.J., Leyland-Jones, B., Shak, S., Fuchs, H., Paton, V., Bajamonde, A., et al. (2001) Use of chemotherapy plus a monoclonal antibody against HER2 for metastatic breast cancert that overexpresses HER2 *N Engl J Med* **344(11)**, 783–92.

4. Czernin, J., Allen-Auerbach, M., Schelbert, H.R. (2007) Improvements in cancer staging with PET-CT: literature-based evidence as of September 2006 *J Nucl Med* **48(1)**, 78S-88S.

5. Phelps, M., Hoffmann, E., Mullani, N., TerPogossian, M. (1975) Application of annihilation coincidence detection to transaxial reconstruction tomography *J Nuc Med* **16**, 210–4.

6. Czernin, J., Phelps, M.E. (2002) Positron emission tomography scanning: current and future applications *Ann Rev Med* **53**, 89–112.

7. Beyer, T., Townsend, D., Brun, T., Kinahan, P., Charron, M., Roddy, R., et al. (2004)

A combined PET-CT scanner for clinical oncology *J Nuc Med* **41**, 1369–79.

8. Rosenberg, R., Hunt, W., Williamson, M., Gilliland, F., Wiest, P., Kelsey, C., et al. (1998) Effects of age, breast density, ethnicity, and estrogen replacement therapy on screening mammographic sensitivity and cancer stage at diagnosis: review of 183,134 screening mammograms in Albuquerque, New Mexico *Radiology* **209**, 511–8.

9. Mandelson, M., Oestreicher, N., Porter, P., White, D., Finder, C., Taplin, S., et al. (2000) Breast density as a predictor of mammographic detection: Comparison of interval -and screen-detected cancers *J Natl Cancer Inst* **92**, 1081–7.

10. Pisano, E., Gatsonis, C., Hendrick, R., Yaffe, M., Baum, J., Acharyya, S., et al. (2005) Diagnostic accuracy of digital versus film mammography for breast cancer screening *N Engl J Med* **353**, 1773–83.

11. Laya, M., Larson, E., Taplin, S., White, E. (1996) Effect of estrogen replacement therapy on the specificity and sensitivity of screening mammography *J Natl Cancer Inst* **88**, 643–9.

12. Wahl, R., Helvie, M., Chang, A., Andersson, I. (1994) Detection of breast cancer in women after augmentation mammoplasty using fluorine-18-fluorodeoxyglucose-PET *J Nucl Med* **3**, 872–5.

13. Bird, R., Wallace, T., Yankaskas, B. (1992) Analysis of cancers missed at screening mammography *Radiology* **184**, 613–7.

14. Orel, S., Kay, N., Reynolds, C., Sullivan, D. (1999) BI-RADS categorization as a predictor of malignancy *Radiology* **211(3)**, 845–50.

15. Wright, C., Mueller, C. (1995) Screening mammography and public health policy: the need for perspective *Lancet* **346**, 29–32.

16. Hall, J., Lee, M., Newman, B., Morrow, J., Anderson, L., Huey, B., et al. (1990) Linkage of early-onset familial breast cancer to chromosome 17q21 *Science* **250**, 1684–9.

17. Warner, E., Plewes, D.B., Hill, K.A., Causer, P.A., Zubovits, J.T., Jong, R.A., et al. (2004) Surveillance of BRCA1 and BRCA2 mutation carriers with magnetic resonance imaging, ultrasound, mammography, and clinical breast examination *JAMA* **292(1)**, 1317–25.

18. Kriege, M., Brekelmans, C.T.M., Boetes, C., Besnard, P.E., Zonderland, H.M., Obdeijn, I.M., et al. (2004) Efficacy of MRI and mammography for breast-cancer screening in women with a familial or genetic predisposition *N Engl J Med* **35(15)**, 427–37.

19. Riedl, C.C., Ponhold, L., Flory, D., Weber, M., Kroiss, R., Wagner, T., et al. (2007) Magnetic resonance imaging of the breast improves detection of invasive cancer, pre-invasive cancer, and premalignant lesions during surveillance of women at high risk for breast cancer *Clin Cancer Res* **13(20)**, 6144–52.

20. Warburg, O., Posener, K., Negelein, E., VIII. (1924) The metabolism of cancer cells *Biochem Zeitschr* **152**, 129–69.

21. Robey, I., Stephen, R., Brown, K., Baggett, B., Gatenby, R., Gillies, R. (2008) Regulation of the Warburg effect in early-passage breast cancer cells *Neoplasia* **10**, 745–56.

22. Hoffman, E.J., Huang, S.C., Phelps, M.E. (1979) Quantitation in positron emission computed tomography *J Comput Assist Tomogr* **3**, 299–308.

23. Buck, A., Schirrmeister, H., Kühn, T., Shen, C., Kalker, T., Kotzerke, J., et al. (2002) FDG uptake in breast cancer: correlation with biological and clinical prognostic parameters *Eur J Nucl Med Mol Imaging* **29(10)**, 1317–23.

24. Avril, N., Rosé, C., Schelling, M., Dose, J., Kuhn, W., Bense, S., et al. (2005) Breast imaging with positron emission tomography and fluorine-18 fluorodeoxyglucose: use and limitations *J Clin Oncol* **18**, 3495–502.

25. Dehdashti, F., Mortimer, J.E., Siegel, B.A., Griffeth, L.K., Bonasera, T.J., Fusselman, M.J., et al. (1995) Positron Tomographic assessment of estrogen receptors in breast cancer: comparison with FDG-PET and in vitro receptor assays *J Nucl Med* **36(10)**, 1766–74.

26. Bos, R., van der Hoeven, J.J.M., van der Wall, E., van der Groep, P., van Diest, P.J., Comans, E.F.I., et al. (2002) Biologic correlates of 18Fluorodeoxyglucose uptake in human breast cancer measured by positron emission tomography *J Clin Oncol* **20(2)**, 379–87.

27. Avril, N., Menzel, M., Dose, J., Schelling, M., Weber, W., Janicke, F., et al. (2001) Glucose metabolism of breast cancer assessed by 18F-FDG PET: histologic and immunohistochemical tissue analysis *J Nucl Med* **42(1)**, 9–16.

28. Oshida, M., Uno, K., Suzuki, M., Nagashima, T., Hashimoto, H., Yagata, H., et al. (1998) Predicting the prognoses of breast carcinoma patients with positron emission tomography using 2-deoxy-2-fluoro[18F]-D-glucose *Cancer* **11**, 2227–34.

29. Mankoff, D.A., Dunnwald, L.K., Gralow, J.R., Ellis, G.K., Schubert, E.K., Tseng, J.,

et al. (2003) Changes in blood flow and metabolism in locally advanced breast cancer treated with neoadjuvant chemotherapy *J Nucl Med* **44(11)**, 1806–14.

30. Schoder, H., Gonen, M. (2007) Screening for cancer with PET and PET-CT: potential and limitations *J Nucl Med* **48(1)**, 4S-18S.

31. Vranjesevic, D., Schiepers, C., Silverman, D.H., Quon, A., Villalpando, J., Dahlbom, M., et al. (2003) Relationship between 18F-FDG uptake and breast density in women with normal breast tissue *J Nucl Med* **44(8)**, 1238–42.

32. Kumar, R., Chauhan, A., Zhuang, H., Chandra, P., Schnall, M., Alavi, A. (2006) Standardized uptake values of normal breast tissue with 2-Deoxy-2-[F-18]Fluoro-D-glucose positron emission tomography: variations with age, breast density, and menopausal status *Mol Imaging Biol* **8(6)**, 355–62.

33. Kubota, K., Matsuzawa, T., Amemiya, A., Kondo, M., Fujiwara, T., Watanuki, S., et al. (1989) Imaging of breast cancer with [f18] Fluorodeoxyglucose and positron emission tomography *J Comput Asst Tomogr* **13**, 1097.

34. Bassa, P., Kim, E.E., Wong, F.C., Korkmaz, M., Yang, D., et al. (1996) Evaluation of pre-operative chemotherapy using PET with flu-orine-18-fluorodeoxyglucose in breast cancer *J Nucl Med* **37**, 931–8.

35. Rostom, A.Y., Powe, J., Kandil, A., Ezzat, A., Bakheet, S., El-Khwsky, F., et al. (1999) Positron emission tomography in breast cancer: a clinicopathological correlation of results *Br J Radiol* **72**, 1064–8.

36. Utech, C., Young, C., Winter, P. (1996) Prospective evaluation of fluorine-18 fluoro-deoxyglucose positron emission tomography in breast cancer for staging of the axilla related to surgery and immunocytochemistry *Eur J Nucl Med* **23**, 1588–93.

37. Noh, D., Yun, I., Kim, J., Kang, H., Lee, D., Chung, J., et al. (1998) Diagnostic value of positron emission tomography for detecting breast cancer *World J Surg* **22**, 223–8.

38. Schirrmeister, H., Kühn, T., Guhlman, A., Santjohanser, C., Hörster, T., Nüssle, K., et al. (2001) Fluorine-18 2-deoxy-2-fluoro-D-glucose PET in the preoperative staging of breast cancer: comparison with the standard staging procedures *Eur J Nuc Med* **28**, 351–8.

39. Tse, N., Hoh, C., Hawkins, R., Zinner, M., Dahlbom, M., Choi, Y., et al. (1992) The application of positron emission tomographic imaging with fluorodeoxyglucose to the eval-uation of breast disease *Ann Surg* **16(1)**, 27–34.

40. Nieweg, O., Kim, E., Wong, W., Broussard, W., Singletary, E., Hortobagyi, G., et al. (1993) Positron emsission tomography with Fluorine-18-deoxyglucose in the detection and staging of breast cancer *Cancer* **71**, 3920–5.

41. Adler, L.P., Crowe, J.P., al-Kaisi, N.K., Sunshine, J.L. (1993) Evaluation of breast masses and axillary lymph nodes with [F-18] 2 deoxy-2-fluoro-D-glucose PET *Radiology* **187**, 743–50.

42. Avril, N., Dose, J., Jänicke, F., Bense, S., Ziegler, S., Laubenbacher, C., et al. (1996) Metabolic characterization of breast tumors with positron emission tomography using F-18 Fluorodeoxyglucose *J Clin Oncol* **14**, 1848–57.

43. Crippa, F., Seregeni, E., Agresti, R., Chiesa, C., Pascali, C., Bogni, A., et al. (1996) Association between [18F]fluorodeoxyglu-cose uptake and postoperative histopathol-ogy, hormone receptor status, thymidine labelling index and p53 in primary breast cancer: a preliminary observation *Eur J Nuc Med* **25**, 1429–34.

44. Noh, D., Yun, I., Kang, H., Kim, Y., Kim, J., Chung, J., et al. (1999) Detection of cancer in augmented breasts by positron emission tomography *Eur J Surg* **165**, 847–51.

45. Avril, N., Rose, C.A., Schelling, M., Dose, J., Kuhn, W., Bense, S., et al. (2000) Breast imaging with positron emission tomography and fluorine-18 fluorodeoxyglucose: use and limitations *J Clin Oncol* **18(20)**, 3495–502.

46. Bleckmann, C., Dose, J., Bohuslavizki, K., Buchert, R., Klutman, S., Mester, J., et al. (1999) Effect of attenuation correction on lesion detectability in FDG PET of breast cancer *J Nuc Med* **40**, 2021–4.

47. Yutani, K., Hojo, S., Tatsumi, M., Shiba, E., Noguchi, S., Nishimura, T. (1999) Correlation of F-18-FDG and Tc-99m-MIBI uptake with proliferative activity in breast cancer *J Nucl Med* **40(5)**, 16P–17P.

48. Boerner, A., Weckesser, M., Herzog, H., Schmitz, T., Audretsch, W., Nitz, U., et al. (1999) Optimal scan time for fluorine-18 fluorodeoxyglucose positron emission tomography in breast cancer *Eur J Nucl Med* **26**, 226–30.

49. Mavi, A., Urhan, M., Yu, J.Q., Zhuang, H., Houseni, M., Cermik, T.F., et al. (2006) Dual time point 18F-FDG PET imaging detects breast cancer with high sensitivity and correlates well with histologic subtypes *J Nucl Med* **47(9)**, 1440–6.

50. Doshi, N., Shao, Y., Silverman, R., Cherry, S. (2000) Design and evaluation of an LSO

PET detector for breast cancer imaging *Med Phys* **27**, 1535–43.

51. Raylman, R., Majewski, S., Smith, M., Proffitt, J., Hammond, W., Srinivasan, A., et al. (2008) The positron emission mammography/tomography breast imaging and biopsy system (PEM/PET): design, construction and phantom-based measurements *Phys Med Biol* **53**, 637–53.

52. Tafra, L., Cheng, Z., Uddo, J., Lobrano, M.B., Stein, W., Berg, W.A., et al. (2005) Pilot clinical trial of 18F-fluorodeoxyglucose positron-emission mammography in the surgical management of breast cancer *Am J Surg* **190(4)**, 628–32.

53. Berg, W.A., Weinberg, I.N., Narayanan, D., et al. (2006) High-resolution fluorodeoxyglucose positron emission tomography with compression ("*positron emission* mammography") is highly accurate in depicting primary breast cancer *Breast J* **12(4)**, 309–23.

54. Berriolo-Riedinger, A., Touzery, C., Riedinger, J-M., Toubeau, M., Coudert, B., Arnould, L., et al. (2007) [18F]FDG-PET predicts complete pathological response of breast cancer to neoadjuvant chemotherapy *Eur J Nucl Med Mol Imaging* **34(12)**, 1915–24.

55. Krag, D., Weaver, D., Ashikaga, T., Moffat, F., Klimberg, V.S., Shriver, C., et al. (1998) The sentinel node in breast cancer -- a multicenter validation study *N Engl J* Med **339(14)**, 941–6.

56. Adler, L., Faulhaber, P., Schnur, K., Al-Kasai, N., Shenk, R. (1997) Axillary lymph node metastases: screening with [F-18]2 deoxy-2-D-glucose (FDG) PET *Radiology* **203**, 323–7.

57. Crippa, F., Agresti, R., Donne V.D., Pascali, C., Bogni, A., Chiesa, C., et al. (1997) The contribution of positron emission tomography (PET) with 18F-fluorodeoxyglucose (FDG) in the pre-operative detection of axillary metastases of breast cancer: the experience of the National Cancer Institute of Milan *Tumori* **83**, 542–3.

58. Crippa, F., Agresti, R., Seregni, E., Greco, M., Pascali, C., Bogni, A., et al. (1998) Prospective evaluation of fluorine -18-FDG PET in presurgical staging of the axilla in breast cancer *J Nucl Med* **39**, 4–8.

59. Smith, I., Ogston, K., Whitford, P., Smith, F., Sharp, P., Norton, M., et al. (1998) Staging of the axilla in breast cancer: accurate in vivo assessment using positron emission tomography with 2-(fluorine-18)-fliuoro-2-deoxy-D-glucose *Ann Surg* **228**, 220–7.

60. Yutani, K., Shiba, E., Tatsumi, M., Uehara, T., Taguchi, T., Takai, S-I., et al. (2000) Comparison of FDG-PET with MIBI-SPECT in the detection of breast cancer and axillary lymph node metastasis *J Comput Assist Tomogr* **24**, 274–80.

61. Wahl, R.L., Siegel, B.A., Coleman, R.E., Gatsonis, C.G. (2004) Prospective multicenter study of axillary nodal staging by positron emission tomography in breast cancer: a Report of the Staging Breast Cancer With PET Study Group *J Clin Oncol* **22(2)**, 277–85.

62. Fuster, D., Duch, J., Paredes, P., Velasco, M., Munoz, M., Santamaria, G., et al. (2008) Preoperative staging of large primary breast cancer with [18F]Fluorodeoxyglucose positron emission tomography/computed tomography compared with conventional imaging procedures *JCO* **17**, 1496.

63. Donegan, W. (1977) The influence of untreated internal mammary metastases upon the course of mammary cancer *Cancer* **39**, 533–8.

64. Eubank, W.B., Mankoff, D.A., Takasugi, J., Vesselle, H., Eary, J.F., Shanley, T.J., et al. (2001) 18-Fluorodeoxyglucose positron emission tomography to detect mediastinal or internal mammary metastases in breast cancer *J Clin* Oncol **19(15)**, 3516–23.

65. Tran, A., Pio, B.S., Khatibi, B., Czernin, J., Phelps, M.E., Silverman, D.H.S. (2005) 18F-FDG PET for staging breast cancer in patients with inner-quadrant versus outer-quadrant tumors: comparison with long-term clinical outcome *J Nucl Med* **45(9)**, 1455–9.

66. Carey, L.A., Metzger, R., Dees, E.C., Collichio, F., Sartor, C.I., Ollila, D.W., et al. (2005) American Joint Committee on Cancer Tumor-Node-Metastasis Stage After Neoadjuvant Chemotherapy and Breast Cancer Outcome *J Natl Cancer Inst* **97(15)**, 1137–42.

67. Mahner, S., Schirrmacher, S., Brenner, W., Jenicke, L., Habermann, C.R., Avril, N., et al. (2008) Comparison between positron emission tomography using 2-[fluorine-18] fluoro-2-deoxy-D-glucose, conventional imaging and computed tomography for staging of breast cancer *Ann Oncol* **19(7)**, 1249–54.

68. Fueger, B., Weber, W., Quon, A., Crawford, T., Allen-Auerbach, M., Halpern, B., et al. (2005) Performance of 2-Deoxy-2-[F-18] fluoro-D-glucose positron emission tomography and integrated PET-CT in restaged breast cancer patients *Mol Imaging Biol* **7**, 369–76.

69. Radan, L., Ben-Haim, S., Bar-Shalom, R., Guralnik, L., Israel, O. (2006) The role of FDG-PET-CT in suspected recurrence of breast cancer *Cancer* **107(11)**, 2545–51.

70. Veit-Haibach, P., Antoch, G., Beyer, T., Stergar, H., Schleucher, R., Hauth, E.A.M., et al. (2007) FDG-PET/CT in restaging of patients with recurrent breast cancer: possible impact on staging and therapy *Br J Radiol* **80(955)**, 508–15.

71. Heusner, T.A., Kuemmel, S., Umutlu, L., Koeninger, A., Freudenberg, L.S., Hauth, E.A.M., et al. (2008) Breast cancer staging in a single session: whole-body PET-CT mammography *J Nucl Med* **49(8)**, *1215–22*.

72. Cook, G., Fogelman, I. (1999) Skeletal metastases from breast cancer: imaging with nuclear medicine *Semin Nucl Med* **29**, 69–79.

73. Cook, G.J.R. (2003) Oncological molecular imaging: nuclear medicine techniques *Br J Radiol* , **76(2)**, S152–8.

74. Puglisi, F., Follador, A., Minisini, A.M., Cardellino, G.G., Russo, S., Andreetta, C., et al. (2005) Baseline staging tests after a new diagnosis of breast cancer: further evidence of their limited indications *Ann Oncol* **16(2)**, 263–6.

75. Kasem, A.R., Desai, A., Daniell, S., Sinha, P. (2006) Bone scan and liver ultrasound scan in the preoperative staging for primary breast cancer *Breast J* **12(6)**, 544–8.

76. Cook, G.J., Houston, S., Rubens, R., Maisey, M.N., Fogelman, I. (1998) Detection of bone metastases in breast cancer by 18FDG PET: differing metabolic activity in osteoblastic and osteolytic lesions *J Clin Oncol* **16(10)**, 3375–9.

77. Specht, J., Tam, S., Kurland, B., Gralow, J., Livingston, R., Linden, H., et al. (2007) Serial 2-[18F] fluoro-2-deoxy-D-glucose positron emission tomography (FDG-PET) to monitor treatment of bone-dominant metastatic breast cancer predicts time to progression (TTP) *Breast Cancer Res Treat* **105(1)**, 87–94.

78. Du, Y., Cullum, I., Illidge, T.M., Ell, P.J. (2007) Fusion of metabolic function and morphology: sequential [18F]Fluorod eoxyglucose positron-emission tomography/computed tomography studies yield new insights into the natural history of bone metastases in breast cancer *J Clin Oncol* **25(23)**, 3440–7.

79. Blau, M., Nagler, W., Bender, M. (1962) Fluorine-18: a new isotope for bone scanning *J Nucl Med* **3**, 332–4.

80. Schirrmeister, H., Guhlmann, A., Kotzerke, J., Santjohanser, C., Kuhn, T., Kreienberg, R., et al. (1999) Early detection and accurate description of extent of metastatic bone disease in breast cancer with fluoride ion and

positron emission tomography *J Clin Oncol* **17(8)**, 2381–9.

81. Even-Sapir, E., Metser, U., Flusser, G., Zuriel, L., Kollender, Y., Lerman, H., et al. (2004) Assessment of malignant skeletal disease: initial experience with 18F-Fluoride PET-CT and comparison between 18F-Fluoride PET and 18F-Fluoride PET-CT *J Nucl Med* **45(2)**, 272–8.

82. Lordick, F., Ott, K., Krause, B-J, Weber, W.A., Becker, K., Stein, H.J., et al. (2007) PET to assess early metabolic response and to guide treatment of adenocarcinoma of the oesophagogastric junction: the MUNICON phase II trial *Lancet Oncol* **8(9)**, 797–805.

83. Weber, W.A., Figlin, R. (2007) Monitoring cancer treatment with PET-CT: does it make a difference *J Nucl Med* **48(1)**, 36S-44S.

84. Minn, H., Soini, I. (1989) [18F]fluorodeoxyglucose scintigraphy in diagnosis and follow up of treatment in advanced breast cancer *Eur J Nucl Med* **15**, 61–6.

85. Wahl, R.L., Zasadny, K., Helvie, M., Hutchins, G.D., Weber, B., Cody, R. (1993) Metabolic monitoring of breast cancer chemohormonotherapy using positron emission tomography: initial evaluation *J Clin Oncol* **11(11)**, 2101–11.

86. Bruce, D., Evans, N., Heys, S., Needham, G., Ben Younes, H., Mikecz, P., et al. (1995) Positron emission tomography: 2-deoxy-2-[18F]-fluoro-D-glucose uptake in locally advanced breast cancers *Eur J Surg Oncol* **21**, 280–3.

87. Dehdashti, F., Flanagan, F.L., Mortimer, J., Katzenellenbogen, J., Welch, M., Siegel, B.A. (1998) Positron emission tomographic assessment of "metabolic flare" to predict response of metastatic breast cancer to antiestrogen therapy *Eur J Nuc Med* **26**, 51–6.

88. Schelling, M., Avril, N., Nahrig, J., Kuhn, W., Romer, W., Sattler, D., et al. (2000) Positron emission tomography using [(18)F]Fluorodeoxyglucose for monitoring primary chemotherapy in breast cancer *J Clin Oncol* **18(8)**, 1689–95.

89. Smith, I.C., Welch, A.E., Hutcheon, A.W., Miller, I.D., Payne, S., Chilcott, F., et al. (2000) Positron emission tomography using [(18)F]-fluorodeoxy-D-glucose to predict the pathologic response of breast cancer to primary chemotherapy *J Clin Oncol* **18(8)**, 1676–88.

90. Wolmark, N., Wang, J., Mamounas, E., Bryant, J., Fisher, B. (2001) Preoperative chemotherapy in patients with operable breast cancer: nine-year results from National Surgical Adjuvant Breast and Bowel Project

B-18 *J Natl Cancer Institute Monogr* **30**, 96–102.

91. Rousseau, C., Devillers, A., Sagan, C., Ferrer, L., Bridji, B., Campion, L., et al. (2006) Monitoring of early response to neoadjuvant chemotherapy in Stage II and III breast cancer by [18F]Fluorodeoxyglucose positron emission tomography *J Clin Oncol* **24(34)**, *5366–72.*

92. Dunnwald, L.K., Gralow, J.R., Ellis, G.K., Livingston, R.B., Linden, H.M., Specht, J.M., et al. (2008) Tumor metabolism and blood flow changes by positron emission tomography: relation to survival in patients treated with neoadjuvant chemotherapy for locally advanced breast cancer *J Clin Oncol* **26(27)**, 4449–57.

93. Dose Schwarz, J., Bader, M., Jenicke, L., Hemminger, G., Janicke, F., Avril, N. (2005) Early prediction of response to chemotherapy in metastatic breast cancer using sequential 18F-FDG PET *J Nucl Med* **46(7)**, 1144–50.

94. Couturier, O., Jerusalem, G., N'Guyen, J-M, Hustinx, R. (2006) Sequential positron emission tomography using [18F] Fluorodeoxyglucose for monitoring response to chemotherapy in metastatic breast cancer *Clin Cancer Res* **12(21)**, 6437–43.

95. Cachin, F., Prince, H.M., Hogg, A., Ware, R.E., Hicks, R.J. (2006) Powerful prognostic stratification By [18F]Fluorodeoxyglucose positron emission tomography in patients with metastatic breast cancer treated with high-dose chemotherapy *J Clin Oncol* **24(19)**, 3026–31.

96. Yap C, Valk P, Ariannejad M, Seltzer M, Phelps M, Gambhir S et al. (2002) FDG-PET influences the clinical management of lymphoma patients *J Nucl Med* **41(5)**:70P

97. Hillner, B.E., Siegel, B.A., Liu, D., Shields, A.F., Gareen, I.F., Hanna, L., et al. (2008) Impact of positron emission tomography/computed tomography and positron emission tomography (PET) alone on expected management of patients with cancer: initial results from the National Oncologic PET Registry *J Clin Oncol* **26(13)**, 2155–61.

98. Shields, A.F., Grierson, J.R., Dohmen, B.M., Machulla, H.J., Stayanoff, J.C., Lawhorn-Crews, J.M., et al. (1998) Imaging proliferation in vivo with [F-18]FLT and positron emission tomography *Nat Med* **4(11)**:1334–6.

99. Bading, J.R., Shields, A.F. (2008) Imaging of cell proliferation: status and prospects *J Nucl Med* **49(2)**, 64S–80S.

100. Toyohara, J., Waki, A., Takamatsu, S., Yonekura, Y., Magata, Y., Fujibayashi, Y. (2002) Basis of FLT as a cell proliferation marker: comparative uptake studies with [3H]thymidine and [3H]arabinothymidine, and cell-analysis in 22 asynchronously growing tumor cell lines *Nucl Med Biol* **29(3)**: 281–7.

101. Smyczek-Gargya, B., Fersis, N., Dittmann, H., Vogel, U., Reischl, G., Machulla, H-J, et al. (2004) PET with [18F]fluorothymidine for imaging of primary breast cancer: a pilot study *Eur J Nucl Med Mol Imaging* **31(5)**, 720–4.

102. Kenny, L.M., Vigushin, D.M., Al-Nahhas, A., Osman, S., Luthra, S.K., Shousha, S., et al. (2005) Quantification of cellular proliferation in tumor and normal tissues of patients with breast cancer by [18F] Fluorothymidine-positron emission tomography imaging: evaluation of analytical methods *Cancer Res* **65(21)**, 10104–12.

103. Pio, B., Park, C., Pietras, R., Hsueh, W-A, Satyamurthy, N., Pegram, M., et al. (2006) Usefulness of 3′-[F-18]Fluoro-3′-deoxythymidine with positron emission tomography in predicting breast cancer response to therapy *Mol Imaging Biol* **8(1)**, 36–42.

104. Peterson, L.M., Mankoff, D.A., Lawton, T., Yagle, K., Schubert, E.K., Stekhova, S., et al. (2008) Quantitative imaging of estrogen receptor expression in breast cancer with PET and 18F-Fluoroestradiol *J Nucl Med* **49(3)**, 367–74.

105. Linden, H.M., Stekhova, S.A., Link, J.M., Gralow, J.R., Livingston, R.B., Ellis, G.K., et al. (2006) Quantitative fluoroestradiol positron emission tomography imaging predicts response to endocrine treatment in breast cancer *J Clin Oncol* **24(18)**, 2793–9.

106. Schneider, B., Sledge, G. (2007) Drug Insight: VEGF as a therapeutic target for breast cancer *Nat Clin Pract Oncol* **4**, 181–9.

107. Miller, K.D., Chap, L.I., Holmes, F.A., Cobleigh, M.A., Marcom, P.K., Fehrenbacher, L., et al. (2005) Randomized Phase III trial of Capecitabine compared with Bevacizumab plus Capecitabine in patients with previously treated metastatic breast cancer *J Clin Oncol* **23(4)**, 792–9.

108. Kenny, L.M., Coombes, R.C., Oulie, I., Contractor, K.B., Miller, M., Spinks, T.J., et al. (2008) Phase I trial of the positron-emitting Arg-Gly-Asp (RGD) peptide radioligand 18F-AH111585 in breast cancer patients *J Nucl Med* **49(6)**, 879–86.

109. Smith-Jones, P.M., Solit, D.B., Akhurst, T., Afroze, F., Rosen, N., Larson, S.M. (2004)

Imaging the pharmacodynamics of HER2
degradation in response to Hsp90 inhibitors
Nat Biotechnol **22**, 701–6.

110. Smith-Jones, P.M., Solit, D.B., Afroze, F.,
Rosen, N., Larson, S.M. (2006) Early tumor
response to Hsp90 therapy using HER2
PET: comparison with 18F-FDG PET *J Nucl
Med* **47(5)**, 793–6.

111. Weber, W., Czernin, J., Phelps, M.,
Herschman, H. (2008) Technology Insight:
novel imaging of molecular targets is an
emerging area crucial to the development
of targeted drugs *Nat Clin Pract Oncol* **5**,
44–54.

112. Haubner, R., Weber, W.A., Beer, A.J.,
Vabuliene, E., Reim, D., Sarbia, M., et al.
(2005) Noninvasive visualization of the activated alphavbeta3 integrin in cancer patients
by positron emission tomography and [(18)
F]Galacto-RGD. *PLoS Med* **2(3)**, e70.

113. Rajendran, J.G., Mankoff, D.A., O'Sullivan,
F., Peterson, L.M., Schwartz, D.L., Conrad,
E.U., et al. (2004) Hypoxia and glucose
metabolism in malignant tumors: evaluation
by [18F]Fluo-romisonidazole and [18F]
Fluorodeoxyglucose positron emission
tomography imaging *Clin Cancer Res.* **10(7)**,
2245–52.

Chapter 10

Gynecological Cancers

Norbert Avril, Sofia Gourtsoyianni, and Rodney Reznek

Abstract

The clinical problems raised in patients presenting with all forms of gynecological malignancy are currently addressed using conventional cross-sectional imaging, usually MRI. In general, F-18 FDG PET-CT has not been shown to have a clinical role in any of these cancers at presentation, although studies are under way to use this form of metabolic imaging to predict prognosis and the response to treatment. Although F-18 FDG PET-CT is superior to conventional imaging techniques, it is only moderately sensitive in demonstrating lymph node metastasis preoperatively, and is inadequate for local staging of patients with endometrial cancer. In ovarian cancer, F-18 FDG PET-CT provides an accurate assessment of the extent of disease, particularly in areas difficult to assess for metastases by CT and MRI such as the abdomen and pelvis, mediastinum, and supraclavicular region.

F-18 FDG PET-CT is a sensitive method of detecting pelvic and para-aortic lymph nodal disease in cervical cancer, and appears to be superior to MRI and CT despite the limitations in identifying small foci of disease. In the main, as elsewhere in patients with cancer, the value of PET-CT is in identifying and defining the extent of recurrent disease, in distinguishing between posttreatment fibrosis and recurrence, and possibly in monitoring response to therapy.

Key words: FDG PET-CT, Diagnosis, Diagnostic imaging, Ovarian cancer, Endometrial cancer, Cervical cancer, Vulvar cancer, Staging, Treatment monitoring

1. Introduction

F-18 FDG PET(-CT) has only a limited role in the diagnosis and staging of disease in patients presenting with gynecological malignancy. The strength of F-18 FDG PET-CT lies in its ability for precise whole body assessment of lymph node spread and distant metastases (1). Therefore, in some patients presenting initially with advanced disease, F-18 FDG PET-CT can contribute to more accurate staging and thus influence the therapeutic decision. Quantitative measurements of uptake expressed as standardized uptake values (SUV) have been correlated with tumor

Malik E. Juweid and Otto S. Hoekstra (eds.), *Positron Emission Tomography*, Methods in Molecular Biology, vol. 727, DOI 10.1007/978-1-61779-062-1_10, © Springer Science+Business Media, LLC 2011

aggressiveness and survival; however, their clinical role has not yet been established and it is unlikely that SUV measurements will provide significant clinical information for individual patients.

F-18 FDG PET-CT is nevertheless a valuable tool for assessing the extent of recurrent disease and may be critical in defining the optimal treatment. PET-CT is clearly superior to conventional CT in depicting disease within the abdominal cavity, as well as in supraclavicular, mediastinal, and inguinal lymph nodes. This is particularly important in patients with suspected ovarian cancer recurrence and especially those with rising CA-125 levels, and negative or indeterminate conventional imaging findings. In recurrent endometrial, cervical, and vulvar cancer, it is of value in optimizing the selection of patients for site-specific treatment, radiotherapy planning, and in predicting resectability. Limitations to F-18 FDG PET-CT in identifying metastatic disease are its inability to detect small lung deposits or diffuse peritoneal carcinomatosis; conversely, false-positive findings occur in acute inflammation, granulomatous processes, tuberculosis, and sarcoidosis.

Further indications for F-18 FDG PET-CT include assessment of response to treatment of localized disease. In cervical cancer, for example, PET-CT performed 3 months after radiotherapy can provide valuable prognostic information. F-18 FDG PET-CT is generally a valuable tool for assessment of treatment response in patients with metastatic gynecological malignancies, particularly in identifying residual viable tumor tissue by its increased metabolic activity.

Prediction of treatment response by comparing the tumor metabolic activity after one or two cycles of treatment with baseline is a promising indication but needs further validation in clinical trials.

2. Technique for Pelvic PET-CT

Gynecological malignancies typically present with focally increased F-18 FDG uptake, whereas benign tumors are generally negative on PET. However, common pitfalls include increased F-18 FDG uptake in normal ovaries during ovulation, as well as normal physiologic activity in bowel, endometrium, and blood vessels; focal retained activity in ureters, bladder diverticula, pelvic kidneys, and urinary diversions (2–4).

Therefore, specific emphasis needs to be directed particularly towards pelvic PET-CT imaging. Ideally, the bladder should be empty to avoid artifacts on PET images from high radioactivity concentration in the bladder. It is suggested that the patient is scanned in a caudal to cranial direction, thus imaging the pelvis at the beginning of the study. The CT portion of PET-CT is often helpful to identify bladder diverticula and focal retained activity in ureters. Pelvic imaging can be improved by intravenous injection of furosemide (20–40 mg) to reduce tracer retention in the urinary system. A technique of hydration, diuretic administration, and pre-imaging voiding will allow avoiding invasive procedures such as bladder drainage in most cases.

The CT portion of PET-CT is also helpful in identifying normal physiologic activity in bowel, endometrium, and blood vessels. Bowel preparation can be performed with oral hydration as well, and some groups recommend the use of oral contrast (3). The administration of butyl-scopolamine (20–40 mg) at the time F-18 FDG injection has been reported to reduce F-18 FDG uptake in the bowel (5).

3. Endometrial Cancer

Endometrial cancer is the most common gynecologic malignancy in the USA and UK, and accounts for 6% of all cancers in women. There were estimated 40,100 new cases and 7,470 deaths from endometrial cancer in the USA in 2008. Well-differentiated cancers tend to be localized to the surface of the endometrium, whereas poorly differentiated tumors are more likely to present with myometrial invasion. The likelihood of lymph node infiltration is related to the histological grade of the tumor, and the presence of deep myometrial and cervical invasion. Distant metastases most commonly involve the lungs, inguinal and supraclavicular nodes, liver, bones, brain, and vagina. The vast majority of patients present with early stage disease and undergo hysterectomy and bilateral salpingo-oophorectomy. However, the staging of endometrial cancer is surgico-pathological and for the full FIGO staging to be performed, the patient should undergo a total hysterectomy, bilateral salpingo-oophorectomy, as well as assessment and sampling of pelvic and para-aortic lymph nodes. This protocol is controversial and carries a risk of morbidity; patients are usually triaged into categories depending on the prognostic factors, so that those at low risk of extrathoracic spread do not undergo a formal lymphadenectomy, whereas those at high risk undergo a full staging. Various combinations of preoperative intracavitary and external-beam radiation therapy (EBRT) with hysterectomy and bilateral salpingo-oophorectomy are used for treatment of stage II endometrial cancer, with biopsy of the para-aortic nodes at the time of surgery. In general, patients with stage III endometrial cancer are treated with surgery and radiation therapy. Patients with inoperable disease may be treated with radiation therapy, often in a combination of intracavitary and EBRT. When distant metastases, especially pulmonary metastases, are present, hormonal therapy can be useful.

Therefore, imaging of primary endometrial cancer patients is targeted in depicting myometrial invasion, invasion of the cervix, and presence of metastatic lymph nodes. Patient selection according to risk of relapse for radical therapy and more conservative treatment for low risk patients is crucial for endometrial cancer patients, since majority of them are postmenopausal women with comorbidity factors. Fewer than 20% of primary endometrial cancer patients have tumor-involved lymph nodes, and an accurate imaging modality to select the ones that should undergo lymphadenectomy is of great importance.

Imaging for staging should only be performed after histopathological confirmation of endometrial cancer. Combination of T2-weighted imaging and dynamic contrast-enhanced MRI has an accuracy ranging from 84 to 93% for depth of myometrial invasion and 90–92% for depicting cervical involvement, while the accuracy of CT in staging endometrial cancer is only 61–76% due to insufficient contrast between tumor and myometrium (6).

Conventional cross-sectional imaging using size criteria lacks sensitivity in identifying nodal infiltration. MRI using a lymph node-specific contrast agent containing ultra-small particles of iron oxide (USPIO) has been used preoperatively to assess detection of lymph node metastases. Rockall et al. (7) studied 44 patients, 15 with endometrial and 29 with cervical cancer. Of 768 pelvic or para-aortic lymph nodes from sampling, 335 were correlated on MRI, and in total 17 malignant nodes were present in 25% of patients. On a node-by-node basis, the sensitivity and specificity by size criteria were 29% and 99%, respectively, while by USPIO criteria the sensitivity ranged from 82 to 93% with a corresponding specificity of 97%. On a patient-by-patient basis, sensitivity and specificity by size criteria were 27% and 94%, respectively, and 91–100% and 87–94%, respectively by USPIO criteria. MRI using USPIO therefore showed an increase in sensitivity for malignant lymph node detection without loss of specificity. Unfortunately, USPIO is currently not available outside clinical trials, and further direct comparison between MRI USPIO and F-18 FDG PET-CT is essential.

3.1. F-18 FDG PET-CT in Primary Endometrial Cancer

Primary endometrial cancer usually shows an increased F-18 FDG uptake. However, F-18 FDG PET-CT cannot reliably determine the depth of myometrial invasion. This is due to the approximately 4–5-mm spatial resolution of current PET scanner technology, as well as an inherent limitation to define tumor borders precisely on PET images. Two recent studies preoperatively assessed the lymph node status with F-18 FDG PET-CT in 12 and 40 patients, respectively (8, 9). Both studies found a comparable sensitivity of 53% and a specificity of 99%, sensitivity substantially less than that of MRI or transvaginal ultrasound. In the latter study by Kitajima et al., the accuracy of PET-CT was 97.8% (8).

The sensitivity for detecting metastatic lesions 4 mm or less in diameter was 16.7%, for lesions between 5 and 9 mm 66.7%, and for lesions 10 mm or larger 93.3%. These findings have led to the conclusion that although F-18 FDG PET-CT is superior to conventional imaging techniques, it is only moderately sensitive in predicting lymph node metastasis preoperatively, and it is inadequate for local staging of patients with endometrial cancer.

3.2. F-18 FDG PET-CT in Recurrent Endometrial Cancer

Radiation therapy may be an effective palliative treatment for patients with localized recurrences to pelvic and para-aortic lymph nodes or distant metastases in selected sites. Patients positive for estrogen and progesterone receptors respond best to progestin therapy. Only less than one-third of patients respond to chemotherapy with doxorubicin and paclitaxel being the most active anticancer agents.

In a study, 31 women underwent F-18 FDG PET-CT for suspected recurrence (10). Twelve patients had a documented recurrence by surgical biopsy or clinical follow-up, and 19 patients had no evidence of recurrence. Overall sensitivity, specificity, and accuracy of F-18 FDG PET-CT were 100%, 94.7%, 92.3%, respectively. PET-CT results modified the treatment plan in seven (22.6%) patients, resulting in five patients undergoing previously unplanned therapeutic procedures and eliminating previously planned diagnostic procedures in two patients (6.5%). Patients with negative PET-CT showed significantly better progression-free survival than those presenting with positive tumor F-18 FDG uptake.

4. Ovarian Cancer

The majority of ovarian cancers are of epithelial origin (85%), with serous adenocarcinoma being the most common type. Unusually, germ cell tumors (e.g., teratomas) and sex cord stromal tumors (e.g., thecomas) occur. In 2008, there was an estimated 21,650 new cases and 15,520 deaths from ovarian cancer in USA. Ovarian cancer typically spreads via the peritoneum, usually resulting in local invasion of serosal surfaces of the bowel. The incidence of positive nodes at primary surgery has been reported to be 24% in patients with stage I disease, 50% in patients with stage II disease, 74% in patients with stage III disease, and 73% in patients with stage IV disease. Most patients with ovarian cancer have widespread disease at presentation. Treatment includes debulking surgery followed by intravenous platinum-based combination therapy.

Ultrasound (usually transvaginal) is the most appropriate first imaging test in patients suspected of having an adnexal mass. Ultrasound is highly sensitive but lacks specificity in the diagnosis of malignancy, whereas MRI has a similar sensitivity but much higher specificity. MRI is indicated in cases of indeterminate ovarian masses or where the CA-125 is normal, particularly in younger women.

4.1. F-18 FDG PET-CT in Primary Ovarian Cancer

Primary ovarian cancer is often positive on F-18 FDG PET. However, the cellular composition of tumors has a significant effect on the level of F-18 FDG uptake. Tumors containing large cystic components as well as mucinous tumors will often not be metabolically active. It is important to note that most PET studies for detection of primary ovarian cancer were performed more than 10 years ago using a previous generation of PET scanner technology with lower spatial resolution and no direct co-registration with CT. Generally, the number of false-positive F-18 FDG PET findings in the abdomen and pelvis is low. However, in patients with suspicious ovarian masses a number of benign conditions can cause a significant false-positive rate, for example, in benign cystadenomas, teratomas, schwannomas, endometriomas, and in inflammatory processes. Menstruating women can present with increased F-18 FDG uptake of follicular cysts and corpus luteal cysts between days 10 and 25 of the menstrual cycle (11).

F-18 FDG PET for demonstration and characterization of adnexal masses has a sensitivity that ranges between 58% and 86% and a specificity that ranges between 54% and 86%, respectively (12, 13), and is substantially less than MRI. Fenchel et al. (14) compared preoperative F-18 FDG PET with ultrasound and MRI in 101 patients presenting with asymptomatic adnexal masses. F-18 FDG PET correctly classified 7 out of 12 adnexal masses as malignant and 66 of 87 as benign, resulting in a sensitivity of 58% and a specificity of 80%. Sensitivity and specificity for ultrasound were 92% and 60%, and for MRI 83% and 84%, respectively. When all three modalities were combined, the sensitivity was 92% with a corresponding specificity of 85%. All false-negative results by F-18 FDG PET were either invasive stage I tumors or tumors of low malignant potential. The authors concluded that the addition of MRI and/or F-18 FDG PET may improve the diagnostic accuracy of ultrasound in the identification of ovarian cancer. However, in case of an asymptomatic adnexal mass, none of these imaging modalities can definitely rule out the presence of early stage ovarian cancer or a borderline malignancy. Nevertheless, in practice in most institutions, transvaginal ultrasound, conducted with the required level of expertise, is regarded as having a sufficient sensitivity and negative predictive value in excluding malignant disease. Thus, when the ultrasound indicates the presence of benign disease there is seldom any need for further investigation, unless there are other features such as an elevated CA125 or symptomatology suggestive of other pathology.

The standard treatment in patients with advanced peritoneal carcinomatosis from ovarian cancer is primary optimal debulking surgery followed by chemotherapy. However, in many institutions, particularly where the imaging suggests that optimal debulking is unlikely to be achieved, patients undergo primary chemotherapy and in these circumstances it is important to identify the exact extend of disease, as optimal debulking is associated with more favorable response to postoperative chemotherapy and therefore prolonged survival. Accuracy of staging improved from 53% with CT alone to 87% with F-18 FDG PET-CT (15). Both, the F-18 FDG PET and the CT component of PET-CT were insensitive to the small peritoneal implants; however, F-18 FDG PET was able to show malignant involvement in normal sized para-aortic lymph nodes. In a more recent study, the sensitivity and specificity of F-18 FDG PET-CT to detect malignant or borderline malignant pelvic tumors were 71.4% and 81.3%, and 100% and 85% to detect ovarian cancer, respectively. Kawahara et al. found borderline ovarian tumors and mucinous adenocarcinoma of the ovary false-negative on F-18 FDG PET-CT (16).

The use of F-18 FDG PET-CT as a staging tool in newly diagnosed advanced stages of ovarian cancer has not yet been fully determined; however, PET-CT provides an accurate assessment of the extent of disease, particularly in areas difficult to assess for metastases by CT and MRI such as the abdomen and pelvis, mediastinum, and supraclavicular region.

4.2. F-18 FDG PET-CT in Recurrent Ovarian Cancer

The majority of patients with advanced stage ovarian cancer will have persistent disease or develop recurrent disease, even after complete clinical response following primary therapy. The treatment of choice for recurrent disease is chemotherapy, although secondary cytoreduction surgery is often employed. Clinical recurrences that take place within 6 months of completion of a platinum-containing regimen are considered platinum-refractory or platinum-resistant recurrences.

Elevated CA-125 tumor marker levels are relatively reliable indicators of the presence of persistent or recurrent disease. However, CA-125 is not elevated in all patients with ovarian cancer, and in others may not adequately reflect the volume of disease. Cross-sectional imaging is used to localize recurrent ovarian cancer. Although ultrasound is extremely useful in the primary evaluation of an adnexal mass, it is not reliable for the evaluation of persistent or recurrent disease as diffuse abdominal and pelvic tumor implants are not well visualized. In a series of 58 ovarian cancer patients who were clinically disease-free by physical examination and CA-125 measurements, CT prior to second-look surgery provided a sensitivity of only 47% for the detection of disease (17). It is particularly difficult to identify small tumor deposits adjacent to the bowel by CT. MRI has a low accuracy for lesions <2 cm and metastatic lesions in the peritoneum and mesentery.

In an early study of 106 F-18 FDG PET examinations done following surgery and chemotherapy, metabolic imaging correctly identified recurrent disease in 73 out of 88 cases and correctly ruled out disease in 15 out of 18 cases (18). Sensitivity and specificity were both 83%. However, the sensitivity was 94% in patients with suspected disease, while only 65% in clinically disease-free patients, likely to be due to the limited ability of PET to detect small peritoneal tumor deposits. On the other hand, sensitivity and specificity were as high as 95% and 87.5%, respectively, when F-18 FDG PET was performed in patients with increased serum CA 125 levels but negative or equivocal conventional imaging results (19).

When comparing CT with PET-CT, the overall sensitivity increased from 72.7 to 92.3% with the addition of PET to CT and the specificity from 75 to 100% (20). Similar results were reported by others with an increase in sensitivity from 70 to 83% and in specificity from 83% to 92% (21) (see Figs. 1 and 2). Thrall et al. (22) found F-18 FDG PET-CT most helpful in the clinical setting of rising CA-125 levels and negative or indeterminate conventional CT imaging. Of note, F-18 FDG PET-CT revealed unsuspected disease either outside the abdomen or in surgically inaccessible areas in 28.6% of the cases, and thus the treatment plan was changed. In another study, F-18 FDG PET combined with contrast-enhanced CT resulted in a change of management in 39% of the cases compared to 12% for contrast-enhanced CT alone, and 2% for F-18 FDG PET combined with a low-dose CT (8). This indicates an advantage of employing contrast-enhanced CT's with F-18 FDG PET-CT, particularly for recurrent ovarian cancer.

4.3. F-18 FDG PET-CT for Monitoring Therapy Response in Ovarian Cancer

Although a substantial number of ovarian cancer patients respond to chemotherapy, there is the possibility to individualize cancer treatment, which requires recruitment of modalities that allow prediction of treatment response early in the course of therapy. Ovarian cancer patients not responding to initial chemotherapy tend to have a poor prognosis.

Prediction of treatment response refers to early identification of treatment effectiveness by comparing the level of radiotracer uptake before and after one cycle of systemic therapy. Assessment of treatment response means evaluation after completion of a full course of treatment. The concept of using F-18 FDG PET for predicting therapeutic response is based on early changes in tumor glucose utilization and the close correlation of changes in F-18 FDG uptake with the effectiveness of treatment (23, 24). Changes in tumor glucose metabolism have been shown to precede changes in tumor size and to accurately reflect treatment response in various types of tumors. At least two sequential F-18 FDG PET scans are currently necessary for prediction of treatment response; one prior to treatment serving as baseline and one after initiation of chemotherapy, for example, after the first or second cycle.

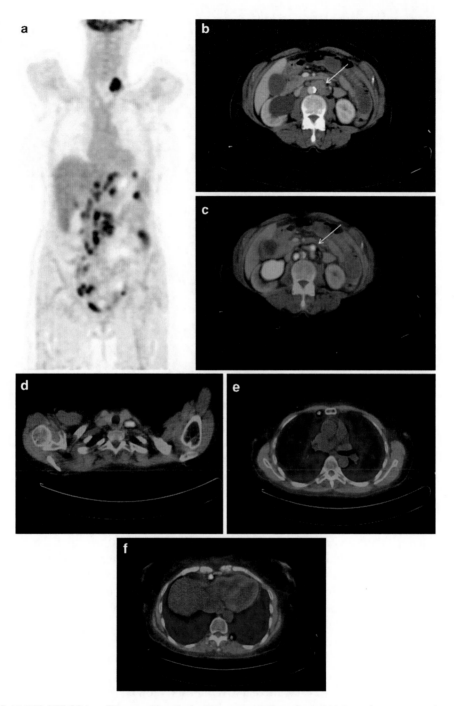

Fig. 1. F-18 FDG-PET-CT in a 67-year-old patient with recurrent disseminated high grade serous ovarian cancer. (**a**) Maximum intensity projection showing widespread metabolically active foci of disease. (**b**) Contrast-enhanced CT showing left para-aortic lymph node enlargement (arrow) and right sided hydronephrosis. (**c**) Fused PET-CT image showing metabolic activity in the enlarged node. (**d**, **e**, **f**) Fused PET-CT image showing activity in left supraclavicular (**d**), right internal mammary (**e**) and paracardial (**f**) lymph nodes.

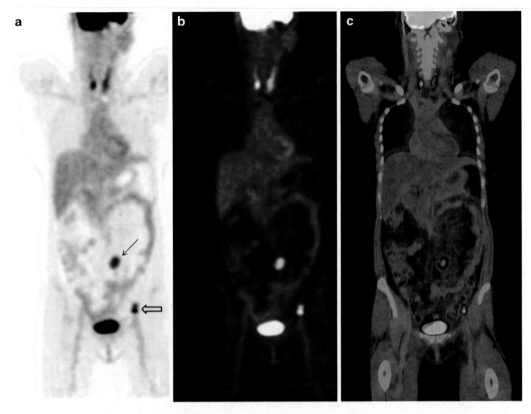

Fig. 2. A 50-year-old patient with history of stage 4 serous papillary ovarian carcinoma, previously treated with neo-adjuvant chemotherapy and debulking surgery shown on follow-up to have a CA 125 of 300. MIP and fused PET-CT images (**a, b, c**) show metabolically active recurrent disease in the left para-aortic (arrow) and left external iliac nodes (open arrow).

In advanced stage ovarian cancer treated with neoadjuvant chemotherapy, the metabolic information from F-18 FDG PET has been found to be superior to clinical response, changes in CA-125, and histopathology (25). A significant correlation was found between F-18 FDG PET metabolic response after the first and third cycle of chemotherapy and overall survival. By using a threshold for decrease in SUV from baseline to 20% after the first cycle, median overall survival was 38 months 3 weeks in meta-bolic responders compared with 23 months 1 week in metabolic nonresponders. At a threshold of 55% decrease in SUV after the third cycle median overall survival was 38 months 9 weeks in met-abolic responders compared with 19 months 7 weeks in nonresponders.

The use of sequential F-18 FDG PET to predict early response to systemic therapy is an appealing application of metabolic imaging. However, further clinical trials would have to validate defined F-18 FDG PET criteria with which treatment can be safely changed.

5. Cervical Cancer

Carcinoma of the cervix is the third most common gynecological malignancy, and during the last 50 years there has been a steep decline in deaths from cervical cancer. The majority of cervical cancers (90%) are squamous cell carcinomas; other histological types include adenocarcinoma, adenosquamous carcinoma, and sarcoma. There were estimated 11,070 new cases and 3,870 deaths from cervical cancer in USA in 2008. The prognosis for patients with cervical cancer is markedly affected by the extent of disease at the time of diagnosis with para-aortic and pelvic lymph node status, tumor size, and patient age being most relevant. Lymphovascular invasion of cervical cancer results in metastatic lymphadenopathy that can extend from internal iliac lymph nodes to retrocrural, mediastinal, and supraclavicular lymph node involvement, particularly when bulky disease in the pelvis is present.

The most important issue in assessing patients presenting with cervical cancer, both clinically and on imaging, is the identification of parametrial spread. Surgery and chemoradiation are equally successful in treating early cervical cancer, but in younger women, surgery is the treatment of choice where there is no parametrial invasion. Patients with more advanced stages of disease are treated with primary radiation therapy with an overall survival advantage for cisplatin-based therapy given concurrently with radiation therapy.

MRI is now the most accurate imaging technique in identifying or excluding parametrial invasion, in defining the true volume of the tumor and its relationship to the remainder of the uterus. MRI has an overall accuracy of 90% in staging cervical cancer, a very high negative predictive value approaching 95% for parametrial invasion, and is accurate to within 5 mm of surgical size in evaluating the size of the tumor.

CT plays a limited role in assessing the primary tumor, as cervical cancer is isodense to normal cervix and it cannot distinguish cancer from surrounding normal cervical tissue. However, contrast-enhanced CT may be useful in staging advanced disease to demonstrate pelvic sidewall extension, ureteral obstruction, advanced bladder and rectal invasion, adenopathy, and extrapelvic spread of disease. CT can also be used to guide biopsy of enlarged nodes, for radiation therapy planning, and to monitor patients for tumor recurrence. Transvaginal ultrasound has limited application in the assessment of cervical cancer.

5.1. F-18 FDG PET-CT in Primary Cervical Cancer

An early F-18 FDG PET study identified all 21 primary tumors when patients voided just prior to imaging but only 16 (76%) of the primary tumors when there was activity in the bladder (26). In a series of 101 patients, F-18 FDG PET detected 99% of primary tumors, using hydration and diuretics, and bladder drainage for reducing urinary activity (31). Similar results were shown in several smaller series (27–29). The level of metabolic activity of primary cervical tumors has been reported to be a predictor of survival (30). However, since the F-18 FDG uptake and subsequent SUV measurements are influenced by many factors such as tumor size, blood glucose level, time interval, and mode of PET data acquisition, as well as PET image reconstruction and analysis, there is currently no clinical use.

Quantitative assessment of tumor volume by F-18 FDG PET was found to correlate with prognosis (26). However, this information was also available by MRI, which in contrast to F-18 FDG PET provides detailed anatomic information that allows assessment of local invasion and radiation treatment planning. While F-18 FDG PET is generally positive in patients with primary cervical cancer, the lack of anatomical information, even in conjunction with CT, limits the clinical utility for initial local assessment of extent of disease.

In 35 patients, Reinhart et al. compared the diagnostic accuracy of MRI with F-18 FDG PET for detection of metastatic lymph node involvement prior to radical hysterectomy and pelvic lymphadenectomy (29). Histology revealed pN0-stage cancer in 24 patients and pN1-stage cancer in 11 patients. F-18 FDG PET had a sensitivity of 91% with a corresponding specificity of 100%, compared to 73% and 83%, respectively for MRI. In another study of 22 patients, F-18 FDG PET found nine unsuspected extrapelvic nodal sites (six para-aortic, two mediastinal and one supraclavicular node) (27). However, F-18 FDG PET missed eight microscopic pelvic nodal metastases. It is important to note that although F-18 FDG PET can visualize increased metabolic activity in normal size tumor-involved lymph nodes, it cannot detect microscopic tumor deposits – a limitation which holds true for any imaging modality.

Narayan et al. assessed whether F-18 FDG PET or MRI could obviate the need for nodal sampling in patients with locally advanced cervical carcinoma prior to radiotherapy (28). Imaging findings were compared to surgical staging in 27 patients. In 24 patients evaluable for pelvic nodal status, sensitivity and specificity for F-18 FDG PET were 83% and 92%, respectively. MRI detected only 6 of 12 (50%) patients with confirmed pelvic nodal disease, all of which were also seen by CT and F-18 FDG PET and had an overall accuracy of 75%.

The lymph node status as assessed by F-18 FDG PET can be a predictor of disease-free survival (31). For pelvic lymph node status, the 2-year disease-free survival was 84% for CT and F-18 FDG PET-negative patients, 64% for CT-negative and F-18 FDG PET-positive patients, and 48% for CT- and F-18 FDG PET-positive patients. The para-aortic lymph node status as assessed by

F-18 FDG PET was the strongest predictor of survival in a multivariate regression analysis. No patients with positive supraclavicular lymph nodes on F-18 FDG PET survived for 2 years (32). The cause-specific survival for patients with FIGO stage IIIb carcinoma was found to be highly dependent upon the extent of lymph node metastasis demonstrated by F-18 FDG PET at the initial presentation. Three-year estimates of cause-specific survival were 73% for patients with no lymph node metastasis, 58% for those with only pelvic lymph node metastasis, 29% for those with pelvic and para-aortic lymph node metastasis, and 0% for those with pelvic and para-aortic and supraclavicular lymph node metastasis (33).

In summary, F-18 FDG PET-CT is a sensitive method of detecting pelvic and para-aortic lymph nodal disease in cervical cancer, and appears to be superior to MRI and CT. Despite the limitations of F-18 FDG PET in identifying small foci of disease, there appears to be an important role for F-18 FDG in the selection of patients for radiation therapy without the need for histological confirmation of lymph node involvement.

5.2. F-18 FDG PET-CT in Recurrent Cervical Cancer

About one-third of patients with cervical cancer experience disease recurrence within 2 years after completion of treatment, and in our experience close to 80% of these recurrences will occur in the first year (see Figs. 3 and 4). Predictors of recurrence are stage and lymph node status at time of disease presentation. The key question on identifying recurrence is whether the mass is suitable for exenteration. CT and MRI are limited in their ability to differentiate recurrent disease from treatment-related fibrosis.

In an early study of 20 patients, F-18 FDG PET accurately detected 18 patients with recurrent disease, 12 patients with local recurrences, 16 patients with pelvic lymph node metastases, 14 patients with para-aortic lymph node metastases, and 4 patients with distant metastases of other sites (34). The sensitivity and specificity of F-18 FDG PET was 86% and 92% for local recurrence and 100% and 94%, respectively for pelvic lymph node metastases. Sensitivity and specificity were 100% for para-aortic lymph node metastases and for distal metastases. In another study of 36 patients, locally or distant recurrent cervical cancer was detected by CT with a sensitivity, specificity, and accuracy of 77.8%, 83.3%, and 80.5%, respectively, while for F-18 FDG PET, the corresponding figures were 100%, 94.4%, and 97.2% (35). In a series of 38 patients, F-18 FDG PET accurately diagnosed recurrent disease in 13 patients with false-negative or equivocal conventional imaging results (27). Ten patients with a negative F-18 FDG PET were still in complete remission after a minimal follow-up time of 12 months.

The largest study reported to date included 249 patients with previously treated cervical cancer (36). Sensitivity and specificity

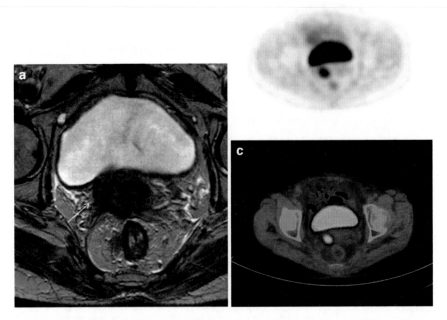

Fig. 3. F-18 FDG PET-CT in a 67-year-old patient with residual cervical cancer following chemoradiotherapy. (**a**) Axial T2 weighted sequence on MRI showing the low signal intensity cervix containing an intermediate – high signal intensity focus (arrow). (**b** and **c**) The PET/CT shows an area of very high activity corresponding to the residual MRI abnormality certifying that this reflects active disease on the MIP (**b**) and fused images (**c**).

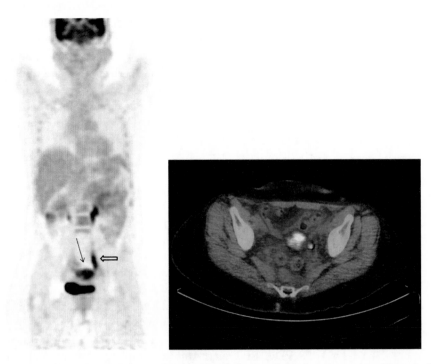

Fig. 4. This 48-year-old patient treated 3 years previously with chemoradiation for a large stage 1B grade 3 cervical cancer, presented with PVB. A biopsy showed the presence of SCC. F-18 FDG-PET-CT showed a large central, metaboli-cally active recurrent mass (arrow). Demonstration of a dilated left ureter down in the level of the recurrence (open arrow) indicated extension to the left pelvic sidewall, contributing to the decision against performing an exenteration.

of F-18 FDG PET for detection of recurrent disease were 90% and 76%, respectively. Sakurai et al. (37) reported an overall accuracy of F-18 FDG PET in the assessment of recurrent cervical carcinoma after radiation therapy of 87%. Sensitivity for extrapelvic lymph node metastases was 100%. F-18 FDG PET seems to be a reliable method for detecting recurrent cervical cancer. The use of combined PET-CT imaging to determine the localization of recurrent tumors may improve the diagnostic utility in the future, and the assessment of patients in whom an exenteration is being contemplated.

5.3. F-18 FDG PET-CT for Monitoring Therapy Response in Cervical Cancer

The role of F-18 FDG PET in therapy monitoring for cervical cancer has yet to be determined. One study looked at the role of F-18 FDG in assessing response to radiotherapy (38). This group followed 20 patients with pre-therapy F-18 FDG PET and compared the results to posttreatment F-18 FDG PET findings. Recurrence was confirmed by biopsy or clinical follow-up. Recurrent disease was accurately identified in three out of five patients. False-positive F-18 FDG PET findings were related to inflammatory changes after radiation therapy. In contrast, Grigsby found that post-radiotherapy F-18 FDG PET provides valuable prognostic information in cervical cancer (39). The timing is of crucial importance and F-18 FDG PET in the latter study was performed 3 months after the completion of therapy. Particularly, complete metabolic response was associated with excellent survival outcome with a 3-year cause-specific survival of 100%. Partial metabolic response was associated with intermediate survival outcome (3-year cause-specific survival 51%) and decreased progression-free survival (3-year progression-free survival 35%). New sites of increased metabolic activity on post-therapy F-18 FDG PET were associated with poor survival outcome (3-year cause-specific survival 17%).

These findings indicate a potentially important role of F-18 FDG PET and PET-CT for assessment of therapy response in recurrent cervical cancer.

6. Vulvar Cancer

Vulvar cancer is a rare cancer of the female genital tract (5%) and is primarily a disease of elderly women. There were estimated 3,460 new cases and 870 deaths from vulvar cancer in USA in 2008. Histopathology is most commonly squamous cell carcinoma (40). Survival depends largely on the pathologic status of the inguinal lymph nodes. In patients with operable disease without nodal involvement, the overall survival rate is 90%; however, in patients with nodal involvement, the 5-year overall survival rate is approximately 50–60%. Overall, about 30% of patients with operable disease have nodal lymph node metastases.

The diagnosis of vulvar carcinoma and the assessment of superficial inguinal nodes are done clinically. MRI is not used for tumor detection but rather for local staging and in order to determine the relationship with adjacent anatomical structures such as the anal sphincter, and to plan surgery. Nodal involvement is a key prognostic determinant.

Inguinal and femoral lymph nodes are first involved followed by pelvic lymph nodes. A 90% survival is expected in patients with negative groin lymph nodes, while there is a 50% survival in patients with positive groin lymph nodes (41). Nodal staging is of high importance for vulvar cancer staging. The MRI criterion for distinguishing between involved and noninvolved lymph nodes is

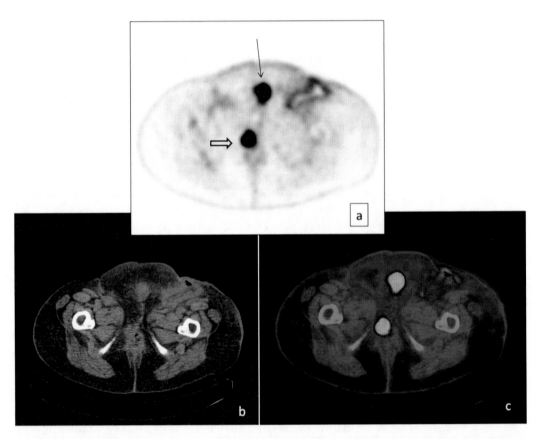

Fig. 5. This 77-year-old patient had previously undergone a wide local excision for a G2 SCC vulvar cancer. She presented with evidence strongly suggestive of recurrent disease in MRI examination. F-18 FDG PET-CT shows metabolically active areas indicative of recurrence to the left of mons pubis (arrow) and to the right side of the introitus (open arrow). The slight F-18 FDG activity in left inguinal region is due to the residual abnormality following drainage of a previously demonstrated lymphocele.

a short axis of 10 mm diameter, which provides a sensitivity of only 40% and a specificity of 97% (42). MRI studies have been performed with USPIO lymph node-specific contrast material to increase sensitivity and specificity (7, 43). Ultrasound with FNAC has also been shown to be promising. However, the most promising diagnostic test for depicting inguinal lymph node status in vulvar cancer appears to be the sentinel node identification using Tc99m colloids (44).

6.1. F-18 FDG PET-CT Imaging of Vulvar Cancer

There are scant studies reporting PET results in vulvar cancer staging (45–47). As described for other gynecological malignancies, F-18 FDG PET-CT can visualize metastatic lymph nodes when they are still of normal size according to conventional cross-sectional imaging, thus showing promising results also for vulvar cancer lymph node staging, which requires further investigation and validation (see Fig. 5).

7. Conclusion

The clinical problems raised in patients presenting with all forms of gynecological malignancy are currently addressed using conventional cross-sectional imaging, usually MRI. In general, F-18 FDG PET-CT has not been shown to have a clinical role in any of these cancers at presentation, although studies are under way to use this form of metabolic imaging to predict prognosis and the response to treatment. In the main, as elsewhere in patients with cancer, the value of PET-CT is in the identification and defining the extent of recurrent disease, in distinguishing between posttreatment fibrosis and recurrence, and possibly in monitoring response to therapy. Further study into an extended role is awaited.

References

1. Fletcher, J.W., Djulbegovic, B., Soares, H.P., Siegel, B.A., Lowe, V.J., Lyman, G.H., et al. (2008) Recommendations on the use of 18F-FDG PET in oncology *J Nucl Med* **49**, 480–508.

2. Weber, W.A., Avril, N., Schwaiger, M. (1999) Relevance of positron emission tomography (PET) in oncology *Strahlenther Onkol* **175**, 356–73.

3. Subhas, N., Patel, P.V., Pannu, H.K., Jacene, H.A., Fishman, E.K., Wahl, R.L. (2005) Imaging of pelvic malignancies with in-line F-18 FDG PET-CT: case examples and common pitfalls of FDG PET *Radiographics* **25**, 1031–43.

4. Short, S., Hoskin, P., Wong, W. (2005) Ovulation and increased FDG uptake on PET: potential for a false-positive result *Clin Nucl Med* **30**, 707.

5. Stahl, A., Weber, W.A., Avril, N., Schwaiger, M. (2000) Effect of N-butylscopolamine on intestinal uptake of fluorine-18-fluorodeoxyglucose in PET imaging of the abdomen *Nuklearmedizin* **39**, 241–5.

6. Barwick, T.D., Rockall, A.G., Barton, D.P., Sohaib, S.A. (2006) Imaging of endometrial adenocarcinoma *Clin Radiol* **61**, 545–5.

7. Rockall, A.G., Sohaib, S.A., Harisinghani, M.G., Babar, S.A., Singh, N., Jeyarajah, A.R.

(2005) Diagnostic performance of nanoparticle-enhanced magnetic resonance imaging in the diagnosis of lymph node metastases in patients with endometrial and cervical cancer *J Clin Oncol* **23**, 2813–21.

8. Kitajima, K., Murakami, K., Yamasaki, E., Domeki, Y., Kaji, Y., Fukasawa, I., et al. (2008) Performance of integrated FDG PET/contrast-enhanced CT in the diagnosis of recurrent ovarian cancer: comparison with integrated FDG-PET/non-contrast-enhanced CT and enhanced CT *Eur J Nucl Med Mol Imaging* **35**, 1439–48.

9. Nayot, D., Kwon, J.S., Carey, M.S., Driedger, A. (2008) Does preoperative positron emission tomography with computed tomography predict nodal status in endometrial cancer? A pilot study *Curr Oncol* **15**, 123–5.

10. Chung, H.H., Kang, W.J., Kim, J.W., Park, N.H., Song, Y.S., Chung, J.K., et al. (2008) The clinical impact of [(18)F]FDG PET-CT for the management of recurrent endometrial cancer: correlation with clinical and histological findings *Eur J Nucl Med Mol Imaging* **35**, 1081–8.

11. Kim, S.K., Kang, K.W., Roh, J.W., Sim, J.S., Lee, E.S., Park, S.Y. (2005) Incidental ovarian 18F-FDG accumulation on PET: correlation with the menstrual cycle *Eur J Nucl Med Mol Imaging* **32**, 757–63.

12. Hubner, K.F., McDonald, T.W., Niethammer, J.G., Smith, G.T., Gould, H.R., Buonocore, E. (1993) Assessment of primary and metastatic ovarian cancer by positron emission tomography (PET) using 2-[18F]deoxyglucose (2-[18F]FDG) *Gynecol Oncol* **51**, 197–204.

13. Kumar, R., Alavi, A. (2004) PET imaging in gynecologic malignancies. *Radiol Clin North Am* **42**, 1155–67, ix.

14. Fenchel, S., Grab, D., Nuessle, K., Kotzerke, J., Rieber, A., Kreienberg, R., et al. (2002) Asymptomatic adnexal masses: correlation of FDG PET and histopathologic findings *Radiology* **223**, 780–8.

15. Yoshida, Y., Kurokawa, T., Kawahara, K., Tsuchida, T., Okazawa, H., Fujibayashi, Y., et al. (2004) Incremental benefits of FDG positron emission tomography over CT alone for the preoperative staging of ovarian cancer *AJR Am J Roentgenol* **182**, 227–33.

16. Kawahara, K., Yoshida, Y., Kurokawa, T., Suzuki, Y., Nagahara, K., Tsuchida, T., et al. (2004) Evaluation of positron emission tomography with tracer 18-fluorodeoxyglucose in addition to magnetic resonance imaging in the diagnosis of ovarian cancer in selected women after ultrasonography *J Comput Assist Tomogr* **28**, 505–16.

17. De Rosa, V., Mangoni di Stefano, M.L., Brunetti, A., Caraco, C., Graziano, R., Gallo, M.S., et al. (1995) Computed tomography and second-look surgery in ovarian cancer patients. Correlation, actual role and limitations of CT scan *Eur J Gynaecol Oncol* **16**, 123–9.

18. Zimny, M., Siggelkow, W., Schroder, W., Nowak, B., Biemann, S., Rath, W., et al. (2001) 2-[Fluorine-18]-fluoro-2-deoxy-d-glucose positron emission tomography in the diagnosis of recurrent ovarian cancer *Gynecol Oncol* **83**, 310–5.

19. Chang, W.C., Hung, Y.C., Kao, C.H., Yen, R.F., Shen, Y.Y., Lin, C.C. (2002) Usefulness of whole body positron emission tomography (PET) with 18F-fluoro-2-deoxyglucose (FDG) to detect recurrent ovarian cancer based on asymptomatically elevated serum levels of tumor marker *Neoplasma* **49**, 329–33.

20. Nakamoto, Y., Saga, T., Ishimori, T., Mamede, M., Togashi, K., Higuchi, T., et al. (2001) Clinical value of positron emission tomography with FDG for recurrent ovarian cancer *AJR Am J Roentgenol* **176**, 1449–54.

21. Picchio, M., Sironi, S., Messa, C., Mangili, G., Landoni, C., Gianolli, L., et al. (2003) Advanced ovarian carcinoma: usefulness of [(18)F]FDG-PET in combination with CT for lesion detection after primary treatment *Q J Nucl Med* **47**, 77–84.

22. Thrall, M.M., DeLoia, J.A., Gallion, H., Avril, N. (2007) Clinical use of combined positron emission tomography and computed tomography (FDG-PET-CT) in recurrent ovarian cancer *Gynecol Oncol* **105**, 17–22.

23. Weber, W.A. (2006) Positron emission tomography as an imaging biomarker *J Clin Oncol* **24**, 3282–92.

24. Avril, N.E., Weber, W.A. (2005) Monitoring response to treatment in patients utilizing PET *Radiol Clin North Am* **43**, 189–204.

25. Avril, N., Sassen, S., Schmalfeldt, B., Naehrig, J., Rutke, S., Weber, W.A. (2005) Prediction of response to neoadjuvant chemotherapy by sequential F-18-fluorodeoxyglucose positron emission tomography in patients with advanced-stage ovarian cancer *J Clin Oncol* **23**, 7445–53.

26. Miller, T.R., Grigsby, P.W. (2002) Measurement of tumor volume by PET to evaluate prognosis in patients with advanced cervical cancer treated by radiation therapy *Int J Radiat Oncol Biol Phys* **53**, 353–9.

27. Belhocine, T., Thille, A., Fridman, V., Albert, A., Seidel, L., Nickers, P., et al. (2002) Contribution of whole-body (18)FDG PET imaging in the management of cervical cancer *Gynecol Oncol* **87**, 90–7.

28. Narayan, K., Hicks, R.J., Jobling, T., Bernshaw, D., McKenzie, A.F. (2001) A comparison of MRI and PET scanning in surgically staged loco-regionally advanced cervical cancer: potential impact on treatment *Int J Gynecol Cancer* **11**, 263–71.

29. Reinhardt, M.J., Ehritt-Braun, C., Vogelgesang, D., Ihling, C., Hogerle, S., Mix, M., et al. (2001) Metastatic lymph nodes in patients with cervical cancer: detection with MR imaging and FDG PET *Radiology* **218**, 776–82.

30. Xue, F., Lin, L.L., Dehdashti, F., Miller, T.R., Siegel, B.A., Grigsby, P.W. (2006) F-18 fluorodeoxyglucose uptake in primary cervical cancer as an indicator of prognosis after radiation therapy *Gynecol Oncol* **101**, 147–51.

31. Grigsby, P.W., Siegel, B.A., Dehdashti, F. (2001) Lymph node staging by positron emission tomography in patients with carcinoma of the cervix *J Clin Oncol* **19**, 3745–9.

32. Tran, B.N., Grigsby, P.W., Dehdashti, F., Herzog, T.J., Siegel, B.A. (2003) Occult supraclavicular lymph node metastasis identified by FDG-PET in patients with carcinoma of the uterine cervix *Gynecol Oncol* **90**, 572–6.

33. Singh, A.K., Grigsby, P.W., Dehdashti, F., Herzog, T.J., Siegel, B.A. (2003) FDG-PET lymph node staging and survival of patients with FIGO stage IIIb cervical carcinoma *Int J Radiat Oncol Biol Phys* **56**, 489–93.

34. Sun, S.S., Chen, T.C., Yen, R.F., Shen, Y.Y., Changlai, S.P., Kao, A. (2001) Value of whole body 18F-fluoro-2-deoxyglucose positron emission tomography in the evaluation of recurrent cervical cancer *Anticancer Res* **21**, 2957–61.

35. Park, D.H., Kim, K.H., Park, S.Y., Lee, B.H., Choi, C.W., Chin, S.Y. (2000) Diagnosis of recurrent uterine cervical cancer: computed tomography versus positron emission tomography *Korean J Radiol* **1**, 51–5.

36. Ryu, S.Y., Kim, M.H., Choi, S.C., Choi, C.W., Lee, K.H. (2003) Detection of early recurrence with 18F-FDG PET in patients with cervical cancer *J Nucl Med* **44**, 347–52.

37. Sakurai, H., Suzuki, Y., Nonaka, T., Ishikawa, H., Shioya, M., Kiyohara, H., et al. (2006) FDG-PET in the detection of recurrence of uterine cervical carcinoma following radiation therapy – tumor volume and FDG uptake value *Gynecol Oncol* **100**, 601–7.

38. Nakamoto, Y., Eisbruch, A., Achtyes, E.D., Sugawara, Y., Reynolds, K.R., Johnston, C.M., et al. (2002) Prognostic value of positron emission tomography using F-18-fluorodeoxyglucose in patients with cervical cancer undergoing radiotherapy *Gynecol Oncol* **84**, 289–95.

39. Grigsby, P.W., Siegel, B.A., Dehdashti, F. (2001) Lymph node staging by positron emission tomography in patients with carcinoma of the cervix *J Clin Oncol* **19**, 3745–9.

40. Griffin, N., Grant, L.A., Sala, E. (2008) Magnetic resonance imaging of vaginal and vulval pathology *Eur Radiol* **18**, 1269–80.

41. Ghurani, G.B., Penalver, M.A. (2001) An update on vulvar cancer *Am J Obstet Gynecol* **185**, 294–9.

42. Sohaib, S.A., Richards, P.S., Ind, T., Jeyarajah, A.R., Shepherd, J.H., Jacobs, I.J., et al. (2002) MR imaging of carcinoma of the vulva *AJR Am J Roentgenol* **178**, 373–7.

43. Harisinghani, M.G., Saini, S., Weissleder, R., Hahn, P.F., Yantiss, R.K., Tempany, C., et al. (1999) MR lymphangiography using ultrasmall superparamagnetic iron oxide in patients with primary abdominal and pelvic malignancies: radiographic-pathologic correlation *AJR Am J Roentgenol* **172**, 1347–51.

44. Selman, T.J., Luesley, D.M., Acheson, N., Khan, K.S., Mann, C.H. (2005) A systematic review of the accuracy of diagnostic tests for inguinal lymph node status in vulvar cancer *Gynecol Oncol* **99**, 206–14.

45. Imperiale, A., Heymann, S., Claria, M., Cimarelli, S., Sellem, D.B., Goetz, C., et al. (2007) F-18 FDG PET-CT in a rare case of Bartholin's gland undifferentiated carcinoma managed with chemoradiation and interstitial brachytherapy *Clin Nucl Med* **32**, 498–500.

46. Husain, A., Akhurst, T., Larson, S., Alektiar, K., Barakat, R.R., Chi, D.S. (2007) A prospective study of the accuracy of 18Fluorodeoxyglucose positron emission tomography (18FDG PET) in identifying sites of metastasis prior to pelvic exenteration *Gynecol Oncol* **106**, 177–80.

47. De Hullu, J.A., Pruim, J., Que, T.H., Aalders, J.G., Boonstra, H., Vaalburg, W., et al. (1999) Noninvasive detection of inguinofemoral lymph node metastases in squamous cell cancer of the vulva by L *Int J Gynecol Cancer* **9**, 141–6.

Chapter 11

Sarcoma

Sarah Ceyssens and Sigrid Stroobants

Abstract

Sarcomas are a diverse group of malignancies originating in the connective tissue. The approach of a patient with a mass suspect for sarcoma starts with performing a biopsy to obtain tissue for evaluation by pathology. The main role of the current imaging modalities, in general, is to recognize patients with typically benign disease, in whom further invasive staging can be omitted, and select patients with a suspected malignancy, who should be referred for biopsy. Since soft tissue sarcoma tends to be large and heterogeneous, there is growing interest in using imaging modalities to guide these biopsies. Together with pathology, imaging modalities are the basis for accurate staging, evaluation of locoregional extent of the primary lesion, screening for occult metastases, evaluation of response to cancer treatment, and the detection of tumor recurrence. In this chapter, an overview is given of the use of 18F-FDG PET in these settings, its strengths as well as its limitations.

Key words: Sarcoma, FDG PET, Biopsy, Staging, Metastases, Response, Recurrence

1. Introduction

Sarcomas are a diverse group of mesodermal malignancies originating in the connective tissue. Based on the Surveillance, Epidemiology, and End Results (SEER) database, approximately 12,700 new cases of sarcoma, both soft tissue and bone, will be diagnosed in 2008 in USA (1). Sarcomas can be grouped into two wide-ranging groups, soft tissue sarcoma (STS) and primary bone sarcoma, each of which different in staging and treatment approaches.

Although each STS has distinctive histological characteristics, on the whole they share many clinical and pathological features and are treated in similar ways. The three most important prognostic variables are grade, size, and location of the primary tumor (2). Surgical resection is the cornerstone of curative treatment.

Malik E. Juweid and Otto S. Hoekstra (eds.), *Positron Emission Tomography*, Methods in Molecular Biology, vol. 727,
DOI 10.1007/978-1-61779-062-1_11, © Springer Science+Business Media, LLC 2011

However, it is still under debate how extensive that surgical excision should be, and whether it should be preceded or followed by chemotherapy and/or irradiation. Since lymphatic spread is uncommon in the natural course of STS with the exception of selected subtypes (angiosarcoma, epithelioid sarcoma, and rhabdomyosarcoma), elective lymphadenectomy seems not to be warranted (3). Nevertheless, in case of tumor spread to regional lymph nodes, some investigators believe that aggressive treatment can bring about long-term survivors (2), while others consider it an expression of disseminated disease, and any treatment of these lymph nodes palliative (4).

The approach to a patient with a sarcoma starts with a biopsy in order to obtain adequate tissue for diagnosis. Tumor grade has significant prognostic and management implications. Since STS tends to be large and heterogeneous, there is a risk of sampling error, with possible underestimation of the actual tumor grade. Therefore, it is plausible that there is a growing interest in using imaging modalities (e.g., biologically most active zone as shown on F-18 FDG PET) to guide biopsies. Together with pathology, imaging modalities are the basis for accurate staging, evaluating locoregional extent of the primary lesion and screening for occult metastases.

2. Characterization and Grading

Soft tissue masses can be benign or malignant, and the ratio of benign to malignant lesions is more than 100:1. Accurate differentiation between a benign or malignant tumor is crucial to define the therapeutic strategy. While resection with a limited margin of normal tissue is generally sufficient for benign tumors, a wide resection is required in STS in order to obtain local control. Besides the confirmation of the diagnosis of a sarcoma, it is essential to know the exact histology and the grading of the primary tumor. Important factors for patient outcome are tumor size, anatomic depth, and the location of the primary lesion (determining the ability to perform a complete resection) as well as histological grade of the tumor (reflecting the biological behavior and, more specifically, the metastatic potential). All these factors are grouped into the AJCC staging system of STS (5).

Conventional radiography still remains the first-line imaging modality in the diagnostic workup of sarcoma in general. Although radiography is used for initial detection and characterization of skeletal sarcoma, its value in the evaluation of STS is rather limited due to its poor resolution compared with cross-sectional modalities. However, it is often used for the assessment of calcifications in the tumoral mass, which can aid the characterization of the tumor (6).

As a result of its high contrast resolution, magnetic resonance imaging (MRI) is excellent to establish the local extent of the mass. On the other hand, there is still much controversy regarding its value in differentiating benign from malignant soft tissue masses. Only few benign soft tissue masses (such as lipomas, hemangiomas, and myositis ossificans) have a typical appearance on MRI and can be correctly diagnosed as benign. Nevertheless, for the lesions whose appearance is nonspecific, MRI seems frequently deficient in its ability to discriminate benign from malignant masses (7). Several imaging parameters are associated with malignancy such as lesion size >5 cm, high signal intensity on T2-weighted images and heterogeneity on T1 images, ill-defined margins, peri-tumoral edema, involvement of adjacent bone, extra-compartmental distribution, and encasement of the neurovascular structures (8, 9). Additionally, most of the STS have a tendency to display a greater rate of contrast enhancement than benign lesions, and tend to exhibit an initial peripheral enhancement, as well as an early onset of contrast enhancement followed by a rapid increase in intensity to an early maximum shifting to a stable level, or a slight decrease in signal intensity, as can be demonstrated on dynamic contrast-enhanced subtraction MRI (CDE-MRI) (10). However, for lesions whose imaging appearance is nonspecific, there is a considerable overlap between benign and malignant lesions in all of these findings, and no single characteristic or a combination of characteristics can reliably differentiate benign from malignant lesions (7, 11). In these cases, a biopsy is still warranted.

Computed tomography (CT) offers a better spatial resolution, but an inferior contrast resolution compared to MRI and may be used for initial staging when MRI is contra-indicated. It can provide a clear anatomic delineation of complex areas (e.g., axial skeleton) not well evaluated by radiography (6).

Several studies have already investigated the role of 2-fluoro-2-deoxy-d-glucose, F18-FDG, positron emission tomography (PET) in the characterization and grading of soft tissue masses. Ioannidis et al. published a meta-analysis on the results of PET in the characterization of 441 soft tissue lesions (227 malignant and 214 benign) (12). For diagnosis of malignancy, sensitivity and specificity were 92% and 73% for visual analysis, 87% and 79% for standardized uptake value (SUV) > 2.0, and 70% and 87% for SUV > 3.0. False-negative results were seen in low-grade sarcomas, while false-positive findings were seen in inflammatory lesions or lesions with high cellularity (e.g., giant cell tumor). F-18 FDG uptake correlated with the histological grade of the tumor, with a significant higher uptake in intermediate/high-grade tumors compared to that in low-grade tumors, although there was some overlap. No significant difference was seen between the low-grade malignant and benign lesions. Nearly all intermediate/ high-grade lesions were accurately diagnosed on the basis of qualitative interpretation, and 89% of them had SUV ≥ 2.0, in contrast to only 33% of the low-grade tumors and 19% of the benign masses. Taking into account the uptake pattern (hetero-geneous in high-grade lesions vs. homogeneous in low-grade sarcoma) (13, 14) or increasing the interval between F-18 FDG injection and scanning from 1 to 4 h (where malignant lesions tend to show a steady increase in F-18 FDG uptake with a peak activity reached at approximately 4 h, whereas benign lesions peak already within 30 min followed by a washout) (15, 16) can improve the discrimination between intermediate/high-grade lesions and low-grade/benign lesions. However, F-18 FDG PET may not always offer adequate discrimination between low-grade tumors and benign lesions.

Folpe et al. found in addition to pathological grade, a strong correlation between SUV and Ki-67 labeling index, mitotic figure counts and P53 overexpression, factors known to have prognostic value (17). The impact of pretreatment SUV on final outcome has been investigated by the same group. A SUV > 6.0 was shown to correlate with a significant shorter disease-free survival ($p < 0.001$) and overall survival (OS) ($p < 0.003$). After adjustment for standard clinical prognostic factors such as histology, grade, age, and sex, multivariable analysis pointed out that SUV was an independent predictor of survival and disease progression (18). Also, the heterogeneity in tissue uptake of F-18 FDG was found to be a strong predictor of final outcome (19).

Another advantage of F-18 FDG PET is the information on biological activity of the tumoral parts. Since STS tends to be large and heterogeneous, there is a risk of sampling error when taking a biopsy. The most commonly used tracer in PET, F-18 FDG, is a glucose analog that accumulates in the cells in propor-tion to the rate of glucose metabolism. By identifying the most metabolically active portion of a tumor mass, nuclear medicine techniques can guide biopsy to a site most likely to contain tumor tissue of the highest grade present.

In conclusion, the approach of a patient with a mass suspect for sarcoma remains performing a biopsy to obtain tissue for eval-uation by pathology. The main role of the current imaging modal-ities is to recognize patients with typically benign disease, in whom further invasive staging can be omitted, and select those patients with a suspected malignancy, who should be referred for biopsy (7). Since STS tend to be large and heterogeneous, there is a risk of sampling error, and imaging can help to guide the biopsy toward the most aggressive zone.

3. Evaluation of Disease Extent

STSs originate in the mesenchymal tissues of muscles, fat, blood vessels, nerves, tendons, and synovial tissues. As such, MRI represents an ideal imaging modality to evaluate the anatomical compartments involved by the primary tumor and its relation to adjacent structures, in particular adjacent bone and neurovascular structures.

Literature data on the use of F-18 FDG PET for distant staging in STS is limited. Although most studies focus on the additional value of F-18 FDG PET to conventional imaging (CI), only few reports compare the diagnostic performance of both modalities (20–22). Völker et al. evaluated the impact of F-18 FDG PET for initial staging and therapy planning in 46 pediatric patients. Concerning the detection of lymph node metastases, a superior sensitivity of F-18 FDG PET (95% lesion-based analysis vs. 88% patient-based analysis) was found compared to that of CI (25% lesion-based analysis vs. 62% patient-based analysis) (20). Similar results were found for F-18 FDG PET-CT versus CI in a study of Tateishi et al. on 117 patients (sensitivity of 88% for N-staging PET-CT vs. 53% for CI) (22). The power of F-18 FDG PET in the assessment of nodal involvement resides in its ability to depict tumoral involvement in normal-sized nodes and to exclude disease in reactively enlarged nodes (23). Even so, in view of the fact that lymphatic spread is uncommon in the natural course of STS, the additional value will be minor. Only in case of a higher incidence of lymphatic spread (angiosarcoma, epithelioid sarcoma, and rhabdomyosarcoma), F-18 FDG PET can be useful.

The most common site for distant metastases is the lungs. In the above mentioned study of Völker et al. (22), the sensitivity of CI for lung metastases was significantly higher (100%) than the sensitivity of F-18 FDG PET (25%). Breathing motion and partial volume effect can give rise to false-negative results on F-18 FDG PET. High-resolution CT is the imaging modality of preference to detect lung metastases, although it was shown to be only cost-effective in patients with high-grade T2-lesions or T2 extremity lesions (24).

Liver metastases can be detected as the first sign of dissemination in primary intra-abdominal STS, and are usually visualized on the abdominal CT performed to evaluate the primary mass. No specific literature is yet available on the accuracy of PET for the detection of liver metastases in STS. Delbeke et al. (25) evaluated the value of F-18 FDG PET for the detection of liver metastases in different kinds of tumors, including a few sarcomas. F-18 FDG PET had a sensitivity of 100%, but all lesions were larger than 1 cm. Similar to lung metastases, sensitivity for the detection of liver metastases depends on tumor size, with a sensitivity of 85% for lesions greater than 1 cm compared to only 25% for lesions less than 1 cm (26).

When screening patients for bone metastases, one should best consider the type of the primary lesion: where the sensitivity of F-18 FDG PET and bone scanning are comparable in patients with osteosarcoma (F-18 FDG PET 90%, CIM including bone scanning 90%, bone scan alone 81%), F-18 FDG PET clearly is superior in case of Ewing sarcoma (EWS) (sensitivity PET 89% vs. 57% for CI). The basis for the latter could be found in an infiltration of the bone marrow rather than the mineralized bone by EWS, and by a dominating osteoclastic activity (20). Since tumor spread is rare in STS, the use of bone scintigraphy seems only to be encouraged in symptomatic patients (27).

The main power of F-18 FDG PET(-CT) lies in the ability to screen the entire patient for distant tumor deposits without significantly increasing the radiation burden. The key role of F-18 FDG PET-CT largely lies in detecting metastases at unexpected sites, outside the standard field of view of CT and MRI, and in the exclusion of disease in equivocal results on CI.

4. Response Evaluation

Traditionally, response to cancer treatment in solid tumors by anatomic imaging techniques is defined as a significant decrease in tumor dimensions. The response evaluation criteria in solid tumors (RECIST) response criteria (version 1.0) describe partial response as a decrease of at least 30% in the sum of diameters of the target lesions. However, these criteria are not always capable to distinguish responders from nonresponders to neoadjuvant therapy (28–31). There are important shortcomings in the evaluation of tumor response by volume changes, especially in STS. Accurate measurement of tumor dimensions can be particularly difficult in ill-defined lesions such as bone, bowel, and peritoneal lesions. Since tumor tissue can be substituted by necrotic or fibrotic tissue as an effect of therapy, a reduction in viable tumor cell fraction does not always come into view as a volume reduction. In addition, volume changes are rather late events. In fact, changes measured by computer tomography are rarely significant when performed earlier than 2–3 months after the start of treatment. As a consequence of this, patients can be unnecessarily exposed to ineffective, toxic, or expensive treatments during a prolonged period. In the neoadjuvant setting, it can even reduce the chance of a curative resection by postponing surgery. Finally, the new anti-vascular and cytostatic agents aim at a stabilization of tumor growth rather than tumor shrinkage. Consequently, no major volume changes are to be expected. Recently the RECIST-criteria have been revised (version 1.1) (32) to overcome these limitations, but clinical validation of these newer approaches is still required.

Over the last years, promising results were accomplished with F-18 FDG PET in the evaluation of treatment efficacy. Several studies have shown a good correlation between an early and significant decline in metabolic activity and response to therapy in various tumors, such as lymphoma, esophageal, stomach, colorectal, head and neck, and non-small cell lung cancers, as well as a good correlation between the early decrease in F-18 FDG uptake and patient outcome (33). Because F-18 FDG uptake is related to the number of viable cells and necrotic or fibrotic tissue is usually not F-18 FDG avid, accurate differentiation between responders and nonresponders seems to be possible early after the start of treatment (34, 35).

Evilevich et al. analyzed changes in F-18 FDG uptake and size from a PET-CT scan before and after neoadjuvant chemotherapy in high-grade soft tissue sarcoma, and compared their accuracy for the assessment of histopathological response. Quantitative F-18 FDG PET outperforms the size-based criteria to distinguish responders from nonresponders, defined as ≥95% pathological necrosis on the resected tumor. Using a decrease in tracer uptake of 60% resulted in a sensitivity of 100% and specificity of 71%, whereas a sensitivity of 25% and specificity of 100% was seen for RECIST (36). Similar results were found by Schuetzeo et al. Forty-six patients with high-grade localized sarcomas were evaluated with F-18 FDG PET before and after neoadjuvant chemotherapy. A significant correlation was found between the change in the maximum standardized uptake value (SUV_{max}) and the amount of residual viable tumor in the resected specimens. A SUV_{max} higher than 6 and less than 40% decrease in F-18 FDG uptake were associated with a high risk for systemic disease recurrence. Patients with a ≥40% decline in SUV_{max} after chemotherapy were at a significantly lower risk for recurrent disease and death after complete resection and adjuvant radiotherapy (37).

Changes in F-18 FDG uptake to neoadjuvant chemotherapy have also been investigated in bone sarcoma. In a report of Schulte, 27 patients with osteosarcoma were examined. Tumor-to-background ratio (TBR) of F-18 FDG uptake instead of SUV was determined on F-18 FDG PET, before and after neoadjuvant chemotherapy. With a cutoff level of 0.6 for TBR, all responders and eight out of ten nonresponders could be identified (38). Analogous results were found in another study on 17 patients with primary bone tumors (11 osteosarcomas and 6 Ewing's sarcomas). All good responders had a ≥30% decline in TBR, whereas in patients with poor response, a decrease of less than 30% or even an increase in TBR was seen (39). According to a report of

Ye et al., TBR correlated better with response to neoadjuvant chemotherapy, than did SUV_{max} (40).

F-18 FDG PET performed after neoadjuvant chemotherapy correlates well with histological response of Ewing's sarcoma. Standardized uptake value after therapy was associated with outcome. Patients with a SUV_{max} less than 2.5 after chemotherapy had a significantly higher probability of a 4-year progression-free survival than patients with a $SUV_{max}{}^3 2.5$ (72% (SUV_{max} <2.5) respectively 27% (SUV_{max} ≥2.5) for all patients and 80% (SUV_{max} <2.5) respectively 33% (SUV_{max} ≥ 2.5) for patients with localized disease at diagnosis) (41).

Early clinical trials in gastrointestinal stromal tumors (GISTs) treated with the molecular targeted therapy Imatinib, a receptor tyrosine kinase inhibitor of c-KIT, show a significant improvement in progression-free survival and OS compared to historical controls (41, 42). Subjective tumor response already occurs within a few days of treatment in responding patients, but objective tumor shrinkage is minimal and tends to occur only after several weeks or months. Although patients in partial remission according to RECIST clearly benefit from Imatinib in terms of survival, Imatinib is also beneficial in a substantial subset of patients with stable disease, and even in a subset of patients who undergo an initial increase in tumor volume, which is probably due to intratumoral hemorrhage, edema, or development of myxoid degeneration (43). Metabolic imaging with F-18 FDG PET has proven to be highly sensitive in detecting early tumor response to Imatinib treatment and precedes tumor shrinkage by several weeks to months. A complete normalization of all hypermetabolic foci is seen within a week of treatment and is predictive of favorable outcome (44, 45). However, since PET is costly and still limited in availability, CT criteria other than standard RECIST were also evaluated. Since a cystic-like appearance with "near"-fluid attenuation and loss of contrast-enhancement is the typical appearance of responding lesion on CT, the use of Hounsfield Unit (HU) measurements is proposed as an alternative response marker (46). Using the CHOI criteria, where response is defined as a reduction in HU ≥ 15% and/or a volume reduction ≥10%, the prognostic value of these new CT response criteria is similar to the one obtained with F-18 FDG PET (47). Once GISTs have responded to therapy, careful follow-up with imaging is necessary to detect secondary resistance related to newly acquired KIT mutations. Progressive disease is not only seen as an increase in size of a pre-existing lesion or the appearance of a new metastasis, but also as the development of an intratumoral nodule and/or an increase in "solid" tissue, in the background of a hypodense lesion. Each treated lesion should therefore be carefully analyzed for any new intratumoral changes. Whenever a CT finding is inconsistent with the clinical picture or is inconclusive, F-18 FDG PET may be indicated for further evaluation (48).

5. Detection of Recurrence

The majority of recurrences develop within 2 years of resection of the primary tumor, although there is clinical evidence suggesting that late recurrence (>5 years after treatment) is not uncommon (49, 50). Positive surgical margins are the main predictors for local relapse, whereas grade, size, and tumor-node-metastasis stage predict the development of distant metastases and OS (51). Early detection and treatment of local recurrence are desirable if surgical control is to be achieved, even if this does not necessarily influence the final outcome of the patient.

Currently, MRI is still the technique of choice for the evaluation of suspected local recurrence in the extremities. Both radiotherapy and chemotherapy can induce changes (such as soft tissue trabeculation, increased fatty marrow, focal marrow abnormalities, and hemorrhage), complicating the interpretation of posttreatment MR images. However, by using an organized systematic approach and by following some algorithms, this challenge should be minimized (52, 53).

Several studies have evaluated the performance of F-18 FDG PET in the detection of local recurrence. In the abovementioned meta-analysis of Ioannidis et al., similar diagnostic performance was found for F-18 FDG PET in primary and recurrent lesions (12). Since anatomical imaging techniques such as MRI and CT and F-18 FDG PET are rarely carried out in parallel, only few studies address their comparative performance. In a study by Lucas et al., the performance of F-18 FDG PET was compared to the performance of MRI in 60 patients. It demonstrated both a lower sensitivity (76% vs. 88%) and specificity (94% vs. 96%) for F-18 FDG PET (13).

6. Conclusion

The approach of a patient with a mass suspect for sarcoma starts with a biopsy to confirm the diagnosis of a sarcoma and to determine exact histology and grading of the primary tumor. First, since no imaging technique can surpass pathology in this purpose, the main role of the current imaging modalities is to recognize patients with typically benign lesions, in whom further invasive staging can be omitted, and to select patients with a suspected malignancy, who should be referred for biopsy. Second, since STS tends to be large and heterogeneous, imaging can help to guide the biopsy toward the most aggressive zone.

Conventional radiography, MRI, and CT still remain the first-line imaging modalities in the diagnostic workup of sarcoma in general. Because of its limited spatial resolution and lack of anatomical detail, F-18 FDG PET is of no use in the evaluation of the local extent of the tumor.

However, a fascinating development is the introduction of combined PET-CT-machines. Since this technique unites the anatomical information of the CT and the metabolic information of the PET, it improves diagnostic accuracy, provides surgery and radiation therapy planning, and can guide biopsies by merging the anatomic and metabolic information in one single procedure. Still, studies are required to evaluate the impact of combining these imaging techniques on the overall diagnostic performance in sarcoma.

With regard to the detection of metastases, one must take into account the limitations of F-18 FDG PET. Since breathing motion and partial volume effect can result in false-negative results on F-18 FDG PET, high-resolution CT remains mandatory for the detection of lung metastases of STS of the extremities and head and neck region. Liver metastases can be detected as the first sign of dissemination in primary intra-abdominal STS and are usually visualized on the abdominal CT performed to evaluate the primary mass. Although no specific data are yet available on the accuracy of PET for the detection of liver metastases in STS, the experience in other tumor types showed no significant benefit of PET over spiral CT for the detection of liver metastasis. Concerning bone metastases, F-18 FDG PET clearly is superior in case of EWS compared to CI, although the sensitivity of the former technique is similar to that of bone scanning in case of an osteosarcoma. The key role of F-18 FDG PET-CT is by large an additional role, situated in the detection of metastases at unexpected sites, outside the standard field of view of CT and MRI, and in the exclusion of disease in equivocal results on CI. Furthermore, the amount of F-18 FDG uptake, although correlated with histological grade, seems to be an independent predictor for overall and disease-free survival.

References

1. Source: http://seer.cancer.gov/csr/1975-2005/results_merged/ sect_01_overview.pdf.

2. Pisters, P.W., Leung, D.H., Woodruff, J., Shi, W., Brennan, M.F. (1996) Analysis of prognostic factors in 1041 patients with localized soft tissue sarcomas of the extremities *J Clin Oncol* **14**, 1679–89.

3. Fong, Y., Coit, D.G., Woodruff, J.M., Brennan, M.F. (1993) Lymph node metastases from soft tissue sarcoma in adults. Analysis of data from a prospective database of 1772 sarcoma patients. *Ann Surg* **217**, 72–217.

4. Gaskeer, H.A., Albus-Lutter, C.E., Gortzak, E., Zoetmulder, F.A. (1988) Regional lymph node metastases in patients with soft tissue sarcomas of the extremities: what are the therapeutic consequences *Eur J Surg Oncol* **14**, 151–6.

5. Greene, F.L., Page, D., Fleming, I., eds. (2002) AJCC Cancer Staging Manual, 6th ed. New York: Springer-Verlag.

6. Fadul, D., Fayad, L.M. (2008) Advanced modalities for the imaging of sarcoma *Surg Clin North Ann* **88**, 521–37.

7. Moulton, J.S., Blebea, J.S., Dunco, D.M., Braley, S.E., Biset, G.S., III, Emery, K.H. (1995) MR imaging of soft-tissue masses: diagnostic efficacy and value of distinguishing between benign and malignant lesions *AJR Am J Roentgenol* **164**, 1191–9.

8. De Schepper, A.M., De Bueckeleer, L., Vandevenne, J., Somville, J. (2000) Magnetic resonance imaging of soft tissue tumors *Eur Radiol* **10**, 213–23.

9. Kransdorf, M.J., Murphey, M.D. (2000) Radiologic evaluation of soft-tissue masses: a current perspective *AJR Am J Roentgenol* **175**, 575–87.

10. van der Woude, H.J., Verstraete, K.L., Hogendoorn, P.C., Taminiau, A.H., Hermans, J., Bloem, J.L. (1998) Musculoskeletal tumors: does fast dynamic contrast-enhanced subtraction MR imagining contribute to the characterization *Radiology* **208**, 821–8.

11. Mayerhoefer, M.E., Breitenseher, M., Amann, G., Dominikus, M. (2008) Are signal intensity and homogeneity useful parameters for distinguishing between benign and malignant soft tissue masses on MR images? Objective evaluation by means of texture analysis *Magn Reson Imaging* **26(9)**, 1316–22.

12. Ioannidis, J.P., Lau, J. (2003) 18F-FDG PET for the diagnosis and grading of soft-tissue sarcoma: a meta-analysis *J Nucl Med* **44**, 717–24.

13. Lucas, J.D., O'Doherty, M.J., Cronin, B.F., et al. (1999) Prospective evaluation of soft-tissue masses and sarcomas using fluorodeoxyglucose positron emission tomography *Br J Surg* **86**, 550–6.

14. Schulte, M., Brecht-Krauss, D., Heymer, B., et al. (1999) Fluorodeoxyglucose positron emission tomography of soft tissue tumours: is a non-invasive determination of biological activity possible *Eur J Nucl Med* **26**, 599–605.

15. Lodge, M.A., Lucas, J.D., Marsden, P.K., Cronin, B.F., O'Doherty, M.J., Smith, M.A. (1999) A PET study of 18FDG uptake in soft tissue masses *Eur J Nucl Med* **26**, 22–30.

16. Ferner, R.E., Lucas, J.D., O'Doherty, M.J, et al. (2000) Evaluation of (18)fluorodeoxyglucose positron emission tomography ((18)FDG PET) in the detection of malignant peripheral nerve sheath tumours arising from within plexiform neurofibromas in neurofibromatosis 1 *J Neurol Neurosurg Psychiatry* **68**, 353–7.

17. Folpe, A.L., Lyles, R.H., Sprouse, J.T., Conrad, E.U. III, Eary, J.F. (2000) (F-18) fluorodeoxyglucose positron emission tomography as a predictor of pathologic grade and other prognostic variables in bone and soft tissue sarcoma *Clin Cancer Res* **6**, 1279–87.

18. Eary, J.F., O'Sullivan, F., Powitan, Y., et al. (2002) Sarcoma tumor FDG uptake measured by PET and patient outcome: a retrospective analysis *Eur J Nucl Med Mol Imaging* **29**, 1149–54.

19. Eary, J.F., O'Sullivan, F., O'Sullivan, J., Conrad, E.U. (2008) Spatial heterogeneity in sarcoma 18F-FDG uptake as predictor of patient outcome *J Nucl Med* **49**, 1973–9.

20. Völker, T., Denecke, T., Steffen, I., et al. (2007) Positron emission tomography for staging of pediatric sarcoma patients: results of a prospective multicenter trial *J Clin Oncol* **25**, 5435–41.

21. Tateishi, U., Hosono, A., Makimoto, A., et al. (2007) Accuracy of 18F fluorodeoxyglucose positron emission tomography/computed tomography in staging of pediatric sarcomas *J Pediatr Hematol Oncol* **29**, 608–12.

22. Tateishi, U., Yamaguchi, U., Seki, K., Terauchi, T., Arai, Y., Kim, E.E. (2007) Bone and soft-tissue sarcoma: perspective staging with fluorine 18 fluorodeoxyglucose PET/CT and conventional imaging *Radiology* **245**, 839–47.

23. Dwamena, B.A., Sonnad, S.S., Angobaldo, J.O., Wahl, R.L. (1999) Metastases Fromm non-small cell lung cáncer: mediastinal staging in the 1990s – meta-analytic comparison of PET and CT *Radiology* **213**, 530–6.

24. Porter, G.A., Cantor, S.B., Ahmad, S.A., et al. (2002) Cost-effectiveness of staging computed tomography of the chest in patients with T2 soft tissue sarcomas *Cancer* **94**, 197–204.

25. Delbeke, D., Martin, W.H., Sandler, M.P., Chapman, W.C., Wright, J.K. Jr., Pinson, C.W. (1998) Evaluation of benign vs. malignant hepatic lesions with positron emission tomography *Arch Surg* **133**, 510–5.

26. Fong, Y., Saldinger, P.F., Akhurst, T., et al. (1999) Utility of 18F-FDG positron emission tomography scanning on selection of patients for resection of hepatic colorectal metastases *Ann J Surg* **178**, 282–7.

27. Jager, P.L., Hoekstra, H.J., Leeuw, J., van Der Graaf, W.T., de Vries, E.G., Piers, R. (2000) Routine bone scintigraphy in primary staging of soft tissue sarcomas: is it worthwhile *Cancer* **89**, 1726–31.

28. Stacchiotti, S., Collini, P., Messina, A., et al. (2009) High-grade soft-tissue sarcomas: tumor response assessment – pilot study to assess the correlation between radiologic and pathologic response by using RECIST and Choi criteria *Radiology* **251**, 447–56.

29. Evilevitch, V., Weber, W.A., Tap, W.D. (2008) Reduction of glucose metabolic activity is

more accurate than change in size in predicting histopathologic response to neoadjuvant therapy in high-grade soft-tissue sarcomas *Clin Cancer Res* **14**, 715–20.

30. Ceresoli, G.L., Chiti, A., Zucali, P.A., et al. (2007) Assessment of tumor response in malignant pleural mesothelioma. *Cancer Treat Rev* **33**, 533–41.

31. Goffin, J., Baral, S., Tu, D., Nomikos, D., Seymour, L. (2005) Objective responses in patients with malignant melanoma or renal cell cancer in early clinical studies do not predict regulatory approval *Clin Cancer Res* **11**, 5928–34.

32. Eisenhauer, E.A., Therasse, P., Bogaerts, J., et al. (2009) New response evaluation criteria in solid tumours: revised RECIST guideline (version 1.1) *Eur J Cancer* **45**, 228–47.

33. Juweid, M.E., Cheson, B.D. (2006) Positron emission tomography and assessment of cancer therapy *N Engl J Med* **354**, 496–507.

34. Spaepen, K., Stroobants, S., Dupont, P., et al. (2001) Prognostic value of positron emission tomography (PET) with fluorine-18 fluorodeoxyglucose ([18F]FDG) after first line chemotherapy in non-Hodgkin's lymphoma: is [18F]FDG PET a valid alternative to conventional diagnostic methods *J Clin Oncol* **19**, 414–9.

35. Canellos, G.P. (1988) Residual mass in lymphoma may not be residual disease. *J Clin Oncol* **6**, 931–3.

36. Evilevitch, V., Weber, W.A., Tap, W.D., et al. (2008) Reduction of glucose metabolic activity is more accurate than change in size of predicting histopathologic response to neoadjuvant therapy in high-grade soft-tissue sarcomas *Clin Cancer Res* **14**, 715–20.

37. Scheutze, S.M., Rubin, B.P., Vernon, C., et al. (2005) Use of positron emission tomography in localized extremity soft tissue sarcoma treated with neoadjuvant chemotherapy *Cancer* **103**, 339–48.

38. Schulte, M., Brecht-Krauss, D., Werner, M., et al. (1999) Evaluation of neoadjuvant therapy response of oseogenic sarcoma using FDG PET *J Nucl Med* **40**, 1637–43.

39. Franzius, C., Sciuk, J., Brinkschmidt, C., Jürgens, H., Schober, O. (2000) Evaluation of chemotherapy response in primary bone tumors with F-18 FDG positron emission tomography compared with histologically assessed tumor necrosis *Clin Nucl Med* **25**, 874–81.

40. Ye, Z., Zhu, J., Tian, M., et al. (2008) Response of osteogenic sarcoma to neoadjuvant

therapy: evaluated by 18F-FDG-PET *Ann Nucl Med* **22**, 475–80.

41. Demetri, G.D., von Mehren, M., Blanke, C.D., et al. (2002) Efficacy and safety of imatinib mesylate in advanced gastrointestinal stromal tumors. *N Eng J Med* **347**, 472–80.

42. van Oosterom, A.T., Judson, I., Verweij, J., et al. (2001) European Organization for Research and Treatment of Cancer Soft Tissue and Bone Sarcoma Group. Safety and efficacy of imatinib (ST1571) in metastatic gastrointestinal stromal tumors: a phase I study *Lancet* **358**, 1421–3.

43. Blay, J.Y., Bonvalot, S., Casali, P., et al. (2005). GIST consensus meeting panelists Consensus meeting for the management of gastrointestinal stromal tumors Report of the GIST Consensus Conference of 20–21 March 2004, under the auspices of ESMO *Ann Oncol* **16**, 566–78.

44. Van den Abbeele, A.D., Badawi, R.D. (2002) Use of positron emission tomography in oncology and its potential role to assess response to imatinib mesylate therapy in gastrointestinal stromal tumors (GISTs) *Eur J Cancer* **38**, S60–5.

45. Stroobants, S., Goeminne, J., Seegers, M., et al. (2003) 18 FDG positron emission tomography for the early prediction of response in advanced soft tissue sarcoma treated with imatinib mesylate (Glivec) *Eur J Cancer* **39**, 2012–20.

46. Antoch, G., Kanja, J., Bauer, S., et al. (2004) Comparison of PET, CT, and dual-modality PET/CT imaging for monitoring of imatinib (ST1571) therapy in patients with gastrointestinal stromal tumors *J Nucl Med* **45**, 357–65.

47. Choi, H., Charnsangavej, C., Faria, S.C., et al. (2007) Correlation of computed tomography and positron emission tomography in patients with metastatic gastrointestinal stromal tumor treated at a single institution with imatinib mesylate: proposal of new computed tomography response criteria. *J Clin Oncol* **25**, 1753–9.

48. Demetri, G.D., Benjamin, R.S., Blanke, C.D., et al. (2007) NCCN Task Force Report: management of patients with gastrointestinal stromal tumor (GIST) – update of the NCCN clinical practice guidelines *J Natl Compr Canc Netw* **5(2)**, S1–29.

49. Lewis, J.J., Leung, D., Casper, E.S., Woodruff, J., Hajdu, S.I., Brennan, M.F. (1999) Multifactorial analysis of long-term follow-up (more than 5 years) of primary extremity sarcoma *Arch Surg* **134**, 190–4.

50. Pisters, P.W., Pollock, R.E., Lewis, V.O., et al. (2007) Long-term results of prospective trial of surgery alone with selective use of radiation for patients with T1 extremity and trunk soft tissue sarcomas *Ann Surg* **246**, 675–81.

51. Stefanovski, P.D., Bidoli, E., De Paoli, A., et al. (2002) Prognostic factors in soft tissue sarcomas: a study of 395 patients *Eur J Surg Oncol* **28**, 153–64.

52. Garner, H.W., Kransdorf, M.J., Bancroft, L.W., Peterson, J.J., Berquist, T.H., Murphey, M.D. (2009) Benign and malignant soft-tissue tumors: posttreatment MR imaging *Radiographics* **29**, 119–34.

53. Vanel, D., Shapeero, L.G., Tardivon, A., Western, A., Guinebretiere, J.M. (1998) Dynamic contrast-enhanced MRI with subtraction of aggressive soft tissue tumors after resection *Skeletal Radiol* **27**, 505–10.

Chapter 12

PET and PET/CT in the Management of Thyroid Cancer

Sandip Basu, Muammer Urhan, Joshua Rosenbaum, and Abass Alavi

Abstract

The introduction of PET(-CT) has brought about a major paradigm shift in the management of thyroid carcinoma, especially from the diagnostic standpoint. From the viewpoint of patient management, the areas where it has made significant impact include the following: (1) the detection of disease focus in patients with differentiated thyroid carcinoma with elevated Tg levels and negative radioiodine scan. When localized disease is identified with F-18 FDG–PET-CT, surgery or focused radiotherapy could be utilized to eradicate the tumor; (2) the localization of disease in patients of MTC with elevated serum calcitonin levels; (3) the detection of unsuspected focal F-18 FDG uptake in the thyroid in patients undergoing whole body F-18 FDG PET for a different indication. This would prompt a workup to rule out thyroid carcinoma. The use of I-124 is evolving at this time and has been of great promise with regard to (a) its better efficacy of lesion detection and (b) the ability to provide lesion-specific dosimetry. In addition, F-18 FDG PET appears to be of potential value in patients with thyroid lymphoma in making the initial diagnosis, monitoring therapeutic response, and assessing for residual disease and/or recurrence.

Key words: PET, PET-CT, Thyroid carcinoma, Differentiated thyroid carcinoma, Medullary carcinoma of thyroid, Thyroid lymphoma

1. PET(-CT) in Thyroid Carcinoma: What are the Oncologists' Needs?

At present, a few definitive and unresolved issues exist with regard to the clinical management of patients with thyroid carcinoma. Detection and management of disease in patients with differentiated thyroid carcinoma (DTC) who have elevated Tg levels and negative radioiodine scan continues to be difficult. A sizeable proportion of these patients with noniodine avid disease do not demonstrate evidence of disease with anatomical modalities as well. Neck ultrasound can often be inconclusive and nonspecific in discriminating between malignant foci and nonspecific changes in the postsurgical neck region. It is in these patients that F-18 FDG PET-CT can be of pivotal importance. The ability to detect thyroid

Malik E. Juweid and Otto S. Hoekstra (eds.), *Positron Emission Tomography*, Methods in Molecular Biology, vol. 727,
DOI 10.1007/978-1-61779-062-1_12, © Springer Science+Business Media, LLC 2011

cancer recurrence early is critically important, since the management is considerably improved when localized disease is identified with F-18 FDG PET-CT, where early surgery or focused radiotherapy could be utilized to eradicate the tumor.

A similar situation is encountered in patients with medullary thyroid carcinoma (MTC), where precise localization of recurrent or metastatic disease is important in the management of patients with elevated serum calcitonin levels. This is a major challenge because frequently the disease focus remains undetected even after various structural and functional modalities have been used. In combination with anatomic imaging, PET imaging has the potential to become the most preferred procedure for localizing disease in this group of patients. Being a whole body technique, PET has the advantage of not only detecting disease activity in the operative site but also evaluating for distant organ metastasis. In fact, rising levels of calcitonin, together with negative anatomical or conventional functional imaging studies triggered the PET scan request in MTC patients in different PET centers across the world.

2. Significance of Incidental F-18 FDG Uptake in Thyroid Nodules

An emerging role for F-18 FDG PET is in the assessment of incidental observation of thyroid nodule which, when showing high F-18 FDG uptake, should be assessed further to rule out a possible malignancy. The prevalence of incidental thyroid F-18 FDG uptake on PET (including both focal and diffuse uptake) ranges from 1.8 to 2.9% (1–12) (Tables 1 and 2).

The probability of malignancy in diffuse uptake is low, as these are mostly due to inflammatory pathologies such as thyroiditis. From a diagnostic perspective, when one identifies a gland with diffusely increased F-18 FDG uptake, the differential diagnosis includes Hashimoto disease, lymphoma, and diffuse infiltration with carcinoma (13–16). It is important to be aware of these differential diagnoses (some omitted). While in Hashimoto, the increased uptake is caused by inflammatory lymphocytes, in Grave's disease, the increased uptake is caused by hypermetabolic thyrocytes. Incidental focal F-18 FDG uptake in the thyroid, on the other hand, harbors a 30–50% risk of malignancy. Although there is some variation in the reported probability of malignancy in the incidental focal F-18 FDG uptake in the thyroid, it is higher than that of the 4–12.6% risk in nodules detected by US examination (17). Metastatic cancer to the thyroid is a rare entity, accounting for less than 1% of cases of thyroid malignancy in most clinical series (18). Hence, focal thyroid uptake should not be attributed to metastasis from the known

Table 1
Prevalence and malignancy of incidental focal and diffuse thyroid fluorodeoxyglucose uptake in representative studies (with permission from Chen et al. (82))

Author	Year	Number of patients	Prevalence Total (%)	Focal (%)	Diffuse (%)	Malignancy of focal uptake (%)
Cohen (1)	2001	4,525	102 (2.3)	71 (1.6)	31 (0.7)	7/14 (50)
Kang (2)	2003	1,330	29 (2.2)	21 (1.6)	8 (0.6)	4/15 (27)
Kim (3)	2005	4,136	90 (2.2)	45 (1.1)	45 (1.1)	16/32 (50)
Are (4)	2007	8,800	263 (2.9)	101 (1.1)	162 (1.8)	24/57 (42)
Kurata (5)	2007	1,626	29 (1.8)	4 (0.3)	25 (1.5)	2/4 (50)

Table 2
Prevalence and malignancy of incidental focal thyroid fluorodeoxyglucose uptake in representative studies (with permission from Chen et al. (82))

Author	Year	Number of patients	Prevalence (%)	Risk of malignancy (%)
Chen (6)	2005	4,830	60 (1.2)	7/50 (14)
Yi (7)	2005	140	6 (4.3)	4/7 (57)
Choi (8)	2006	1,763	70 (4.0)	17/44 (39)
Chu (9)	2006	6,241	76 (1.2)	4/14 (29)
King (10)	2007	15,711	22 (0.1)	3/21 (14)
Bogsrud (11)	2007	7,347	79 (1.1)	17/48 (35)
Nam (12)	2007	689	19 (2.8)	5/12 (42)

primary malignancy in patients harboring other malignancy, although in rare circumstances it might occur (19) (Fig. 1).

The role of SUVs in distinguishing cancer from benign disease is unclear at this time. While some authors have suggested that SUVs may be of value, others have shown no difference of SUV between the two groups, with significant overlap of SUV among different lesions (Fig. 2). The varying results concerning the SUV of malignant and benign lesions could be related to several factors such as the partial volume effect, high F-18 FDG uptake in some benign lesions (e.g., Hürthle cell adenoma or autonomous adenoma), the state of thyroid function, TSH levels inflammation in the gland, and the presence of cancer cells (16, 18, 20, 21).

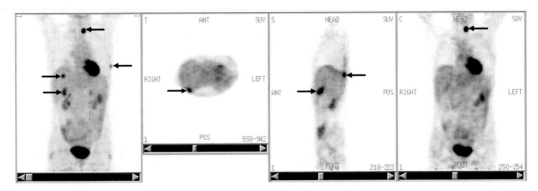

Fig. 1. F-18 FDG PET in a 52-year-old female with melanoma demonstrating a focus of increased F-18 FDG uptake in the right costophrenic angle, corresponding to a lung nodule seen in the same location on the CT scan. There is also increased F-18 FDG uptake in the right hepatic lobe antero-inferiorly and on the left chest along the mid axillary line corresponding to the soft tissue nodularity noted clinically. Another area of intense F-18 FDG uptake is observed in the left lobe of the thyroid gland; SUV_{max} was found to be 18.2. Ultrasonographic examination of the neck showed that this metabolically active lesion corresponded to a 1.1 × 1.3 × 1.5 cm nodule (the largest among several nodules seen in both lobes of the thyroid) in the midportion of the left lobe which was surrounded by a dense calcification. Subsequent histo-pathological examination of the lesion proved it to be a metastasis from malignant melanoma (19).

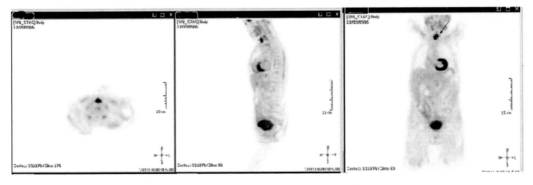

Fig. 2. F-18 FDG PET in an 83-year-old female, a successfully treated case of abdominal diffuse large B-cell lymphoma, demonstrating an F-18 FDG-avid (SUV_{max} 6.9) thyroid incidentaloma. Histopathology revealed adenomatous nodule with Hurthle cell changes. (Permission from Taylor & Francis for Basu et al. (16)).

3. Thyroid Carcinoma: Epidemiology, Variants and their Salient Features

There are approximately 26,000 new cases of thyroid carcinoma diagnosed each year in USA, and the overall incidence continues to rise. Women are more likely to have thyroid carcinoma at a ratio of three to one. In an American Cancer Society estimate, it was proposed that there will be approximately 33,550 new cases of thyroid cancer diagnosed in USA in 2007, and of these new cases, over 70% will be women. The disease can occur in any age group, although it is most common after the age of 30, and its aggressiveness increases significantly in older patients. Overall, thyroid cancer accounts for 1–3% of all human malignancies.

Papillary thyroid cancer (PTC) is the most common of all thyroid cancers, comprising approximately 75% of follicular cell derived cancers, whereas follicular thyroid cancer represents around 15% of all thyroid cancer. PTC can occur in any age group, although its peak incidence in the fourth and fifth decades of life. It is more common in women than in men (a ratio of 2.5:1). The principal risk factors for the development of PTC include a history of childhood head and neck radiation for benign conditions, or a family history of PTC. PTC typically has an excellent prognosis, with the overall 10-year survival rates estimated at 80–90%. Age over 45 years at the time of diagnosis, tumor size over 4 cm, extra-thyroidal extension of tumor, lymph node recurrence, and distant metastases negatively influence survival. On fine needle aspiration (FNA), PTC shows large cells and nuclei, and their cytoplasm has a "ground glass" appearance. Nucleoli are prominent and the nuclei have clefts, grooves, and "holes" due to intranuclear cytoplasmic inclusions. On surgical specimens, the classical histologic appearance of PTC is the papillary structures with no follicles or colloid. Differentiated PTC cells have sodium–iodine symporters that trap iodine, allowing for whole-body imaging with I-131 or I-123. Post-therapy evaluation of patients with positive Tg and negative iodine scans can be done with neck ultrasound, CT and/or MRI, as well as several radiotracers (Tl-201, Tc-99m MIBI/Tetrafosmin). Anaplastic carcinoma, on the other hand, is the most aggressive thyroid tumor, which accounts for about 2% of thyroid cancers and has a 10-year survival rate of only 14% (22, 23). Unlike papillary and follicular thyroid cancers, which arise from thyroid hormone producing follicular cells, MTC is a neuroendocrine tumor (NET) of the parafollicular or C-cells of the thyroid gland. A characteristic feature of this tumor is the production of calcitonin. The C-cells originate from the embryonic neural crest; as a result, MTCs often have the clinical and histologic features of other NETs such as carcinoid and islet-cell tumors. MTC constitutes about 5–10% of all thyroid malignancies. Most MTCs are sporadic. However, some are familial as part of the multiple endocrine neoplasia type 2 (MEN2) syndrome. Overall 10-year survival rates are 90% when all the disease is confined to the thyroid gland, 70% with spread to cervical lymph nodes, and 20% when spread to distant sites is present. Immunostaining for calcitonin reveals nuclei of the tumor cells placed eccentrically, larger and more pleomorphic than those of normal follicular cells. Immunocytologic staining for calcitonin is positive. The background contains many RBC's that nonspecifically take up the stain. When MTC is diagnosed by FNA biopsy, ultrasonography, CT and/or MRI scanning of the neck are indicated to look for cervical lymph node involvement. I-131 metaiodobenzylguanidine (MIBG), In-111 labeled Octreotide, monoclonal anti-CEA antibodies, and Tc-99m pentavalent V-di-mercaptosuccinic acid (DMSA-V) were investigated for evaluation of MTC and are currently used in detection of metastatic/recurrent disease.

3.1. At the Crossroads: From Radioiodine Imaging and Therapy to Molecular Imaging with PET(-CT) (Established Role and Future Possibilities)

The increasing availability of F-18 FDG PET(-CT) has expanded the armamentarium of functional imaging, complementing the well-established radioiodine scans in the management of this disorder. The use of F-18 FDG PET appears invaluable in patients with metastatic thyroid cancer that are thyroglobulin-positive, but radioiodine-negative, rendering traditional I-131 scans and high-dose radioactive iodine therapy ineffective. In these less differentiated or de-differentiated thyroid cancers, the tumor cells lose the expression of sodium iodide symporter and thereby the ability to concentrate radioiodine. The prognosis for most thyroid cancer patients is very good, but the rate of recurrence can be up to 30% and thyroid cancer usually recurs in the neck. The ability to detect thyroid cancer recurrence early is critically important, especially in the setting of rising Tg levels with negative imaging studies. The majority of the studies, hence, have addressed the role of F-18 FDG PET in this setting. The ability of F-18 FDG PET to detect tumors is based on the higher glycolytic metabolism expressed by cancerous cells and higher expression of membrane glucose transporter proteins. Complementing anatomic imaging, PET adds unique metabolic information to the detection and characterization of malignancy.

It has also been shown that malignant tissue can contain both differentiated and undifferentiated features, suggesting that F-18 FDG PET should not be limited to I-131 whole-body scanning (WBS) negative patients (24). Also, it has been shown that F-18 FDG PET can have better sensitivity and specificity than Tg levels, in addition to the ability to localize the recurrent disease (25).

It is important to note that serum Tg was elevated in only 55% of patients with cervical lymph nodes recurrences, while F-18 FDG PET was able to detect 100% of these foci in their series (26). In one series, PET-CT results contributed to changes to the treatment plan in 40% of the patients with a subset of patients having Tg levels >10 ng/ml (27). The other areas where the technique has been explored in fewer studies include: (a) evaluation of the thyroid nodules with or without inconclusive FNA cytology, (b) prognostic evaluation, (c) determination of the extent of disease in high or low-risk patients, (d) assessment of treatment response, (e) evaluation and management of Hurtle cell carcinoma, (f) selection of patients for investigational therapies, (g) determination of extent and relationship of the known metastases to vital structures, and (h) F-18 FDG PET as a method of monitoring response to therapy (28, 29).

3.2. F-18 FDG PET in Papillary and Follicular Thyroid Carcinoma with Elevated Tg and Negative I-131 Whole-Body Scans

While the first report of F-18 FDG PET for thyroid cancer was in 1987, it took almost 10 more years for more studies to become available (30). F-18 FDG PET is becoming more commonly utilized when there is discordance between elevated Tg and negative I-131 WBS (31) (Figs. 3 and 4). It has been suggested that when used in combination, F-18 FDG PET and I-131 WBS may result in tumor foci being missed in as few as 7% of cases, suggesting a complementary role for the two imaging modalities (32–35). A multicentre trial by Grünwald et al. found a higher sensitivity by F-18 FDG PET (75%) compared to I-131 WBS (50%) and Tc-99m sestamibi/Thallium-201 WBS (53%) with comparable specificities. The sensitivity of F-18 FDG PET increased to 85% in

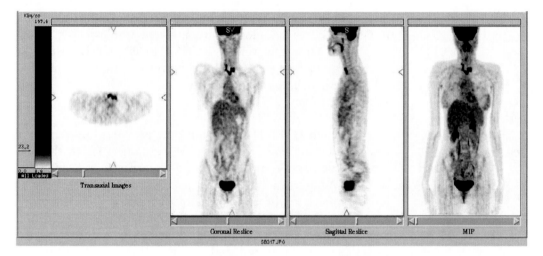

Fig. 3. A 23-year-old female, diagnosed patient of papillary carcinoma of thyroid with serum Tg of 414 ng/ml and normal I-131 whole-body scan. F-18 FDG PET demonstrates multiple diseased nodes in lower neck, confirmed after excision. *Note*: F-18 FDG PET is maximally helpful in this setting, as surgical excision of the diseased nodes is likely to considerably improve the prognosis.

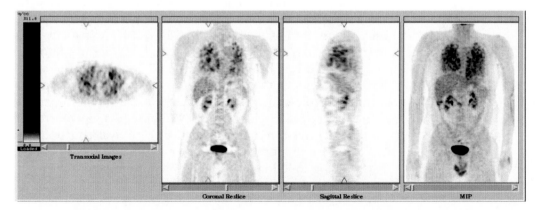

Fig. 4. Patient with follicular carcinoma thyroid and pulmonary metastases, without radioiodine concentration. Serum Tg level was 800 ng/ml. F-18 FDG PET shows extensive F-18 FDG uptake in the noniodine concentrating lesions.

the subgroup of patients with negative I-131 WBS. Discordance appears in some cases between F-18 FDG PET and I-131 WBS, and it has been attributed to the fact that less-DTCs lose the ability to concentrate iodine, due to disruption of the sodium iodide symporter, and tend to utilize more glucose (36, 37). In such cases, F-18 FDG PET can be useful in identifying tumor foci, underscoring its value as an adjunct in tumor detection. It is predicted and has been proven that the sensitivity of F-18 FDG PET is higher when performed during TSH stimulation rather than during TSH suppression, and it is reported in several studies that more F-18 FDG-avid lesion sites are seen with TSH stimulation than with TSH suppression. Majority of these studies are carried out with exogenous rhTSH administration (21, 38–40).

The advent of fusion imaging with hybrid PET-CT scanners has increased diagnostic confidence and reduced equivocal results in either PET or CT alone. Several recent studies have demonstrated the important role of PET-CT in differentiated thyroid cancer, especially those thyroglobulin-positive but iodine-negative cases, altering clinical management in 51% (23 of 60–65) of cases in various studies (27, 41–44).

3.3. F-18 FDG PET and Prognosis of DTC

Imaging with F-18 FDG PET not only provides localization of disease foci but also provides prognostic information that can identify the patients at higher risk of recurrence and metastatic disease. Wang et al. found that patients with F-18 FDG-avid lesions appear to be a more aggressive subset. Furthermore, patients with F-18 FDG-avid, high-volume disease (>125 mL) as assessed with CT and PET have markedly reduced survival (45). These authors predicted that F-18 FDG PET can be utilized as a tool for clinical decision making for either localized or systemic therapy other than I-131 (46). It has also been demonstrated that increased glucose transporter-1 gene expression, which is responsible for enhanced F-18 FDG uptake by the tumor cells, reflects an aggressive clinical course and unfavorable prognosis (47). In part, this is the major reason why promising results are obtained with F-18 FDG PET in patients with Hürthle cell carcinoma. In one of the early studies, the information provided by PET was used to guide or change therapy in 50% of patients with this malignancy, and hence was recommended for the evaluation and clinical management of patients with Hürthle cell carcinoma (48). Robbins et al. documented a significant inverse relationship between survival and both the F-18 FDG avidity of the most active lesion and the number of F-18 FDG-avid lesions. It is hoped that the biologic characterization of these tumors using imaging with F-18 FDG PET or more specific tracers will allow us to noninvasively select the more aggressive subset of patients who will tend to progress in the future (49).

3.4. F-18 FDG PET in the Characterization of Thyroid Nodules

In approximately 20% of the cases, FNA cytology findings are inconclusive and in this scenario the potential role of F-18 FDG PET has been investigated. While a few early reports yielded promising results (e.g., unnecessary surgery could be reduced by 66% using the information provided by F-18 FDG PET imaging in one study), subsequent studies failed to prove its efficacy. In addition, there was no difference between the maximum standardized uptake value of the benign and malignant thyroid nodules (50–55).

3.5. F-18-Fluoride PET in Skeletal Metastases of Thyroid Carcinoma

The conventional skeletal scintigraphy and F-18 FDG PET imaging have been adopted in addition to the radioiodine scan in the evaluation of skeletal metastases (Fig. 5), though it was predicted that these procedures will be completely replaced with F-18 fluoride PET if it becomes widely available (Fig. 6). This tracer is readily extracted from the target and can be used with minimum quality assurance efforts. The cost of producing F-18 fluoride is markedly lower than that of any other PET tracers and will be quite competitive with conventional bone imaging agents. F-18 fluoride PET with its high spatial resolution tomographic images is substantially superior to conventional planar scans for elucidating osseous abnormalities. Schirrmeister et al. suggested that F-18 fluoride PET was more sensitive than radionuclide bone scanning in patients with DTC. We have also obtained similar results in our institute using F-18 fluoride PET (56).

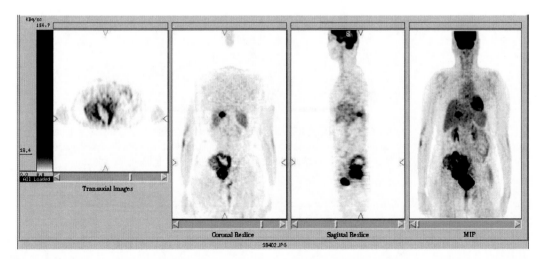

Fig. 5. A 55-year-old female, a known patient of follicular carcinoma of thyroid with skeletal metastasis with serum Tg of >800 ng/ml; the lesions were iodine concentrating. F-18 FDG PET shows avid uptake at the metastatic site in the pelvis with a lytic area.

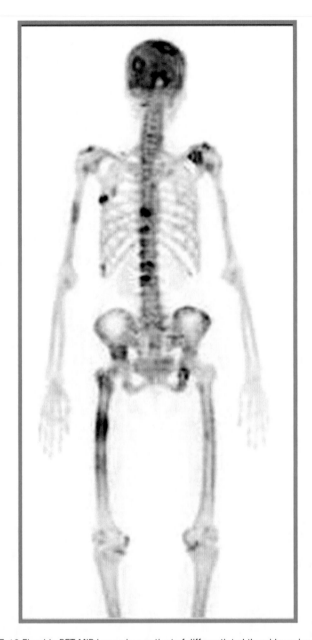

Fig. 6. F-18 Fluoride PET MIP image in a patient of differentiated thyroid carcinoma with skeletal metastases demonstrating excellent resolution, where the small lytic lesions in the skull and osteoblastic lesions in the vertebra are distinctly visualized.

4. Evolving Role of I-124 PET in DTC

The application of I-124 PET is an attractive modality for patients with thyroid carcinoma because it provides high-resolution imaging along with quantitative information, capable of estimating the functional volume of the thyroid tissue being examined. I-124 has a physical half-life of 4.2 days and a decay scheme characterized by 22% of the disintegrations producing positrons of relatively high energies (1,532 and 2,135 keV), as well as a number of high-energy gamma and X-rays. High-energy gamma and positron rays impair the image quality, quantitative accuracy, and spatial resolution of the image generated. Image acquisition by three-dimensional (3D) mode using a narrow energy is preferable to the conventional 2D mode scan, because of down scatter of high-energy photons in the lead or tungsten septa in the latter and subsequent detection of these photons within the PET energy window. The newer PET-CT systems using lutetium oxyorthosilicate and lutetium yttrium orthosilicate with narrower energy window and shorter coincidence-timing window have a discrete advantage over the BGO-based scanner because of the aforementioned reasons. Despite these disadvantages of I-124 PET imaging, it offers certain major advantages compared to the conventional radioiodine scintigraphy and these include: (1) the ability of the technique to predict lesional dosimetry, which serves as a basis for determining the optimal dose for treatment with I-131; (2) the technique is helpful in volume estimations within an imprecision of approximately 20% as demonstrated by Eschmann et al.; (3) I-124 PET-CT is superior to I-131 WBS in detecting recurrent or metastatic disease foci, localizing, and differentiating between the thyroid remnant and cervical lymph node metastases (57) (Fig. 7). Studies with this radioisotope have been relatively limited to date and have investigated: (a) efficacy of lesion detection and (b) lesion-specific and normal organ dosimetry studies.

4.1. Studies Investigating the Efficacy of I-124 PET in Lesion Detection

With the early investigation by Pentlow et al. demonstrating that quantitative imaging with I-124 labeled antibodies appears to be feasible using bismuth germinate (BGO)-based PET scanners, several other investigators have studied the potential of this isotope in the management of thyroid cancer (58). In a recent comparative study investigating the image quality of different iodine isotopes (I-123, I-124, and I-131), I-124 gave the best imaging results (6). In another comparative study of 12 patients with differentiated thyroid cancer who were referred for diagnostic workup, lesion detectability was 100, 87, 83, and 56% for combined I-124 PET-CT, I-124 PET alone, I-131 whole body scintigraphy (WBS), and CT, respectively. These findings indicate that I-124 PET-CT may provide incremental diagnostic value over the other imaging modalities. These authors also concluded that image acquisition can be successfully carried out 24 h after radiotracer administration (59–61).

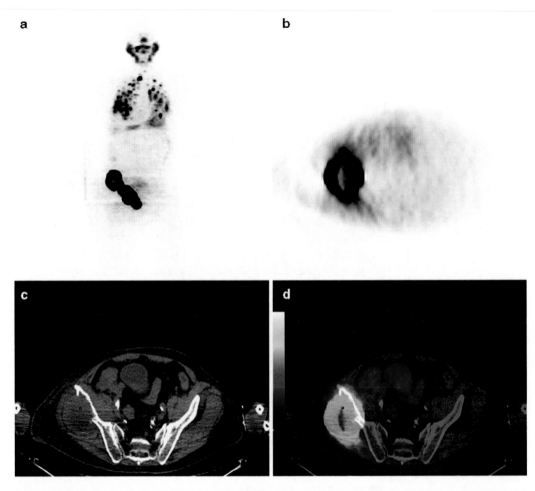

Fig. 7. I-124 PET-CT scan (5.16 mCi follow-up study). (**a**) The MIP image at 48 h again shows iodine-avid disease in the neck, bilateral lungs, and right hemipelvis. The transaxial PET and CT images (**b**, **c**) or the fused PET/CT image (**d**) shows abnormal I-124 uptake in the lytic lesion involving the right iliac bone with extraosseous soft tissue component. (Reproduced with permission from Elsevier Inc. for Grewal et al. (80)).

4.2. Dosimetry Studies with I-124 PET

The feasibility of individualized I-131 therapy dose on the basis of serial I-124 PET dosimetry has been attempted both in adults and pediatric population. I-124-PET dosimetry changed the patient management in terms of therapeutic dose of I-131 administered in 25% of cases, and led to early multi-modality intervention in 32% of patients, compared with and relative to the conventional empiric approaches (62). In another study involving pediatric patients, adult I-124 PET-CT dosimetry protocol appeared to be safe, and informative disease management was modified or disease extent clarified in two out of four patients (63). The study by Eschmann et al. in three thyroid cancer patients showed that higher radiation doses were achieved in thyroid remnants than in metastatic lesions, and considerable variability of the radiation doses exists at the latter sites (57). They also predicted that in differentiated thyroid cancer metastases, the radiation doses would be in the range of 70–170 Gy. Similar substantial variability in intra- and intertumoral absorbed doses in individual patients were also reported by Sgouros et al. and a mean individual absorbed dose in the range of 1.2–540 Gy was noted in their study population (64). In an endeavor to study normal organ dosimetry by I-124 PET imaging and 3D-ID software, it was observed that the highest mean absorbed dose was noted in the right submandibular salivary gland and the lowest mean absorbed dose was seen in the brain (65).

It is likely that future applications of this methodology with I-124 for more accurate localization of disease with the added advantage of more accurate tumor dosimetry to predict dose delivery can substantially improve the management of this malignancy.

5. F-18 FDG PET in Thyroid Lymphoma

Thyroid lymphoma, especially the primary extranodal type, is a relatively rare entity. Primary thyroid lymphomas represent 1–5% of thyroid malignancies and less than 2% of extranodal lymphomas (66, 67). Thyroid lymphoma demonstrates a female preponderance with a reported male: female incidence ratio of 3 to 4:1. The age distribution usually ranges from 50 to 80 years and rarely occurs under the age of 40. The presenting features include a rapidly enlarging neck mass (70%) and compression signs and symptoms, e.g., dysphagia, stridor, hoarseness, and a pressure sensation around the neck. Most patients are usually euthyroid at initial presentation (68–70). In a recently reported retrospective series, the sensitivity of F-18 FDG PET in detection of the disease before treatment was 100% (16). Following successful treatment SUV_{max} declined along with improvement in the disease status (Fig. 8). Disease recurrence was detected earlier by F-18 FDG PET in around 40% of patients compared to CT. The authors concluded that F-18 FDG PET is a useful and sensitive modality for assessing disease activity in thyroid lymphoma. Its ability to detect disease recurrence was found to be superior to CT in two patients. Previously, Lin reported about the efficacy of PET-CT in therapy monitoring in a 57-year-old man with a diffuse large B-cell lymphoma of the thyroid (71).

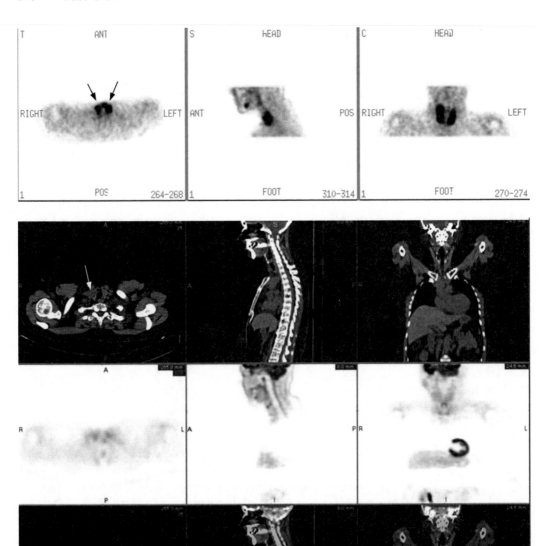

Fig. 8. Pre-chemotherapy F-18 FDG PET-CT (*upper panel*) in a 52-year-old female of non-Hodgkin's lymphoma of the thyroid showing avid F-18 FDG uptake (SUV$_{max}$ 7.6) in both thyroid lobes. *Lower panel* shows complete metabolic response in the F-18 FDG PET following chemotherapy, whereas noncontrast CT shows non F-18 FDG-avid persistent right thyroid nodule (16).

6. PET(-CT) in Medullary Carcinoma of the Thyroid

F-18 FDG PET has shown encouraging results in MTC patients with a higher sensitivity in detecting local recurrent and metastatic disease, when compared with single photon emission tracers. However, F-18 FDG uptake depends on lesion size and to some extent on the grade of differentiation and biologic aggressiveness of the tumor. It appears to be useful mainly in patients with very high calcitonin levels and high progression rate. F-18 FDG PET has been acknowledged for its utility in identifying lymph node metastases in particular, with sensitivity as high as 76% reported in 2000 by Brandt-Mainz et al. (72).

Szakall et al. found that compared with anatomical tomographic imaging methods, F-18 FDG PET detected more cervical, supraclavicular, and mediastinal lymph node lesions (73). In one of the early reports, de Groot et al. observed that F-18 FDG PET detects more lesions than Tc-99m (V) DMSA and In-111-labeled octreotide, as well as bone scintigraphy combined with morphologic imaging such as ultrasound, CT, or MRI (74). To assess the diagnostic role of F-18 FDG PET-CT performed with a hybrid tomograph in the detection of deposits of recurrent MTC, Rubello et al. evaluated 19 MTC patients with elevated serum calcitonin levels (58–1,350 pg/ml). In this study, F-18 FDG PET-CT was the most sensitive imaging modality in detecting metastases in recurrent MTC patients with increased serum calcitonin levels (Fig. 9). Moreover, F-18 FDG PET-CT was useful in some patients for planning an effective second operation (75). However, the role of F-18 FDG PET in MTC has been questioned by some investigators in view of the limited role of F-18 FDG PET in NETs. It appears to be most useful when dedifferentiation takes place and may provide important prognostic information (Fig. 10). Musholt et al. noted that in MTC, there is no increase in expression of the glucose transporter proteins GLUT 1 through GLUT 5, despite the fact that F-18 FDG PET imaging can be useful in the localization of cervicomediastinal MTC metastases (76). From a diagnostic point of view, a multimodality imaging approach is recommended in recurrent MTC, especially based on the combination of anatomical and functional imaging with conventional SPECT tracers and F-18 FDG PET-CT imaging.

Like other NETs, MTC is characterized by the presence of amine uptake mechanism and/or peptide receptors at the cell membrane, allowing the clinical use of specific radiopharmaceuticals that reflect the different metabolic pathways of MTC, and in particular the synthesis, storage and release of hormones (F-18-dihydroxyphenylalanine, F-18-DOPA and F-18-fluorodopamine,

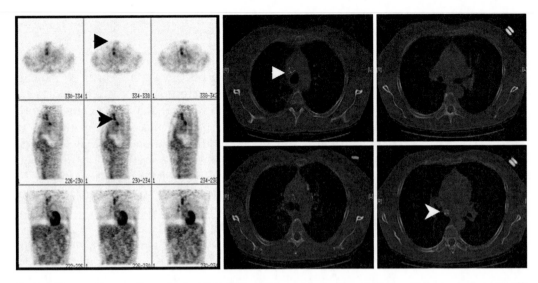

Fig. 9. A 53-year-old man with mediastinal F-18 FDG uptake consistent with metastasis, which was confirmed by CT. (Reproduced with permission from Urhan et al. (81), PET clinics).

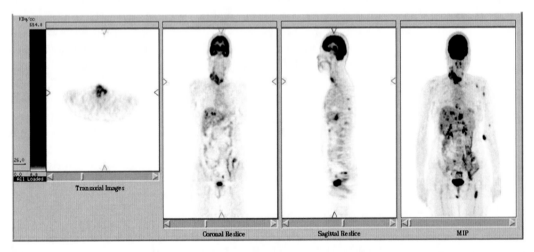

Fig. 10. A 28-year-old female, newly diagnosed to have medullary carcinoma thyroid with serum calcitonin of 17,930 ng/ml. The ultrasonography of the neck had demonstrated the lesion in the right lobe of thyroid with lymph node metastasis. Tc-99m (V) DMSA showed uptake in the primary only. F-18 FDG PET demonstrated numerous foci in liver and skeleton in addition to uptake in the primary.

F-18-FDA), and the expression of receptors (Ga-68 labeled somatostatin analogs). Many of these tracers are currently under investigation, and the clinical results with F-18-DOPA are noteworthy. l-DOPA is a catecholamine precursor that is converted to dopamine by the aromatic amino acid decarboxylase (AADC). Based on its known biochemical pathway and the prior experience with imaging of the dopaminergic system in the brain, amine precursor l-DOPA has been considered a potential candidate to examine endocrine tumors.

Three studies of relatively good statistical strength have been performed to examine the role of FDOPA PET in MCT patients. Koopmans et al. studied the role of F-18 DOPA, F-18 FDG, Tc-99m-DMSA-V, and MRI or CT in assessing patients with recurrent MTC. They evaluated 21 patients: patient and lesion-based sensitivities were determined using a composite reference consisting of all imaging techniques. The investigators concluded that MTC lesions were best detectable when serum calcitonin was >500 ng/L. The results indicated that F-18 DOPA-PET is superior to F-18 FDG PET, DMSA-V, and morphologic imaging. With short calcitonin doubling times (≤12 mo), F-18 FDG PET appeared superior (77). Hoegerle et al. found an overall sensitivity of 63% for F-18 DOPA-PET in 11 patients; this sensitivity was lower than that of CT/MRI but better than those of F-18 FDG PET and SRS (78). In a retrospective analysis of F-18 DOPA-PET in 15 patients with MTC and increased levels of tumor markers, Beuthien-Baumann et al. found similar performances for F-18 FDG and F-18 DOPA; both yielding positive results in 7 of 15 patients, with lesions seen in the neck, mediastinum, abdomen, or bone marrow (79).

References

1. Cohen, M.S., Arslan, N., Dehdashti, F., et al. (2001) Risk of malignancy in thyroid incidentalomas identified by fluorodeoxyglucose-positron emission tomography. *Surgery* **130(6)**, 941–6.

2. Kang, K.W., Kim, S.K., Kang, H.S., et al. (2003) Prevalence and risk of cancer of focal thyroid incidentaloma identified by 18F-fluorodeoxyglucose positron emission tomography for metastasis evaluation and cancer screening in healthy subjects. *J Clin Endocrinol Metab* **88(9)**, 4100–4.

3. Kim, T.Y., Kim, W.B., Ryu, J.S., et al. (2005) 18F-fluorodeoxyglucose uptake in thyroid from positron emission tomogram (PET) for evaluation in cancer patients: high prevalence of malignancy in thyroid PET incidentaloma. *Laryngoscope* **115(6)**, 1074–8.

4. Are, C., Hsu, J.F., Schoder, H., et al. (2007) FDG-PET detected thyroid incidentalomas: need for further investigation. *Ann Surg Oncol* **14(1)**, 239–47.

5. Kurata, S., Ishibashi, M., Hiromatsu, Y., et al. (2007) Diffuse and diffuse-plus-focal uptake in the thyroid gland identified by using FDG-PET: prevalence of thyroid cancer and Hashimoto's thyroiditis. *Ann Nucl Med* **21(6)**, 325–30.

6. Chen, Y.K., Ding, H.J., Chen, K.T., et al. (2005) Prevalence and risk of cancer of focal thyroid incidentaloma identified by 18F-fluorodeoxyglucose positron emission tomography for cancer screening in healthy subjects. *Anticancer Res* **25(2B)**, 1421–6.

7. Yi, J.G., Marom, E.M., Munden, R.F., et al. (2005) Focal uptake of fluorodeoxyglucose by the thyroid in patients undergoing initial disease staging with combined PET/CT for non-small cell lung cancer. *Radiology* **236(1)**, 271–5.

8. Choi, J.Y., Lee, K.S., Kim, H.J., et al. (2006) Focal thyroid lesions incidentally identified by integrated 18FFDG PET/CT: clinical significance and improved characterization. *J Nucl Med* **47(4)**, 609–15.

9. Chu, Q.D., Connor, M.S., Lilien, D.L., et al. (2006) Positron emission tomography (PET) positive thyroid incidentaloma: the risk of malignancy observed in a tertiary referral center. *Am Surg* **72(3)**, 272–5.

10. King, D.L., Stack, B.C. Jr., Spring, P.M., et al. (2007) Incidence of thyroid carcinoma in fluorodeoxyglucose positron emission tomography-positive thyroid incidentalomas. *Otolaryngol Head Neck Surg* **137(3)**, 400–4.

11. Bogsrud, T.V., Karantanis, D., Nathan, M.A., et al. (2007) The value of quantifying 18F-FDG uptake in thyroid nodules found incidentally on whole-body PET-CT. *Nucl Med Commun* **28(5)**, 373–81.

12. Nam, S.Y., Roh, J.L., Kim, J.S., et al. (2007) Focal uptake of (18)F-fluorodeoxyglucose by thyroid in patients with nonthyroidal head and neck cancers. *Clin Endocrinol (Oxf)* **67**(1), 135–9.

13. Boerner, A.R., Voth, E., Theissen, P., et al. (1998) Glucose metabolism of the thyroid in Graves' disease measured by F-18-fluorodeoxyglucose positron emission tomography. *Thyroid* **8**, 765–72.

14. Boerner, A.R., Voth, E., Theissen, P., et al. (2000) Glucose metabolism of the thyroid in autonomous goiter measured by F-18-FDG-PET. *Exp Clin Endocrinol Diabetes* **108**, 191–6.

15. Karantanis, D., Bogsrud, T.V., Wiseman, G.A., et al. (2007) Clinical significance of diffusely increased 18F-FDG uptake in the thyroid gland. *J Nucl Med* **48**, 896–901.

16. Basu, S., Li, G., Bural, G., Alavi, A. (2008) Fluorodeoxyglucose positron emission tomography (FDG-PET) and PET/computed tomography imaging characteristics of thyroid lymphoma and their potential clinical utility. *Acta Radiol* **16**, 1–4.

17. Burguera, B., Gharib, H. (2000) Thyroid incidentalomas: prevalence, diagnosis, significance, and management. *Endocrinol Metab Clin North Am* **29**(1), 187–203.

18. Nakhjavani, M.K., Gharib, H., Goellner, J.R., et al. (1997) Metastasis to the thyroid gland: a report of 43 cases. *Cancer* **79**(3), 574–8.

19. Basu, S., Alavi, A. (2007) Metastatic malignant melanoma to the thyroid gland detected by FDG-PET imaging. *Clin Nucl Med* **32**(5), 388–9.

20. van Tol, K.M., Jager, P.L., Piers, D.A., et al. (2002) Better yield of (18)fluorodeoxyglucose-positron emission tomography in patients with metastatic differentiated thyroid carcinoma during thyrotropin stimulation. *Thyroid* **12**(5), 381–7.

21. Chin, B.B., Patel, P., Cohade, C., et al. (2004) Recombinant human thyrotropin stimulation of fluoro-d-glucose positron emission tomography uptake in well-differentiated thyroid carcinoma. *J Clin Endocrinol Metab* **89**(1), 91–5.

22. Parkin, M.D., Pisani, P., Ferlay, J. (1999) Global cancer statistics. *Cancer J Clin* **49**, 33–64.

23. Hundahl, S.A., Fleming, I.D., Fremgen, A.M., et al. (1998) A National Cancer Data Base report on 53,856 cases of thyroid carcinoma treated in the US, '85–'95. *Cancer* **83**, 2638–48.

24. Iwata, M., Kasagi, K., Misaki, T., et al. (2004) Comparison of whole-body 18F-FDG PET, 99mTc-MIBI SPECT, and post-therapeutic 131I-Na scintigraphy in the detection of metastatic thyroid cancer. *Eur J Nucl Med Mol Imaging* **31**(4), 491–8.

25. Chung, J.-K, So, Y., Lee, J.S., et al. (1999) Value of FDG-PET in papillary thyroid carcinoma with negative 131-I whole-body scan. *J Nucl Med* **40**, 986–92.

26. Yeo, J.S., Chung, J.K., So, Y., et al. (2001) F-18-fluoro-deoxyglucose positron emission tomography as a presurgical evaluation modality for I-131 negative thyroid carcinoma patients with local recurrence in cervical lymph nodes. *Head Neck* **23**, 94–103.

27. Nahas, Z., Goldenberg, D., Fakhry, C., et al. (2005) The role of positron emission tomography/computed tomography in the management of recurrent papillary thyroid carcinoma. *Laryngoscope* **115**, 237–43.

28. Hall, N., Kloos, R.T. (2007) PET Imaging in differentiated thyroid cancer: where does it fit and how do we use it. *Arq Bras Endocrinol Metabol* **51**(5), 793–805.

29. Urhan, M., Mavi, A., Alavi, A., Nanni, C. (2008) Positron emission tomography and thyroid cancer. *PET Clin* **2**, 295–304.

30. Joensuu, H., Ahonen, A. (1987) Imaging of metastases of thyroid carcinoma with fluorine-18 fluorodeoxyglucose. *J Nucl Med* **28**, 910–4.

31. Cohen, J.B., Kalinyak, J.E., McDougall, I.R. (2003) Modern management of differentiated thyroid cancer. *Cancer Biother Radiopharm* **18**(5), 689–705.

32. Feine, U., Lietzenmayer, R., Hanke, J.P., Held, J., Wohrle, H., Muller-Schauenburg, W. (1996) Fluorine-18-FDG and iodine-131-iodide uptake in thyroid cancer. *J Nucl Med* **37**, 1468–72.

33. Grünwald, F., Menzel, C., Bender, H., et al. (1997) Comparison of [18]FDG-PET with [131]iodine and ^{99m}Tc-sestamibi scintigraphy in differentiated thyroid cancer. *Thyroid* **7**, 327–35.

34. Conti, P.S., Durski, J.M., Bacqai, F., Grafton, S.T., Singer, P.A. (1999) Imaging of locally recurrent and metastatic thyroid cancer with positron emission tomography. *Thyroid* **9**, 797–804.

35. Schluter, B., Bohuslavizki, K.H., Beyer, W., Plotkin, M., Buchert, R., Clausen, M. (2001) Impact of FDG PET on patients with differentiated thyroid cancer who present with elevated thyroglobulin and negative ^{131}I scan. *J Nucl Med* **42**, 71–6.

36. Grunwald, F., Kalicke, T., Feine, U., et al. (1999) Fluorine-18 fluorodeoxyglucose positron emission tomography in thyroid cancer:

results of a multicentre study. *Eur J Nucl Med* **26**, 1547–52.

37. McDougal, I.R., Davidson, J., Segall, S.M. (2001) Positron emission tomography of the thyroid, with an emphasis on thyroid cancer. *Nucl Med Commun* **22**, 485–92.

38. van Tol, K.M., Jager, P.L., Piers, D.A., et al. (2002) Better yield of (18)fluorodeoxyglucose positron emission tomography in patients with metastatic differentiated thyroid carcinoma during thyrotropin stimulation. *Thyroid* **715(12)**, 381–7.

39. Moog, F., Linke, R., Manthey, N., et al. (2000) Influence of thyroid-stimulating hormone levels on uptake of FDG in recurrent and metastatic differentiated thyroid carcinoma. *J Nucl Med* **41**, 1989–95.

40. Petrich, T., Borner, A.R., Weckesser, E., et al. (2001) Follow-up of thyroid cancer patients using rhTSH: preliminary results. *Nuklearmedizin* **40**, 7–14.

41. Palmedo, H., Bucerius, J., Joe, A., et al. (2006) Integrated PET/CT in differentiated thyroid cancer: diagnostic accuracy and impact on patient management. *J Nucl Med* **47**, 616–24.

42. Zoller, M., Kohlfuerst, S., Igerc, I., et al. (2007) Combined PET/CT in the follow-up of differentiated thyroid carcinoma: what is the impact of each modality. *Eur J Nucl Med Mol Imaging* **34**, 487–95.

43. Iagaru, A., Kalinyak, J.E., McDougall, I.R. (2007) F-18 FDG PET/CT in the management of thyroid cancer. *Clin Nucl Med* **32**, 690–5.

44. Shammas, A., Degirmenci, B., Mountz, J.M., et al. (2007) ^{18}F-FDG PET/CT in patients with suspected recurrent or metastatic well-differentiated thyroid cancer. *J Nucl Med* **48**, 221–6.

45. Wang, W., Macapinlac, H., Larson, S.M., et al. (1999) [^{18}F]-2-fluoro-2-deoxy-d-glucose positron emission tomography localizes residual thyroid cancer in patients with negative diagnostic (^{131})I whole body scans and elevated serum thyroglobulin levels. *J Clin Endocrinol Metab* **84**, 2291–302.

46. Grünwald, F., Menzel, C., Bender, H., et al. (1998) Redifferentiation therapy-induced radioiodine uptake in thyroid cancer. *J Nucl Med* **39**, 1903–6.

47. Schonberger, J., Ruschhoff, J., Grimm, D., et al. (2002) Glucose transporter-1 gene expression is related to thyroid neoplasm with an unfavorable prognosis: an immunohistochemical study. *Thyroid* **12**, 747–54.

48. Lowe, V.J., Mullan, B.P., Hay, I.D., et al. (2003) 18F-FDG PET of patients with Hürthle cell carcinoma. *J Nucl Med* **44(9)**, 1402–6.

49. Robbins, R.J., Wan, Q., Grewal, R.K., et al. (2006) Real-time prognosis for metastatic thyroid carcinoma based on 2-[^{18}F]fluoro-2-deoxy-d-glucose-positron emission tomography scanning. *J Clin Endocrinol Metab* **91**, 498–505.

50. Reimer, S., Adler, L.P., Bloom, A.D. (1998) Prospective evaluation of PET-FDG in FNA indeterminate thyroid nodules. *J Nucl Med* **39**, 123.

51. Geus-Oei, L.F., Pieters, G.F., Bonenkamp, J.J., et al. (2006) 18FFDG PET reduces unnecessary hemithyroidectomies for thyroid nodules with inconclusive cytologic results. *J Nucl Med* **47**, 770–5.

52. Kim, J.M., Ryu, J.S., Kim, T.Y., et al. (2007) 18F-luorodeoxyglucosepositron emission tomography does not predict malignancy in thyroid nodules cytologically diagnosed as follicular neoplasm. *J Clin Endocrinol Metab* **92(5)**, 1630–4.

53. Kresnik, E., Gallowitsch, H.J., Mikosch, P., et al. (2003) Fluorine-18-fluorodeoxyglucose positron emission tomography in the preoperative assessment of thyroid nodules in an endemic goiter area. *Surgery* **133**, 294–9.

54. Robbins, R.J., Hill, R.H., Wang, W., et al. (2000) Inhibition of metabolic activity in papillary thyroid carcinoma by a somatostatin analogue. *Thyroid* **10**, 177–83.

55. Erdi, Y.E., Macapinlac, H.A., Larson, S.M., et al. (1999) Radiation dose assessment for I-131 therapy of thyroid cancer using I-124 PET imaging. *Clin Positron Imaging* **2**, 41–6.

56. Schirrmeister, H., Guhlman, A., Elsner, K., et al. (1999) Sensitivity in detecting osseous lesions depends on anatomic localization: planar bone scintigraphy versus 18-F PET. *J Nucl Med* **40**, 1623–9.

57. Eschmann, S.M., Reischl, G., Bilger, K., et al. (2002) Evaluation of dosimetry of radioiodine therapy in benign and malignant thyroid disorders by means of iodine-124 and PET. *Eur J Nucl Med Mol Imaging* **29**, 760–7.

58. Pentlow, K.S., Graham, M.C., Lambrecht, R.M., et al. (1991) Quantitative imaging of I-124 using positron emission tomography with applications to radioimmunodiagnosis and radioimmunotherapy. *Med Phys* **18**, 357–66.

59. Pentlow, K.S., Graham, M.C., Lambrecht, R.M., et al. (1996) Quantitative imaging of iodine-124 with PET. *J Nucl Med* **37**, 1557–62.

60. Rault, E., Vandenberghe, S., Van Holen, R., et al. (2007) Comparison of image quality of different iodine isotopes (I-123, I-124, and I-131). *Cancer Biother Radiopharm* **22**, 423–30.

61. Freudenberg, L.S., Antoch, G., Jentzen, W., et al. (2004) Value of I-124-PET/CT in staging of patients with differentiated thyroid cancer. *Eur Radiol* **14**, 2092–8.

62. Freudenberg, L.S., Jentzen, W., Gorges, R., et al. (2007) I-124-PET dosimetry in advanced differentiated thyroid cancer: therapeutic impact. *Nuklearmedizin* **46**, 121–8.

63. Freudenberg, L.S., Jentzen, W., Marlowe, R.J., et al. (2007) 124-iodine positron emission tomography/computed tomography dosimetry in pediatric patients with differentiated thyroid cancer. *Exp Clin Endocrinol Diabetes* **115**, 690–3.

64. Sgouros, G., Kolbert, K.S., Sheikh, A., et al. (2004) Patient-specific dosimetry for I-131 thyroid cancer therapy using I-124 PET and 3-dimensional-internal dosimetry (3D-ID) software. *J Nucl Med* **45**, 1366–72.

65. Kolbert, K.S., Pentlow, K.S., Pearson, J.R., et al. (2007) Prediction of absorbed dose to normal organs in thyroid cancer patients treated with I-131 by use of I-124 PET and 3-dimensional internal dosimetry software. *J Nucl Med* **48**, 143–9.

66. Ansell, S.M., Grant, C.S., Habermann, T.M. (1999) Primary thyroid lymphoma. *Semin Oncol* **26**, 316–23.

67. Honing, M.L., Seldenrijk, C.A., de Maat, C.E. (1998) Primary thyroid lymphoma. *Neth J Med* **52**, 75–8.

68. Derringer, G.A., Thompson, L.D., Frommelt, R.A., et al. (2000) Malignant lymphoma of the thyroid gland: a clinicopathologic study of 108 cases. *Am J Surg Pathol* **24**, 623–39.

69. Ruggiero, F.P., Frauenhoffer, E., Stack, B.C. (2005) Thyroid lymphoma: a single institution's experience. *Otolaryngol Head Neck Surg* **133**, 888–96.

70. Kossev, P., Livolsi, V. (1999) Lymphoid lesions of the thyroid: review in light of the revised European–American lymphoma classification and upcoming World Health Organization classification. *Thyroid* **9**, 1273–80.

71. Lin, E.C. (2007) FDG PET/CT for assessing therapy response in primary thyroid lymphoma. *Clin Nucl Med* **32(2)**, 152–3.

72. Brandt-Mainz, K., Muller, S.P., Gorges, R., et al. (2000) The value of F-18 FDG PET in patients with medullary thyroid cancer. *Eur J Nucl Med* **27**, 490–6.

73. Szakall, S. Jr., Esik, O., Balzik, G., et al. (2002) F-18-PET detection of lymph node metastases in medullary thyroid carcinoma. *J Nucl Med* **43(1)**, 66–71.

74. de Groot, J.W., Links, T.P., Jager, P.L., et al. (2004) Impact of F-18 fluoro-2-deoxy-d-glucose positron emission tomography (FDG-PET) in patients with biochemical evidence of recurrent or residual medullary thyroid cancer. *Ann Surg Oncol* **11(8)**, 786–94.

75. Rubello, D., Rampin, L., Nanni, C., et al. (2008) The role of 18F-FDG PET/CT in detecting metastatic deposits of recurrent medullary thyroid carcinoma: a prospective study. *Eur J Surg Oncol* **34(5)**, 581–6.

76. Musholt, T.J., Musholt, P.B., Dehdashti, F., et al. (1997) Evaluation of fluorodeoxyglucose-positron emission tomographic scanning and its association with glucose transporter expression in medullary thyroid carcinoma and pheochromocytoma: a clinical and molecular study. *Surgery* **122**, 1049–60.

77. Koopmans, K.P., de Groot, J.W., Plukker, J.T., et al. (2008) 18F-dihydroxyphenylalanine PET in patients with biochemical evidence of medullary thyroid cancer: relation to tumor differentiation. *J Nucl Med* **49(4)**, 524–31.

78. Hoegerle, S., Ghanem, N., Altehoefer, C., et al. (2003) ^{18}F-DOPA positron emission tomography for the detection of glomus tumours. *Eur J Nucl Med Mol Imaging* **30**, 689–94.

79. Beuthien-Baumann, B., Strumpf, A., Zessin, J., et al. (2007) Diagnostic impact of PET with ^{18}F-FDG, ^{18}F-DOPA and 3-O-methyl-6-[^{18}F]fluoro-DOPA in recurrent or metastatic medullary thyroid carcinoma. *Eur J Nucl Med Mol Imaging* **34**, 1604–9.

80. Grewal, R.K., Lubberink, M., Pentlow, K.S., Larson, S.M. (2007) The Role of Iodine-124-Positron Emission Tomography Imaging in the Management of Patients with Thyroid Cancer. *PET Clinics* **2(3)**, 313–20.

81. Urhan, M., Alavi, A., Nanni, C. (2007) The Evolving Role of Positron Emission Tomography in Patients with Medullary Thyroid Carcinoma. *PET Clinics* **2(3)**, 305–11.

82. Chen, W., Li, G., Parsons, M., Zhuang, H., Alavi, A. (2007) Clinical Significance of Incidental Focal Versus Diffuse Thyroid Uptake on FDG-PET Imaging. *PET Clinics* **2(3)**, 321–29.

Chapter 13

PET in Testicular Cancer

Alexander Becherer

Abstract

Testicular cancer is a rare tumor, subdivided into seminomatous and nonseminomatous tumors. Whereas there are no serum tumor markers in the first group, they are present in nonseminomatous tumors, and are also important prognostic factors. Overall, the prognosis for testicular cancers is good, which makes the choice of accurate treatment intensity between under- and overtreatment often difficult. Residual masses in advanced clinical stages occur frequently but are nonvital tissue.

PET with F-18 FDG has no defined role in imaging of primary tumors where CT is the first-choice imaging modality. For assessing the success of chemotherapy in the presence of residual masses, especially in pure seminoma, F-18 FDG PET is an important tool. In nonseminomatous tumors, it is hampered by the false-negative results in mature teratoma, for which reason false-negative results are a common problem. F-18 FDG PET performs best in predicting relapse in seminoma residuals larger than 3 cm. So far, no alternative to F-18 FDG for PET imaging of testicular cancer has been found. PET-CT has not yet been proven to be superior to PET alone in testicular cancer.

Key words: Testicular cancer, Germ cell tumors, F-18 FDG, Positron emission tomography

1. Epidemiology and Classification

Testicular cancer is a heterogeneous entity of rare malignant tumors, although it represents the most frequent malignant condition in young men. The worldwide incidence ranges from 0.5 to 9.9 cases per 100,000 men per year, with wide regional differences. While the incidence is highest among Caucasians, it is very low in Africans and Asians.

According to the WHO classification, testicular cancer is divided into two major groups: germ cell tumors (GCT), accounting for 90% of testicular cancer, and nongerm cell tumors. The GCT group

Malik E. Juweid and Otto S. Hoekstra (eds.), *Positron Emission Tomography*, Methods in Molecular Biology, vol. 727, DOI 10.1007/978-1-61779-062-1_13, © Springer Science+Business Media, LLC 2011

consists of seminoma, deriving from the mother cells of sperms and accounting for 40% of GCT, and of nonseminomatous germ cell tumors (NSGCT). The latter group consists of not only embryonal carcinoma, teratoma, yolk sac tumors, choriocarcinoma, and other rare tumor types, but also testicular tumors that display more than one histological type, including mixed tumors with seminomatous components. Only tumors of pure seminomatous histology may be designated as seminoma (Table 1).

In the second major group, the nongerm cell tumors, Leydig cell tumor is the most frequent type (3%). Because of the rareness of nongerm cell testicular tumors, only anecdotal data about the use of PET with or without CT exist; thus these tumors are not further covered in this chapter.

Table 1
WHO classification of testicular germ cell tumors

Intratubular germ cell neoplasia, unclassified
Others

Tumors of one histological type (pure forms)
  Seminoma
  Subtype: Seminoma with syncytiotrophoblastic cells
  Spermatocytic seminoma
  Subtype: Spermatocytic seminoma with sarcoma
  Embryonal carcinoma
  Yolk sac tumor

Trophoblastic tumors
 	
  Choriocarcinoma
  Trophoblastic neoplasms other than choriocarcinoma
  Monophasic choriocarcinoma
  Placental site trophoblastic tumor

Teratoma
  Dermoid cyst
  Monodermal teratoma
  Teratoma with somatic type malignancies

Tumors of more than one histological type (mixed forms)
  Mixed embryonal carcinoma and teratoma
  Mixed teratoma and seminoma
  Choriocarcinoma and teratoma/embryonal carcinoma
  Others

2. Risk Factors

While the distinct causes of testicular cancer are not known, several risk factors could be identified from anamnestic data: history of testicular cancer, either individual (contralateral testis) or familiar (first-degree relatives), maldescensus testis, cryptorchism, infertility, testicular atrophy, and intersexual disorders (e.g., testicular feminization and Klinefelter's syndrome). Trauma and mumps orchitis are not risk factors.

2.1. Testicular Intraepithelial Neoplasia

An important premalignant condition is testicular intraepithelial neoplasia (TIN; synonymous: carcinoma in situ, CIS). TIN in the contralateral testis is present in up to 9% of patients with testicular cancer. The presence of TIN is associated with a 70% cumulative risk for developing a second germ cell cancer within the following 7 years (1). For patients with testicular volumes less than 12 ml in combination with age under 40 years, the risk of TIN exceeds one-third (2, 3). The condition is best diagnosed by open biopsy and this option should be offered to patients at risk, best performed simultaneously with surgery for the primary tumor. No imaging modality including ultrasound is suitable for noninvasive diagnosis of TIN.

For classification of testicular cancer according to the TNM system (Table 2), radical surgery is essential because invasion of tunica vaginalis, vasculature and lymphatic system, and spermatic cord is the criterion for T-staging. For diagnosing scrotal invasion, the criterion for T4 tumor diagnosis, surgery is not mandatory if not indicated otherwise, because this diagnosis can be accurately established by clinical measures. TIN can be diagnosed without radical surgery as well. In all other cases, Tx is used if no radical orchidectomy has been performed.

3. Prognostic Factors

Derived from the TNM stage, there are two clinical stages with different prognosis and management: Clinical stage (CS) I includes the following subtypes: Stage 1A, pT1, N0, M0, and S0; Stage 1B, pT2-4, N0, M0, and S0; and stage 1S, any T, N0, M0, and S1-3. Serum tumor markers are only of importance in nonseminomatous tumors, which generally have a less favorable prognosis in comparison to seminomas. In pure seminomas, size of the primary tumor with a 4-cm cutoff and infiltration of the *rete testis* play a major prognostic role for the presence of metastases (4). In patients with nonseminomatous histology, infiltration of

Table 2
TNM classification (UICC 2002)

T	Primary tumor
pTx	Primary tumor cannot be assessed
pT0	No evidence of primary tumor
pTis	Intratubular germ cell neoplasia (TIN, carcinoma in situ)
pT1	Tumor limited to testis and epididymis, may invade tunica albuginea but not tunica vaginalis, no vascular/lymphatic invasion (VI)
pT2	Like pT1 but with invasion of tunica vaginalis or VI
pT3	Invades spermatic cord with or without VI
pT4	Invades scrotum with or without VI
N	Regional lymph nodes clinical (c) or pathological (p)
Nx	Regional lymph nodes cannot be assessed
N0	No regional lymph node metastasis
cN1	Single or multiple regional nodes, ≤2 cm diameter
pN1	≤5 regional nodes, ≤2 cm diameter
cN2	Single or multiple regional nodes, >2 cm but ≤5 cm
pN2	Regional lymph node mass >2 cm but ≤5 cm, or >5 nodes positive, or extranodal tumor extension
N3	Regional lymph node mass >5 cm
M	Distant metastasis
Mx	Distant metastasis cannot be assessed
M0	No distant metastasis
M1	Distant metastasis
M1a	Non-regional lymph node(s) or lung
M1b	Other sites
S	Serum tumor markers; LDH (U/l), HCG (U/l), AFP (ng/ml)
Sx	Serum marker studies not available
S0	Not elevated
S1	LDH < 1.5× upper limit of normal range, HCG < 5,000, AFP < 1000
S2	LDH 1.5–10× upper limit of normal range, HCG 5,000–50,000, AFP 1,000–10,000
S3	LDH > 10× upper limit of normal range, HCG > 50,000, AFP > 10,000

venous blood vessels and lymphatic infiltration are the most important predictors for the presence of occult metastases. Relapse will occur in almost 50% of these patients if they do not receive adjuvant treatment (5). In metastatic disease, the size of retroperitoneal lymph nodes and again vascular infiltration are the most important prognostic factors.

4. Imaging

4.1. General Considerations

Germ cell tumors are usually malignancies with slow tumor growth, which often do not show up with very high uptake of F-18-2-fluoro-2-desoxyglucose (F-18 FDG) (Fig. 1). Not all lesions, even large ones, can be imaged as clearly as in Fig. 2. Therefore, PET scans have to be interpreted accurately, best with knowledge about the clinical situation and concomitant radiological imaging. Possible positive findings should be compared with the corresponding CT slices since lots of sources of nonspecific F-18 FDG uptake exist especially in the abdomen

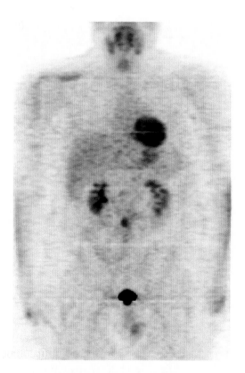

Fig. 1. Small interaortocaval vital post-chemotherapy residual seminoma bulk with moderate F-18 FDG uptake but good contrast against background. Scan with attenuation correction, 2D-mode, iterative reconstruction.

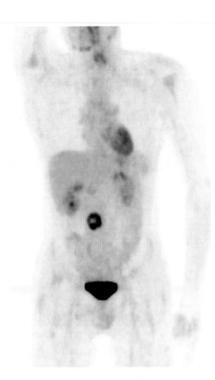

Fig. 2. Seminomatous tumor paracaval with high F-18 FDG uptake and central cold spot, representing necrosis. Scan with attenuation correction, 2D-mode, iterative reconstruction.

and retroperitoneal space. Bowel activity can appear nonlinear and sometimes very intense, and the renal excretion of F-18 FDG in contrast to glucose might cause focal tracer accumulation not only in the renal pelvis but also in the ureter, sometimes also appearing as "hot spots" similar to that of malignant lesions. Thus patients have to by hydrated well before scanning, either orally or with intravenous infusion. The scans have to be reviewed for unclear findings before the patient leaves the department. Sometimes a second image of a questionable region after additional administration of 20 mg of furosemide to flush the urinary tract can be helpful (Fig. 3a, b). The general recommendation in PET scanning to start scan acquisition over the proximal thighs and to proceed toward head is of very high importance in GCT to keep bladder activity low.

All factors lowering F-18 FDG uptake of tumors have to be avoided. One factor is elevated blood glucose (6). PET scans in diabetics and after inadequate fasting are of lower quality with less pronounced delineation of lesions. Therefore, at least 4 h fasting (better overnight) is mandatory. Another factor that has a negative influence on F-18 FDG uptake is previous chemotherapy, when the time interval between completion of the last cycle and the PET scan does not exceed 2 weeks.

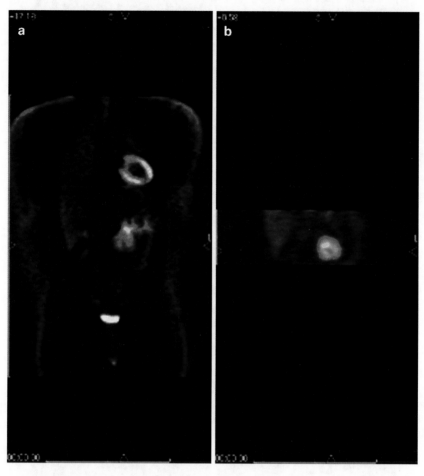

Fig. 3. (a) Scan in a patient with seminoma. Known pararenal residual bulk on the left side. Scan without attenuation correction, 2D-mode, filtered back projection. Note the intense uptake in the level of the kidney which cannot be differentiated from tracer retention in the left kidney pelvis. (b) Local scan over the kidney level after administration of additional fluid and furosemide i.v. with attenuation correction, 2D-mode, filtered back projection. After emptying the left kidney pelvis, the vital tumor is clearly visualized.

Although modern positron emission tomography-computed tomography (PET-CT) scanners are able to acquire a whole body scan in less than 20 min, comfortable patient positioning is important for minimizing artifacts. Especially in small lesions with low tracer uptake, every small patient movement might result in an equivocal or even false-negative result. As shown later in this chapter, patient movement can also cause problems in exact anatomic allocation of lesions (Fig. 4).

In former times, insufficient technical equipment might have caused false-negative results due to reconstruction artifacts in the neighborhood of hot regions, in particular bladder and kidneys. Modern PET scanners reconstruct the data iteratively, which makes the images less influenced by high differences in local activity (Fig. 3).

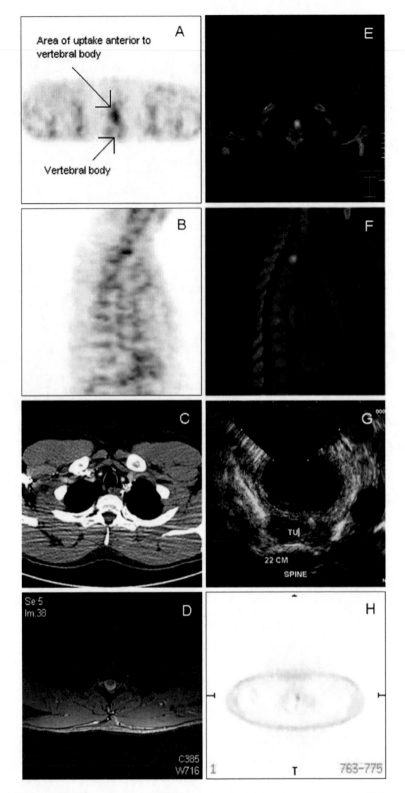

Fig. 4. (**a** and **b**) Axial and sagittal views of F-18 FDG PET scan of a patient showing regional F-18 FDG uptake anterior to the vertebral body. (**c**) CT scan of the positive region identified on the PET scan. (**d**) MRI of the thoracic spine in the region identified on the PET scan. (**e** and **f**) Axial and sagittal views of PET-CT scan of the patient showing that the lesion with 18-FDG uptake was within the vertebral body. (**g**) Endoscopic ultrasound image showing the tumor anterior to the vertebral body. (**h**) Nonattenuated PET scan image from the PET-CT scan.

4.2. Primary Staging of Germ Cell Tumors and PET

Imaging in the primary setting is mainly based on CT imaging, although false-positive findings due to small pulmonary or pleural nodules may occur (7). On the other hand, small retroperitoneal lymph nodes are the source of false negatives in a significant proportion of patients, which makes the clinical differentiation between the stages I and IIA difficult (8). Of the patients staged with nonmetastatic tumors (i.e., CS I), 18% show relapse after orchiectomy in para-aortic lymph nodes (9). Magnetic resonance imaging (MRI) does not provide additional information and should be restricted to patients with contraindication for iodinated contrast agents (10). Bone scans are indicated at clinical suspicion for bone metastasis; the same applies to brain imaging in analogy (8).

4.3. Nonseminomatous Germ Cell Tumors

Nonseminomatous germ cell tumors with low risk (without vascular invasion) are usually followed by CT after radical orchiectomy at 3 and 12 months (11). The relapse rate is low and approximately 80% of patients do not need any further treatment after orchiectomy (12), and in patients relapsing under surveillance, chemotherapy achieves a cure rate of >99% (8). Even in high-risk patients (i.e., with the presence of vascular invasion), despite a high relapse rate of almost 50%, properly carried out surveillance is an option because most relapses are detected in time and 98% of patients are cured at relapse (8). F-18 FDG PET cannot improve the sensitivity of CT alone. In high-risk CS I and II patients with seminomatous and nonseminomatous testicular tumors, identification of small metastases by PET was not possible, although it seems to be more accurate than CT (13, 14). Nevertheless, the good prognosis for both stages with regard to survival does not make the exact determination of the stage in small-volume diseases an issue of major importance if serum markers are within the normal range.

In a multicentric trial on 72 patients with newly diagnosed NCGCT, CS I/II, with metastases to lymph nodes in 26%, F-18 FDG PET was tested against CT in primary staging. Histological diagnosis after surgery was used as reference standard (15). PET was superior in terms of correct lymph node staging, yielding 83% compared to CT with 71%.

Sensitivity/specificity/NPV/PPV was 66%/98%/78%/95% for PET and 41%/95%/67%/87% for CT. The authors concluded that PET is useful in case of a questionable scan. Nevertheless, one must keep in mind that CT had more false-negative cases than PET and that this algorithm implies that no PET had been performed in all false-negative CT scans.

In a similar setting but with a surveillance strategy, 87 patients with negative PET scans were observed to determine the 2-year relapse rate (16). The study was stopped due an unacceptable high relapse rate of 37% after a median interval of 12 months, although PET identified some diseased patients not found by CT.

4.4. Pure Seminoma   In seminoma CS I, up to 32% of patients show relapse if no adjuvant therapy is given, although they have normal CT scans (4), which, on the other hand, leaves the cure rate still close to 100%. Risk stratification in this group after orchiectomy is rather based on the size of primary tumor and *rete testis* infiltration (*see* Subheading 3) than on imaging results. The current standard for patients at high risk for relapse is adjuvant therapy with one cycle of carboplatin or adjuvant radiotherapy on the infradiaphragmal para-aortal/paracaval lymph nodes with a total dose of 20 Gy, depending on the experience of the treatment center (17). For patients with good prognostic factors, surveillance without any adjuvant treatment is an option, because up to 88% of them can be cured by orchiectomy alone after 5 years when risk factors are absent (4). Some centers also propose adjuvant carboplatin or radiotherapy for this group. However, independent of the intended treatment, there is no definite indication for a PET scan in initial staging except in clinical studies, as stated in a recent consensus (8). This opinion is supported by a study with a subset of 12 patients undergoing F-18 FDG PET for initial staging (18), but there is also a contradictory publication (19). In 46 patients with NSGCT CS I, PET was added to conventional CT-based staging. In ten relapsing patients, at the time of relapse, PET was positive in all ten patients and CT in six patients but PET was already positive initially, predicting the relapse correctly up to 8 months prior to relapse. There was no false-positive PET in 36 patients. PET-CT data are unavailable so far in the issue of staging.

The main problems of F-18 FDG PET are the false negatives in micrometastases and in mature teratoma, which are a frequent component of nonseminomatous tumors, and in turn, the false positives in inflammatory masses. In one older study with 54 patients, 27 seminomas and 27 NSGCT, F-18 FDG PET detected micrometastases in only one of seven patients with NSGCT in a lymph node within inflammatory changes, representing an accidentally true positive case. Twenty-one patients with pure seminoma were in CS I, where PET did not add information to CT scans (20). In 4 patients with pure seminomas that underwent retroperitoneal lymph node dissection following chemotherapy, F18 FDG PET correctly predicted absence of tumor in 3 out of these 4, and in the remaining patient the benign nature of a persistent large tumor after two cycles of polychemotherapy was correctly identified which eventually turned out to be a ganglion-euroma. In 20 patients with NSGCT CS II and III, there was one false-positive lesion due to an inflammatory tissue reaction after chemotherapy. However, PET was able to show absence of vital lesions after chemotherapy in seven patients, while it did not detect persistent mature teratoma in five patients. F-18 FDG PET was not found to be suitable yet to be included in the work-up of either seminomatoustumors or NSGCT. The lack of F-18 FDG uptake in mature teratoma was already described earlier (21).

Another study used F-18 FDG PET in seminomas and NSGCT either after initial diagnosis or within 2 weeks after completion of chemotherapy, or at least to weeks but not later than 1 year after chemotherapy (22). PET was significantly more accurate than CT in the latter group due to its specificity of 90% vs. 55%, while no difference was found in the first two groups. There was no significant difference in sensitivity between the different groups. With regard to histology, overall accuracy in NSGCT was significantly better than that in seminoma, where a nonsignificant advantage of PET over CT was observed. Nevertheless, mean SUV in seminomatous lesions was significantly higher than that in nonseminomatous tumors: 9.2 in seminoma, 3.0 in teratocarcinoma, 4.2 in chorionic carcinoma, 4.7 in embryonic carcinoma, and 2.0 in combined tumor. Based on these results, it was stated that the advantage of PET over CT was not discernible at that time, but that further studies should focus on seminoma because of the higher F-18 FDG uptake.

4.5. F-18 FDG PET for Follow-up and Prognosis of Residual Lesions

In higher stages with metastasis to the retroperitoneal lymph nodes, residual masses after completion of treatment are frequent findings. Up to 80% patients with bulky seminoma present with radiographically detectable residual masses after platinum-based chemotherapy (23). Many centers had performed surgery for masses >3 cm if there was no shrinking during follow-up (24–26). Surgery in this indication, however, is difficult due to post-therapeutic tissue alterations, the so-called desmoplastic reaction and fibrosis, and may lead to an increased complication rate (27).

In the issue of differentiation of viable masses from necrosis/fibrosis/scar, most studies with F-18 FDG PET showed a useful role of the method. To investigate the prediction of outcome after high-dose chemotherapy in relapsed GCT, 23 patients (21 with NSGCT, 2 with seminoma) underwent PET and CT/MRI after two to three cycles of induction chemotherapy but before high-dose chemotherapy and compared the prediction of the disease status 6 months after high-dose therapy (28). Parallel to imaging, serum tumor markers were determined. At 6 months, 9 patients had remained progression free and 14 patients progressed. After the 6-month period, only three additional patients showed relapse. PET made a correct prediction in 21/23 patients (91%); CT/MRI was available in 22 patients and made a correct prediction in 13/22 patients (59%); and serum tumor markers could be used for prognosis in 21 patients since 2 patients never had elevated markers, with a correct prediction in 10 patients (48%). When PET was compared with the combined results from radiological imaging and tumor marker decline, data from 20 patients were available. PET made a correct prediction in 19 of them (95%) vs. 12 patients (60%) with CT/MRI plus tumor markers.

Sensitivity/specificity/NPV/PPV was as follows: PET, 100%/78%/100%/88%; CT/MRI, 43%/88%/47%/86%; and tumor markers, 15%/100%/42%/100%. The authors drew the conclusion that F-18 FDG PET could aid in the selection of patients suited for high-dose chemotherapy since it can identify patients not responding to this expensive and possibly toxic treatment.

Another prospective multicentric study on patients with pure seminoma (the SEMPET trial) was able to show the high prognostic contribution of F-18 FDG PET. In the first part of the study, 33 patients with 37 residual post-chemotherapy masses of at least 1 cm diameter on CT were studied (29). PET results obtained 4–12 weeks after completion of chemotherapy were correlated with either histology when the lesion was resected or with clinical outcome after long-term follow-up. To classify a lesion as negative without histology, it had to remain stable or shrink during a follow-up period of at least 2 years; in nine patients histology was available. Of 37 lesions, 14 were larger than 3 cm. F-18 FDG PET was false negative in the smaller lesion of a patient with two lesions of 1.1 and 1.9 cm, which increased in size accompanied by the development of a new supraclavicular metastasis. The remaining 22 lesions ≤3 cm were correctly classified by PET as nonvital, as well as all lesions >3 cm (seven positive, seven negative). In an update of this trial published 3 years later, the patient sample size could be increased to 51 subjects with 19 lesions >3 cm and 37 lesions ≤3 cm (30). The results were still convincing in favor of F-18 FDG PET. It showed a sensitivity/specificity/NPV/PPV of 80%/100%/100%/96%, while CT had only 70%/74%/92%/34% for the discrimination of tumor size (again >3 cm vs. ≤3 cm). The advantage of PET could be demonstrated on a patient base as well as on a lesion base (31). The documentation of response to therapy of F-18 FDG-positive lesions by PET is excellent (Fig. 5a, b). F-18 FDG PET was included in the follow-up algorithm for bulky seminoma in a recent consensus paper on the management and treatment of germ cell cancer (32).

There were also critical voices about the accuracy of F-18 FDG PET in treatment monitoring. At Indiana University, 29 patients with seminoma were prospectively studied and evaluated initially at the time of diagnosis (group A, $N=19$), and after relapse and at the time of salvage chemotherapy (group B, $N=10$). In group A, all patients had a negative PET scan and no patient showed relapse. In group B, five relapses occurred, none of them predicted by PET. The only PET-positive lesion was observed in the posterior mediastinum and turned out to be solely necrosis (33).

4.6. Positron Emission Tomography-Computed Tomography

So far, there are no systematic trials on studies on PET-CT in germ cell cancer. Without doubt, PET-CT will be used more frequently in the near future because virtually every new PET scanner will be delivered as a PET-CT system. The method however has two advantages: much faster data acquisition than

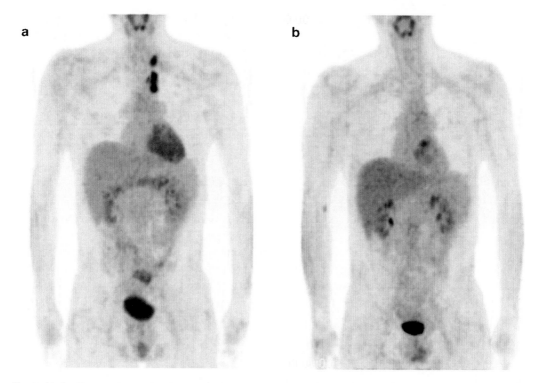

Fig. 5. Mediastinal lymph node relapse before (**a**) and after (**b**) second line chemotherapy. The slight myocardial uptake in scan B must not be mixed up with a lymphatic lesion. Scan with attenuation correction, 2D-mode, iterative reconstruction.

that of older scanner types, which is attractive primarily for patients; and the coregistered anatomic map, which makes the method more attractive for the treating physicians.

A possible special indication might be the inclusion of PET information about tumor metabolism in combination with CT in planning of radiotherapy in analogy to other carcinomas, where recent studies show promising results in a more accurate definition of gross tumor volumes by PET-CT (34–37).

4.7. Pitfalls

The most frequently described pitfall in imaging of NSGCT is mature teratoma, which often presents without any increased F-18 FDG uptake in conventional static PET imaging (13). One study described that kinetic analysis enables the differentiation of teratoma from necrosis or scar (38). However, this method is not feasible in clinical routine as it is time consuming due to the fact that it takes over 60 min only for the dynamic scanning part of PET imaging, without whole body imaging. Teratoma is an important reason for false-negative F-18 FDG PET in NSGCT.

Another problem is the increased association between testicular cancer and sarcoidosis. Compared with other tumors, sarcoidosis has a significant association with testicular cancer.

Compared with the general population, the incidence is increased 100-fold (39). This has been identified as a problem in PET imaging, since sarcoidotic lesions are a well-known pitfall in mimicking malignant foci. Several case reports about false-positive F-18 FDG result, particularly in the mediastinal lesions (40, 41). Sarcoidosis is not a unique problem for PET; it is also a source of false-positive CT scans (42). When reading PET studies, one has to be aware of the possibility of sarcoidosis, especially when sudden mediastinal "metastases" appear in low-risk tumors.

Performing PET-CT, misregistration of the two imaging components might be a problem in small lesions close to structure borders, e.g., soft tissue to bone (43). In this case report, a scan is described where a patient underwent PET-CT with F-18 FDG because of a rise in tumor markers of unknown origin several years after initial treatment. An F-18 FDG-positive lesion projected itself in the anterior part of the vertebral body. Neither CT alone nor MRI could verify the presence of a bony lesion or another suspicious lesion. Eventually, a tumor with the largest diameter of 1.9 cm was found by transesophageal ultrasound and resected. Histology confirmed relapsed NSGCT between esophagus and vertebra body (Fig. 4).

4.8. Other Tracers

In patients with brain metastases, PET with radiolabeled amino acids might be useful. Recently a report showed that L-C-11 methionine was diagnostic in two patients albeit with metastases from nongerminomatous germ cell cancers, one of the patients being female (44). L-C-11 tyrosine (TYR) was studied in NSGCT in order to image tumor proliferation (45). In ten patients, no lesion demonstrated positive visualization; in two large lesions, even decreased uptake of the tracer was noted. The amino acid transport in most GCT is obviously too low to enable increased uptake of TYR. From these results, it can be concluded that imaging attempts with the fluorinated analogon of TYR, F-18-fluoroethyl-L-tyrosine, were futile. One can further expect that the same is true for 11C-thymidine and 18F-thymidine due to the very low proliferation rate in GCT.

4.9. Summary

In GCT to date, PET solely with the glucose analogon F-18 FDG has a certain indication but not with other tracers: In pure seminoma with bulky tumor and residuals <3 cm diameter after platinum-based chemotherapy, F-18 FDG PET is able to differentiate between nonvital and vital lesions. This is helpful in assigning the PET-negative patients to a lower risk group in which surveillance is justified, and saving surgery for patients who will show relapse from their residual tumors. The role of F-18 FDG in NSGCT is not that clear. Mature teratoma components often produce false-negative results. In primary staging, F-18 FDG PET is recommended to be performed only in selected cases or as part of clinical studies for better definition of its diagnostic performance.

Whether PET-CT provides advantages over PET and CT alone remains to be studied. So far, no systematic study in this issue exists in the body of literature. Planning of radiation therapy might become a field for PET-CT in the future.

References

1. Hoei-Hansen, C.E., Rajpert-De Meyts, E., Daugaard, G., Skakkebaek, N.E. (2005) Carcinoma in situ testis, the progenitor of testicular germ cell tumours: a clinical review *Ann Oncol* **16(6)**, 863–8.

2. Dieckmann, K.P., Loy, V. (1996) Prevalence of contralateral testicular intraepithelial neoplasia in patients with testicular germ cell neoplasms *J Clin Oncol* **14(12)**, 3126–32.

3. Harland, S.J., Cook, P.A., Fossa, S.D., et al. (1998) Intratubular germ cell neoplasia of the contralateral testis in testicular cancer: defining a high risk group *J Urol* **160(4)**, 1353–7.

4. Warde, P., Specht, L., Horwich, A., et al. (2002) Prognostic factors for relapse in stage I seminoma managed by surveillance: a pooled analysis *J Clin Oncol* **20(22)**, 4448–52.

5. Albers, P., Siener, R., Hartmann, M., et al. (1999) Risk factors for relapse in stage I non-seminomatous germ-cell tumors: preliminary results of the German Multicenter Trial. German Testicular Cancer Study Group *Int J Cancer* **83(6)**, 828–30.

6. Lindholm, P., Minn, H., Leskinen-Kallio, S., Bergman, J., Ruotsalainen, U., Joensuu, H. (1993). Influence of the blood glucose concentration on FDG uptake in cancer – a PET study *J Nucl Med.* **34(1)**, 1–6.

7. White, P.M., Adamson, D.J., Howard, G.C., Wright, A.R. (1999) Imaging of the thorax in the management of germ cell testicular tumours *Clin Radiol* **54(4)**, 207–11.

8. Krege, S., Beyer, J., Souchon, R., et al. (2008) European consensus conference on diagnosis and treatment of germ cell cancer: a report of the second meeting of the European Germ Cell Cancer Consensus group (EGCCCG): part I *Eur Urol* **53(3)**, 478–96.

9. Sternberg, C.N. (1998) The management of stage I testis cancer *Urol Clin North Am* **25(3)**, 435–49.

10. Krug, B., Heidenreich, A., Dietlein, M., Lackner, K. (1999) The lymph node staging of malignant testicular germ-cell tumors *Rofo* **171(2)**, 87–94.

11. Rustin, G.J., Mead, G.M., Stenning, S.P., et al. (2007) Randomized trial of two or five computed tomography scans in the surveillance of patients with stage I non-seminomatous germ cell tumors of the testis: Medical Research Council Trial TE08, ISRCTN56475197 – the National Cancer Research Institute Testis Cancer Clinical Studies Group *J Clin Oncol* **25(11)**, 1310–5.

12. Klepp, O., Dahl, O., Flodgren, P., et al. (1997) Risk-adapted treatment of clinical stage 1 non-seminoma testis cancer *Eur J Cancer* **33(7)**, 1038–44.

13. Albers, P., Bender, H., Yilmaz, H., Schoeneich, G., Biersack, H.J., Mueller, S.C. (1999) Positron emission tomography in the clinical staging of patients with Stage I and II testicular germ cell tumors *Urology* **53(4)**, 808–11.

14. Bender, H., Schomburg, A., Albers, P., Ruhlmann, J., Biersack, H.J. (1997) Possible role of FDG-PET in the evaluation of urologic malignancies *Anticancer Res* **17(3B)**, 1655–60.

15. de Wit, M., Brenner, W., Hartmann, M., et al. (2008) [18F]-FDG-PET in clinical stage I/II non-seminomatous germ cell tumours: results of the German multicentre trial *Ann Oncol* **19(9)**, 1619–23.

16. Huddart, R.A., O'Doherty, M.J., Padhani, A., et al. (2007) 18-fluorodeoxyglucose positron emission tomography in the prediction of relapse in patients with high-risk, clinical stage I nonseminomatous germ cell tumors: preliminary report of MRC Trial TE22 – the NCRI Testis Tumour Clinical Study Group *J Clin Oncol* **25(21)**, 3090–5.

17. Oliver, R.T., Mason, M.D., Mead, G.M., et al. (2005) Radiotherapy versus single-dose carboplatin in adjuvant treatment of stage I seminoma: a randomised trial *Lancet* **366(9482)**, 293–300.

18. Spermon, J.R., De Geus-Oei, L.F., Kiemeney, L.A., Witjes, J.A., Oyen, W.J. (2002) The role of (18)fluoro-2-deoxyglucose positron emission tomography in initial staging and re-staging after chemotherapy for testicular germ cell tumours *BJU Int* **89(6)**, 549–56.

19. Lassen, U., Daugaard, G., Eigtved, A., Hojgaard, L., Damgaard, K., Rorth, M. (2003) Whole-body FDG-PET in patients with stage I non-seminomatous germ cell tumours *Eur J Nucl Med Mol Imaging* **30(3)**, 396–402.

20. Muller-Mattheis, V., Reinhardt, M., Gerharz, C.D., et al. (1998) Positron emission tomography with [18 F]-2-fluoro-2-deoxy-D-glucose (18FDG-PET) in diagnosis of retroperitoneal lymph node metastases of testicular tumors *Urologe A* **37(6)**, 609–20.

21. Reinhardt, M.J., Muller-Mattheis, V.G., Gerharz, C.D., Vosberg, H.R., Ackermann, R., Muller-Gartner, H.W. (1997) FDG-PET evaluation of retroperitoneal metastases of testicular cancer before and after chemotherapy *J Nucl Med* **38(1)**, 99–101.

22. Cremerius, U., Effert, P.J., Adam, G., et al. (1998) FDG PET for detection and therapy control of metastatic germ cell tumor *J Nucl Med* **39(5)**, 815–22.

23. Quek, M.L., Simma-Chiang, V., Stein, J.P., Pinski, J., Quinn, D.I., Skinner, D.G. (2005) Postchemotherapy residual masses in advanced seminoma: current management and outcomes *Expert Rev Anticancer Ther* **5(5)**, 869–74.

24. Puc, H.S., Heelan, R., Mazumdar, M., et al. (1996) Management of residual mass in advanced seminoma: results and recommendations from the Memorial Sloan-Kettering Cancer Center *J Clin Oncol* **14(2)**, 454–60.

25. Horwich, A., Paluchowska, B., Norman, A., et al. (1997) Residual mass following chemotherapy of seminoma *Ann Oncol* **8(1)**, 37–40.

26. Motzer, R., Bosl, G., Heelan, R., et al. (1987) Residual mass: an indication for further therapy in patients with advanced seminoma following systemic chemotherapy *J Clin Oncol* **5(7)**, 1064–70.

27. Mosharafa, A.A., Foster, R.S., Koch, M.O., Bihrle, R., Donohue, J.P. (2004) Complications of post-chemotherapy retroperitoneal lymph node dissection for testis cancer *J Urol* **171(5)**, 1839–41.

28. Bokemeyer, C., Kollmannsberger, C., Oechsle, K., et al. (2002) Early prediction of treatment response to high-dose salvage chemotherapy in patients with relapsed germ cell cancer using [(18)F]FDG PET *Br J Cancer* **86(4)**, 506–11.

29. De Santis, M., Bokemeyer, C., Becherer, A., et al. (2001) Predictive impact of 2-18fluoro-2-deoxy-D-glucose positron emission tomography for residual postchemotherapy masses in patients with bulky seminoma *J Clin Oncol* **19(17)**, 3740–4.

30. De Santis, M., Becherer, A., Bokemeyer, C., et al. (2004) 2-18fluoro-deoxy-d-glucose positron emission tomography is a reliable predictor for viable tumor in postchemotherapy seminoma: an update of the prospective multicentric SEMPET trial *J Clin Oncol* **22(6)**, 1034–9.

31. Becherer, A., De Santis, M., Karanikas, G., et al. (2005) FDG PET is superior to CT in the prediction of viable tumour in postchemotherapy seminoma residuals *Eur J Radiol* **54(2)**, 284–8.

32. Krege, S., Beyer, J., Souchon, R., et al. (2008) European consensus conference on diagnosis and treatment of germ cell cancer: a report of the second meeting of the European Germ Cell Cancer Consensus Group (EGCCCG): part II *Eur Urol* **53(3)**, 497–513.

33. Ganjoo, K.N., Chan, R.J., Sharma, M., Einhorn, L.H. (1999) Positron emission tomography scans in the evaluation of postchemotherapy residual masses in patients with seminoma *J Clin Oncol* **17**:3457–60.

34. Guido, A., Fuccio, L., Rombi, B., et al. (2008) Combined (18)F FDG-PET/CT imaging in radiotherapy target delineation for head-and-neck cancer *Int J Radiat Oncol Biol Phys* **73(3)**, 759–63.

35. Deantonio, L., Beldi, D., Gambaro, G., et al. (2008) FDG-PET/CT imaging for staging and radiotherapy treatment planning of head and neck carcinoma *Radiat Oncol* **3**, 29.

36. Newbold, K.L., Partridge, M., Cook, G., et al. (2008) Evaluation of the role of 18FDG-PET/CT in radiotherapy target definition in patients with head and neck cancer *Acta Oncol* **47(7)**, 1229–36.

37. Yu, H.M., Liu, Y.F., Hou, M., Liu, J., Li, X.N., Yu, J.M. (2008) Evaluation of gross tumor size using CT, (18)F-FDG PET, integrated (18)F-FDG PET/CT and pathological analysis in non-small cell lung cancer *Eur J Radiol* **72(1)**, 104–13.

38. Sugawara, Y., Zasadny, K.R., Grossman, H.B., Francis, I.R., Clarke, M.F., Wahl, R.L. (1999) Germ cell tumor: differentiation of viable tumor, mature teratoma, and necrotic tissue with FDG PET and kinetic modeling *Radiology* **211(1)**, 249–56.

39. Rayson, D., Burch, P.A., Richardson, R.L. (1998) Sarcoidosis and testicular carcinoma *Cancer* **83(2)**, 337–43.

40. Karapetis, C.S., Strickland, A.H., Yip, D., van der Walt, J.D., Harper, P.G. (2001) PET and PLAP in suspected testicular cancer relapse: beware sarcoidosis *Ann Oncol* **12(10)**, 1485–8.

41. Muggia, F.M., Conti, P.S. (1998) Seminoma and sarcoidosis: a cause for false positive mediastinal uptake in PET *Ann Oncol* **9(8)**, 924.

42. Waterston, A., Seywright, M., White, J. (2006) A salutary tale of mistaken identity in testicular cancer *Urol Oncol* **24(5)**, 407–9.

43. Wang, J., Cook, G., Frank, J., et al. (2007) Case report: PET/CT, a cautionary tale *BMC Cancer* **7**, 147.

44. Nakamura, H., Makino, K., Kuratsu, J.I. (2009) Carbon 11-labeled methionine positron emission tomography for detection of residual viable tumor cells after adjuvant therapy in nongerminomatous malignant germ cell tumors in 2 cases including an autopsy case *Surg Neurol* **71(1)**, 83–8.

45. Kole, A.C., Hoekstra, H.J., Sleijfer, D.T., Nieweg, O.E., Schraffordt Koops, H., Vaalburg, W. (1998) L-[1-carbon-11]tyrosine imaging of metastatic testicular nonseminoma germ-cell tumors *J Nucl Med* **39(6)**, 1027–9.

Chapter 14

Pancreatic and Hepatobiliary Cancers

Andreas K. Buck, Ken Herrmann, Florian Eckel, and Ambros J. Beer

Abstract

Morphology-based imaging modalities have replaced classical conventional nuclear medicine modalities for detection of liver or pancreatic lesions. With positron emission tomography and the glucose analog F-18 fluorodeoxyglucose (FDG), a sensitive and specific modality for the detection of hepatic metastases and extrahepatic tumor deposits from hepatocellular or pancreatic cancer is available. F-18 FDG PET can increase the accuracy of staging primary tumors of the liver or the pancreas, and can be used for response monitoring. Radiopharmaceuticals such as Ga-68 DOTATOC and F-18 DOPA allow the specific detection of neuroendocrine pancreatic tumors and their metastatic deposits. Hybrid scanners such as PET-CT integrate morphologic and metabolic information, and allow to increase the sensitivity and specificity of noninvasive imaging in many tumor entities. The development of specific radiopharmaceuticals and technical innovations such as SPECT-CT has increased the reliability of conventional scintigraphic imaging. This chapter focuses on the use of PET-CT in hepatobiliary and pancreatic cancers.

Key words: Pancreatic cancer, Neuroendocrine cancer, Primary liver cancer, Staging, Differential diagnosis, Positron emission tomography, Hybrid imaging techniques

1. PET(-CT) Using F-18 FDG

The glucose analog $2'$-[^{18}F]-fluoro-$2'$-deoxy-D-glucose (F-18 FDG) represents the most important radiopharmaceutical for PET imaging of the liver and the pancreas. With the exclusion of several rarely observed entities, benign tumors usually do not present with increased glucose utilization. However, false-positive findings can originate from inflammatory lesions (e.g., caused by bile duct stents) or infectious diseases (e.g., liver abscesses or liver manifestations of *Echinococcus multilocularis*).

PET-CT hybrid scanners combine morphologic and metabolic imaging, thereby increasing not only the sensitivity of CT for the detection of liver or pancreatic lesions but also its specificity

Malik E. Juweid and Otto S. Hoekstra (eds.), *Positron Emission Tomography*, Methods in Molecular Biology, vol. 727, DOI 10.1007/978-1-61779-062-1_14, © Springer Science+Business Media, LLC 2011

due to better lesion characterization. Coregistration of CT also allows elimination of several shortcomings of PET. Most importantly, the number of uncertain PET findings can be significantly reduced and all PET lesions can be assigned to a definite anatomic structure. To use its full diagnostic capabilities, the CT scan can be performed with oral and/or i.v. contrast enhancement (1). Pancreatic and liver lesions frequently do not show up at low-dose CT. Therefore, if diagnostic CT within 14 days prior to PET-CT imaging is not available, acquisition of a diagnostic CT with i.v. contrast enhancement is recommended for imaging tumors of the pancreas or the liver. Recently, it has been reported that contrast-enhanced PET-CT enables detection of a higher number of hepatic lesions compared to non-enhanced PET-CT. Lower detection rates regarding small liver lesions <10 mm in size are also a well-known limitation of PET imaging. The reduced sensitivity in small liver or pancreatic lesions is caused predominantly by partial volume effects and respiratory motion artifacts. The application of oral contrast agents aids in the differentiation of the pancreatic head and the duodenum or mesenteric lymph nodes from adjacent small bowel loops (1). When a water-equivalent contrast agent is used, contrast-associated artifacts at PET can be avoided. If PET-CT is performed for response monitoring, functional data are more relevant for therapy assessment than anatomic information. Accordingly, an imaging protocol comprising a low-dose CT is recommended.

2. Ga-68 DOTATOC-PET and Ga-68 DOTATOC-PET-CT

Compared to F-18 FDG, Ga-68 DOTA-DPhe-Tyr-octreotide (Ga-68 DOTATOC) is highly specific for somatostatin receptor expressing tumors. Ga-68 DOTATOC is a recently introduced compound originating from the somatostatin analog In-111 DTPA-DPhe-octreotide. The major difference is the replacement of the gamma emitter In-111 by the positron emitter Ga-68, therefore enabling imaging with PET. A second discrepancy is the modification of the carrier molecule DTPA-DPhe-octreotide to DOTA-DPhe-Tyr-octreotide, resulting in a higher affinity of the radiotracer to the somatostatin receptor 2 (2). This causes a significantly higher sensitivity for the detection of somatostatin receptor-positive tumors (3). The sensitivity is also higher compared to that of other morphologic diagnostic modalities including contrast-enhanced CT. The combined performance of Ga-68 DOTATOC-PET and CT is useful since Ga-68 DOTATOC does not present anatomic landmarks and therefore the anatomic referencing of lesions may be difficult.

3. F-18 DOPA-PET(-CT)

Neuroendocrine tumors have the ability for decarboxylation of 5′-hydroxytryptamine and L-3,4-dihydroxyphenylalanine (L-DOPA). Therefore, it is possible to visualize neuroendocrine tumors with PET or PET-CT using the radiopharmaceutical 6-F-18 fluoro-L-DOPA. The tracer uptake is highly dependent on the histological subtype or the tumor grading. The number of clinical studies is still small. However, it has been demonstrated that F-18 DOPA-PET has a sensitivity of about 80% for the detection for liver metastases from neuroendocrine tumors, which is slightly higher compared to the performance of somatostatin receptor scintigraphy using In-111 DTPA-octreotide. On the contrary, the specificity is reduced due to false-positive findings. In summary, F-18 DOPA is a promising radiotracer that needs further evaluation.

4. Other PET-Radio-pharmaceuticals for Imaging Hepatobiliary and Pancreatic Cancers

A high number of innovative radiopharmaceuticals with a potential for visualizing and quantifying specific pathophysiologic processes are currently under evaluation. For hepatobiliary cancers, nucleoside analogs such as 3′-deoxy-3′-F-18 fluorothymidine (F-18 FLT) may be used to image the proliferative activity of primary pancreatic or liver cancers specifically (4). This approach may aid in differential diagnosis of benign and malignant tumors and early response monitoring (5). Imidazole derivatives such as F-18 misonidazole (FMISO) can be used for specific imaging of hypoxic tumor tissue, potentially leading to more efficient radiotherapy by increasing the radiation dose to the hypoxic fraction of tumors. The radiotracer F-18 galacto-RGD is a pentapeptide binding to the integrin $\alpha v \beta_3$ which plays an important role in angioneogenesis and metastasis (6). These radiopharmaceuticals are able to quantify specific metabolic processes or the expression of certain receptors in vivo. Yet the role of these PET tracers for imaging hepatobiliary or pancreatic cancers remains to be determined.

5. Pancreatic Cancer

With about 34,000 new pancreatic cancers diagnosed in USA in 2006, the incidence of pancreatic cancer is lower compared to that of the most common tumor entities. Cure is possible only at very early stages of the disease. Since most patients are diagnosed at a late stage preventing curative surgery, the vast majority of patients die from their disease. In 2006, approximately 32,000 deaths from pancreatic cancer were expected in USA. Recently, an increase in the incidence of pancreatic cancer has been reported, presumably arising from an increased life expectancy of the population. Of the pancreatic cancers, 80% are derived from ductal origin and represent adenocarcinomas, and 5–10% originate from islet cells. The most frequent localization is the pancreatic head with about 70%; tumors in the pancreatic corpus or the tail of the pancreas appear in 20% and 10%, respectively. The early diagnosis of pancreatic cancer is still challenging despite the progress in diagnostic technologies. The most relevant modalities comprise ultrasound of the abdomen, CT, and tumor markers such as CEA and Ca 19-9. Besides CT, magnetic resonance imaging (MRI) and MR-based illustration of the bile duct system/pancreatic duct (MRCP), endoscopic retrograde cholangiopancreatography (ERCP), and endoscopic ultrasound (EUS) are frequently performed. Endoscopic ultrasound is frequently combined with fine-needle aspiration biopsy (7). Angiography using contrast enhancement is another technique for the detection and characterization of hepatobiliary tumors, but this invasive technique is less frequently performed.

With a median survival of 17 months, the outcome of patients with pancreatic cancer is poor (8, 9). The only curative approach so far used is the total resection of the tumor, usually performed as pancreatoduodenectomy (Whipple's procedure). Total pancreatectomy or resection of the pancreatic tail is less common. Only the tumor stages T1 and T2 are regarded as resectable tumors, whereas locally advanced or metastasized tumors are regarded as incurable. The benefit of preoperative, neoadjuvant chemoradiotherapy is currently under investigation. After surgery, adjuvant chemoradiotherapy can be applied to increase cure rates. However, the impact of this approach on patient outcome, quality of life, and overall survival remains to be determined (10).

5.1. Conventional Imaging of Pancreatic Tumors

Imaging of the pancreas remains challenging. Besides initial tumor staging, monitoring response to treatment and diagnosis of recurrent disease are increasingly performed indications for imaging. Especially, sensitive detection of early cancers and lymph node metastases, differential diagnosis of pancreatic cancer and chronic, mass-forming pancreatitis, and the noninvasive assessment of tumor resectability remain challenging. In patients with newly diagnosed pancreatic tumors, the sensitivity of helical CT for detecting pancreatic cancer is 65–90% and the specificity 46–85%. The positive predictive values (PPVs) and negative predictive values (NPVs) were reported to be as high as 79–87% and 31–61%, respectively (11). For prediction of resectability with CT, heterogenous results have been reported with a PPV of 89% and an NPV of 28% (12). In a recent meta-analysis, Bipat and colleagues reported sensitivity and specificity values of 81% or 82%, respectively (11). With the availability of modern multi-slice CT scanners using more advanced imaging protocols such as dynamic multiphase CT, the accuracy of CT imaging is steadily increasing. Abdominal ultrasound is available and less costly but insufficient for assessment of resectability. Endoscopic ultrasound has been shown to be significantly more sensitive. Detection rates of pancreatic cancer are reported between 93% and 98% (13–15). The resectability can be predicted correctly in 88% of the patients. T-staging at EUS was reported to be correct in 67% and nodal staging in 44%.

Magnetic resonance imaging offers superior tissue contrast compared to CT and other imaging modalities. Regarding detection of pancreatic cancer, MRI has a sensitivity of 84–88% and a specificity of 78%, respectively (11, 13). In multicenter studies, an accuracy value of 70% and a PPV of 88% have been reported for the differentiation of resectable and unresectable cancer. However, the corresponding NPV was as low as 23% (12). Therefore, MRI is not regarded as a method of choice for initial staging and assessment of resectability of pancreatic cancer (16). Novel, diffusion-weighted imaging protocols have the potential to increase the accuracy of MRI; however, data regarding this are lacking in the literature.

5.2. PET(-CT) for Differentiating Benign from Malignant Pancreatic Tumors

Bares and colleagues were one of the first to demonstrate the opportunity to differentiate benign from malignant pancreatic tumors based on an increased glucose utilization in malignant lesions. Of 13 pancreatic cancers, 12 presented with increased focal F-18 FDG uptake (sensitivity 92%), whereas two benign tumors were negative at F-18 FDG PET (17). Table 1 summarizes publications addressing sensitivity and specificity values of PET(-CT) regarding detection of pancreatic cancer and differential diagnosis of pancreatic masses (18–32). For F-18 FDG PET, meta-analyses comprising more than 1,000 patients report a median sensitivity of 91% and a median specificity of 78%, respectively. However, there is a wide range of reported sensitivity and specificity values in individual studies (sensitivity, 64–96%; specificity, 64–94%). These numbers are somewhat lower compared to those published for other solid cancers. This observation is presumably related to increased blood sugar values which can be frequently observed in patients with pancreatic tumors. In a series of Zimny and colleagues, 25% of the study collective had diabetes (32). Whereas in patients with normal blood sugar values, the sensitivity of PET was adequate with a value of 98% (46/47), the sensitivity dropped to 68% (17/27) in patients with hyperglycemia. The tumoral uptake (F-18 FDG-SUV) in patients with normal

Table 1

Differential diagnosis of pancreatic tumors (cancer vs. inflammatory lesions or benign tumors) with PET(-CT) (*, cystic pancreatic tumors)

	Number of patients studied	Imaging modality	Sensitivity (%)	Specificity (%)
(73)(*)	68	PET	57	85
(31)	109	PET-CT	91	87
(28)	86	PET-CT	88	88
(22)	95	PET-CT	89	69
(26)	104	PET	89	64
(25)	86	PET	91	76
(27)	47	PET	96	75
(29)	42	PET	71	64
(19)	65	PET	92	85
(20)	152	PET	86	78
(32)	106	PET	85	84
(23)	46	PET	94	82
(21)	80	PET	94	88
(24)	24	PET	93	78
(18)	40	PET	93	85

blood glucose values was significantly higher with 6.9 ± 3.7 compared to 5.5 ± 3.4 in patients with hyperglycemia at the time point of PET imaging. Recently, it has been suggested that treatment with insulin should be performed in hyperglycemic patients to increase the sensitivity of PET. Delbeke and colleagues applied insulin i.v. (2–10 i.e.) every 15 min to achieve blood sugar values below 150 mg/dl (19). This approach resulted in a sensitivity value of 80% in diabetic patients. A recent guideline of the Society of Nuclear Medicine (SNM) admits the use of insulin for this purpose (33). However, it is recommended that the time point of F-18 FDG injection should be delayed to reduce unspecific tracer uptake in muscle tissue. The second drawback of the use of F-18 FDG in pancreatic cancer is a frequently observed coexistence of malignant tumors with inflammatory processes such as acute or chronic active pancreatitis. Diederichs and colleagues showed that the specificity of F-18 FDG PET significantly drops if C-reactive protein (CRP) is elevated or an increased leukocyte count can be measured in the peripheral blood (34). The specificity was as low as 40% compared to 87% in patients with normal CRP values or normal white blood cell count.

5.3. PET(-CT) for Staging Pancreatic Cancer

In patients with pancreatic cancer, detection of locoregional lymph node and distant metastases is an important challenge for noninvasive imaging modalities. Many studies have shown that the performance of PET for lymph node staging is poor (Table 2), with sensitivity values of 17%–33%, Table 2: 32% (19, 22, 26). Also, integrated PET-CT imaging does not lead to a significant increase in sensitivity, as recently reported by Heinrich and colleagues (22). Better sensitivity values of PET(-CT) have been reported for the detection of liver, peritoneal, or extra-abdominal metastases (Fig. 1). In the study by Heinrich, the sensitivity of PET regarding detection of liver metastases was 81% (13/16), which was significantly higher than that of contrast-enhanced CT (56%, 9/16). The specificity of CT regarding detection of liver metastases was 95% compared to 100% of PET-CT.

Due to the sensitive detection of distant metastases, two publications reported a significant impact of PET and PET-CT regarding patient management. In the series of Delbeke et al., the therapeutic regimen was changed in 8/56 (13%) patients due to the detection of previously unknown metastases (19). Heinrich reported an impact of PET-CT on therapeutic decision making in 16%, predominantly due to prevention of surgery in patients with distant metastases detected exclusively at F-18 FDG PET(-CT) (22). Cost effectiveness of PET(-CT) has been addressed by only one study (22). Due to the prevention of futile surgery, there was a gain of 62,900 US$ compared to the theoretical approach of conventional preoperative staging without PET. However, additional costs for chemo or radiochemotherapy in patients not

Table 2
N-Staging of pancreatic cancer with PET(-CT)
(*, software-based image fusion)

	Number of patients studied	Imaging modality	Sensitivity (%)	Specificity (%)
(22)	95	PET-CT	21 (3/14)	
(26)	104	PET-CT (*)	32 (10/31)	
(19)	65	PET	17 (2/12)	
(32)	106	PET	46 (12/26)	
(18)	40	PET	61 (19/31)	

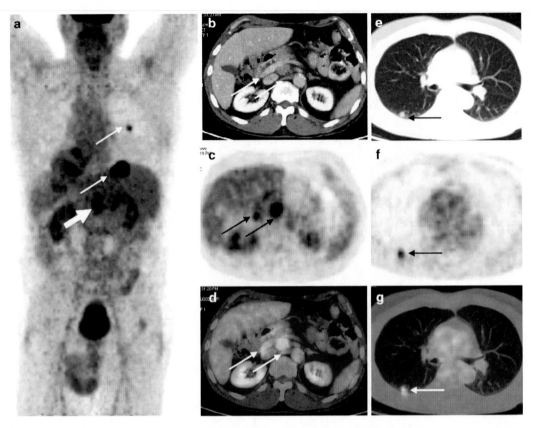

Fig. 1. Detection of metastatic disease in a 54-year-old patient with pancreatic cancer using F-18 FDG PET-CT. (a) Intense focal F-18 FDG uptake in the malignant primary tumor (*large arrow*); small arrows indicate liver metastases and a solitary lung metastasis. (b) Enlarged retroperitoneal lymph nodes are present at helical CT and are indicative of locoregional lymph node metastases. (c) F-18 FDG PET reveals intense glucose uptake corresponding to enlarged lymph nodes. (d) Image fusion (PET-CT) demonstrates the typical finding of locoregional lymph node metastases with high glucose utilization. (e) Solitary pulmonary nodule is present at helical CT (*arrow*). (f) Intense focal F-18 FDG uptake in the right lower lobe is highly suspicious for metastatic disease. (g) Image fusion demonstrates a solitary lung metastasis with intense glucose utilization.

undergoing surgery have not been calculated. Therefore, the additional value of functional imaging with PET(-CT) for staging pancreatic cancer needs to be addressed in future multicenter trials (Table 3).

5.4. Recurrent Disease

Ruf and colleagues assessed 31 patients with clinical suspicion of local relapse (35). The patients were included due to increased tumor marker levels (Ca 19-9) or clinical signs of recurrence. PET was able to detect 96% of local recurrences (22/23), which was significantly higher than that detected by CT or MRI (9/23). Also, distant recurrence in the abdomen could be detected exclusively at PET (7/7) vs. 0/7 with CT and MRI, whereas CT and MRI performed better for the detection of small liver metastases

Table 3
M-Staging of pancreatic cancer with PET(-CT) (*, software-based image fusion)

	Number of patients studied	Imaging modality	Sensitivity (%)	Specificity (%)
(22)	95	PET-CT	81 (13/16)	100 (43/43)
(74)	34	PET	93 (28/30)	
(26)	104	PET-CT (*)		100 (14/14)
(15)	35	PET	78 (7/9)	
(19)	65	PET	81 (17/21)	
(75)	168	PET	68 (15/22)	95 (138/146)
(32)	106	PET	51 (16/31)	
(18)	40	PET	54 (7/13)	

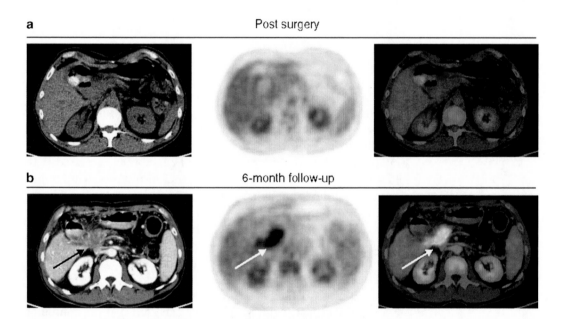

Fig. 2. F-18 FDG PET-CT for detection of recurrent pancreatic cancer. In a follow-up study performed 6 months after resection of the primary tumor (**a**), CT (*left*), PET (*middle*), and PET-CT (*right*) do not reveal evidence for local recurrence, or lymph node or distant metastases. At a further 6-month follow-up (**b**), a soft tissue mass in the region of the pancreatic head is evident at helical CT (*left*); F-18 FDG PET indicates intense focal F-18 FDG uptake of the suspicious lesion. Fused PET-CT image (*right*) indicates local recurrence of pancreatic cancer.

(92%, 11/12 vs. 42%, 5/12). However, numbers are small and the added value of PET imaging needs to be addressed on a larger series. Figure 2 demonstrates the typical appearance of local recurrence from pancreatic cancer at PET-CT follow-up.

5.5. Response Monitoring and Prognostic Utility of PET in Pancreatic Cancer

Several studies have indicated an association of tumoral F-18 FDG uptake and individual prognosis. All publications showed that the F-18 FDG uptake was inversely correlated with overall survival. In the study by Zimny et al., the tumor marker Ca 19-9 and F-18 FDG SUV were the only independent predictors using multivariate analysis. In patients with an SUV <6.1, overall survival was 5 months compared to 9 months in patients with an SUV ≥6.1 (36). Lyshchik and coworkers assessed the prognostic utility of dual-phase F-18 FDG PET in 65 patients (37). To date, only a few studies comprising a limited number of patients have been performed. As shown for other cancers, functional imaging with PET was able to discriminate responding from nonresponding tumors already 2 months after the start of therapy, whereas no significant change in tumor size was observed at spiral CT (38). In another small series comprising 11 patients, Maisey assessed the effect of treatment with 5-fluorouracil in combination or without mitomycin C and identified 6 patients without residual F-18 FDG uptake, which was associated with significantly longer overall survival (319 days vs. 139 days, respectively) (39).

6. Neuroendocrine Tumors of the Pancreas

Because of the usually slow tumor growth and a nonsignificantly increased glucose metabolism, neuroendocrine tumors (NETs) usually do not present with focal F-18 FDG uptake (40). Only rapidly growing, undifferentiated NETs exhibit an increased F-18 FDG uptake. On the contrary, somatostatin receptor scintigraphy is an established, highly specific, and sensitive technique for the diagnosis of primary NETs of the pancreas and detection of metastases. With Ga-68 DOTATOC, there is a corresponding PET tracer, which has led to a significant increase in the diagnostic accuracy of functional tumor imaging. For detecting lesions of NET, PET using Ga-68 DOTATOC as the tracer exceeds the performance of morphology-based imaging modalities regarding sensitivity and specificity (Fig. 3). It can be expected that the combined examination with contrast-enhanced CT and PET (PET-CT) using Ga-68 DOTATOC will be a standard approach for tumor screening and staging/restaging of NETs of the pancreas, because integrated imaging allows also the definite localization of PET lesions.

7. Hepatocellular Carcinoma

Primary hepatobiliary tumors are among the leading causes of cancer death worldwide. Hepatocellular carcinoma (HCC) represents the most frequent histological subtype with >60% of primary liver

a   Before surgery

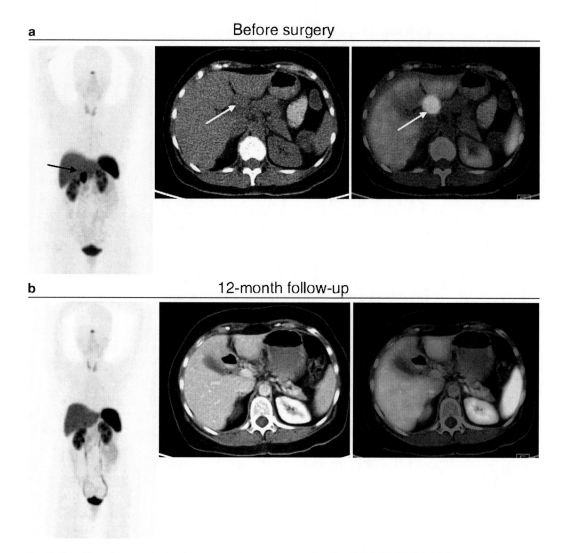

b   12-month follow-up

Fig. 3. Detection of a neuroendocrine pancreatic carcinoma using Ga-68 DOTATOC-PET-CT. The whole body view (**a**) indicates an intense focal uptake of Ga-68 DOTATOC in the area of the pancreatic head, representing a somatostatin receptor (sstr2)-expressing tumor. The CT indicates the malignant primary tumor (*arrow, middle*); the fused image indicates intense tracer uptake of the neuroendocrine pancreatic carcinoma. A 12-month follow-up study (**b**) showed normal CT findings (*middle*). There is also no evidence for local recurrence or lymph node/distant metastases at whole-body view of Ga-68 DOTATOC-PET (*left*) or fused image (*right*).

cancers. In endemic regions such as Southeastern Asia or central areas of Africa, HCC represents one of the most common malignant tumors, with an overall incidence of 1,000,000 new cases every year. In USA and Europe, the incidence of HCC is <3% of all cancers. The prognosis of liver cancer is poor with approximately 11 months of median survival of untreated patients. As mentioned above for pancreatic cancers, surgical resection of the primary tumor is the only kind of treatment with the potential of cure. This is feasible only in a minority of patients. Most patients suffer from liver cirrhosis and present with reduced liver function, preventing extensive surgery. Locoregional treatment strategies include percutaneous thermal tumor ablation (e.g., radiofrequency ablation and laser-induced thermotherapy) or selective internal radiotherapy (SIRT). Transarterial chemoembolization has the potential to induce necrosis of the liver tumor but has not been demonstrated to increase survival.

7.1. Conventional Imaging of Primary Liver Tumors

Standard diagnostic procedures include ultrasound (US) of the liver, CT, and MRI, whereas CT is usually performed as three-phase helical CT. Recently, screening for the presence of HCC has been suggested in patients with liver cirrhosis. Sensitivity values for the detection of HCC with US have been reported between 35% and 84% (41). CT is the standard imaging modality for further assessment of liver lesions detected at US. Sensitivity of spiral CT ranges between 92% and 95% (42). MRI is also frequently used for imaging of hepatic lesions. The sensitivity is slightly higher compared to that of CT, with values between 75% and 94% (42). Diagnosis of HCC is very likely in tumors larger than 20 mm and with markedly increased AFP serum levels (>400 µg/L). In lesions <20 mm, specificity of AFP is insufficient for the diagnosis of HCC, and a biopsy is recommended (42).

Tumors leading to biliary obstruction can be additionally imaged using magnetic resonance cholangiopancreatography (MRCP) or ERCP. Sensitivity and specificity values for differentiation of malignant from benign causes of biliary obstruction were reported to be 81% and 70% for MRCP and 74% and 70% for ERCP, respectively (43). Delayed contrast CT has been reported to increase tumor detection with sensitivity and specificity values of 74% and 82%, respectively. MRI is a sensitive modality for the detection of cholangiocellular carcinoma (CCC), usually presenting with mild or moderate rim enhancement followed by a concentric filling with the contrast agent.

7.2. PET and PET-CT for Imaging and Staging of Hepatocellular Carcinoma

PET using the glucose analog F-18 FDG does not have a high sensitivity for the detection of HCC, since highly differentiated tumors have the ability to accomplish gluconeogenesis and, therefore, can convert F-18 FDG-6-phosphate to F-18 FDG (44–46). Consecutively, the trapping of the radiopharmaceutical is reduced, resulting in a low sensitivity. The sensitivity of F-18 FDG PET can be increased to a yield of 62.5% if a delayed acquisition of PET data after 2–3 h is performed (47). Therefore, the current role F-18 FDG PET in HCC applies only to the detection of extrahepatic tumor deposits in patients with F-18 FDG-avid primary lesions (Fig. 4). In a pilot study, a change in the therapeutic management has been observed in 26% of the patients due to the detection of extrahepatic tumor deposits (48). However, the role of F-18 FDG PET(-CT) for staging and management of

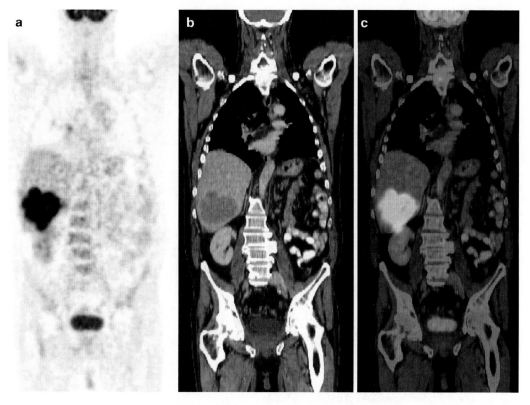

Fig. 4. Demonstration of F-18 FDG-avid hepatocellular carcinoma in the right liver lobe. (**a**) Intense focal F-18 FDG uptake of the malignant primary tumor (F-18 FDG PET, coronary section); (**b**) corresponding coronal section of helical CT; (**c**) fused PET-CT image indicating intense glucose utilization of the primary tumor. There is no evidence for distant metastases at PET-CT.

patients with HCC needs to be evaluated in prospective studies comprising a higher number of included patients.

The sensitivity of PET imaging may be increased with more innovative tracers enabling molecular tumor imaging. Recently, Ho and coworkers indicated that HCC negative at F-18 FDG PET may be visualized with PET and C-11 acetate, which is a substrate for ß-oxidation and a precursor for the biosynthesis of amino acids and fatty acids (49). The authors have demonstrated F-18 FDG uptake predominantly in poorly differentiated HCC, whereas C-11 acetate accumulated in well-differentiated cancers. C-11 acetate was also specific for HCC and did not accumulate in metastatic liver lesions or CCC. Another study by the same group demonstrated a high sensitivity, specificity, and accuracy for detecting extrahepatic metastases from HCC (98%, 86%, and 96%, respectively) (50). There was also a change in patient management due to the detection of metastases not described with standard imaging modalities. C-11 choline has also been suggested for imaging of HCC, whereas the use of C-11 choline is hampered by physiologically high uptake of the radiotracer in the liver (51).

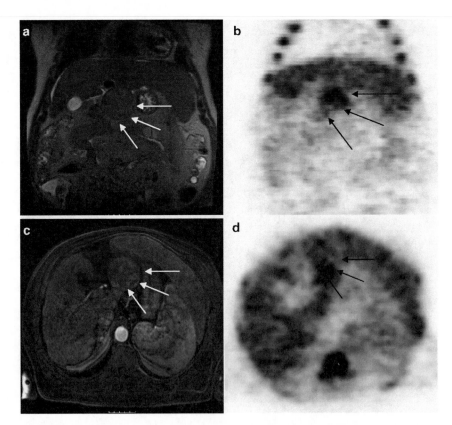

Fig. 5. Demonstration of the proliferation fraction of hepatocellular carcinoma (HCC) using PET with the radionucleoside 3'-deoxy-3'-F-18-fluorothymidine (F-18 FLT) for tumor detection. (**a, c**) coronal and transaxial MRI sections demonstrating exact lesion size of the malignant primary tumor (*arrow*); (**b, d**) corresponding sections of F-18 FLT PET showing intense focal tracer uptake in HCC. Additional, diffuse F-18 FLT uptake can be seen in the vertebral column, representing physiologically increased proliferation fraction of bone marrow; moderately intense background uptake of F-18 FLT in the liver due to glucuronidation of the radiotracer.

The in vivo proliferation marker F-18 FLT may be used for noninvasive characterization of the proliferation fraction of HCC (Fig. 5). In a small series of our own group, sensitivity of F-18 FLT PET was 70% (13/18), Eckel et al. [72] for the detection of primary cancers (unpublished data). Whether increased tracer uptake can be used for identification of more aggressive tumors potentially responding to chemotherapy or targeted drugs remains to be determined.

7.3. PET(-CT) for Response Assessment in Hepatocellular Carcinoma and Detection of Recurrence

Magnetic resonance imaging has become the standard imaging modality for monitoring local response of HCC, with very high sensitivity and specificity values reported in the literature (52). To date, there is no publication indicating a potential role of integrated PET-CT imaging for monitoring response to treatment in HCC.

However, there may be a role of PET and PET-CT for the detection of recurrent HCC. Recently, Chen and coworkers reported an acceptable sensitivity, specificity, and accuracy of F-18 FDG PET for detecting recurrent HCC (73.3%, 100%, and 74.2%, respectively) (53). However, the patient number (26) was rather small. The clinical utility of PET(-CT) regarding response monitoring and detection of recurrence needs to be investigated in studies comprising larger patient numbers.

8. Cholangiocellular Carcinoma and Gallbladder Carcinoma

Compared to HCC, CCC and gallbladder carcinoma represent rare tumor entities. Usually, CCC presents with increased F-18 FDG uptake (54, 55). F-18 FDG is not secreted by the biliary system and, therefore, every uptake in the bile duct system has to be interpreted as pathologic uptake. Compared to HCC, F-18 FDG PET has a relatively high sensitivity for the detection of CCC. In a retrospective study comprising 36 patients with CCC and 14 patients with gallbladder cancer, unspecific F-18 FDG uptake has been observed in inflammatory lesions, especially in granulomas and sclerosing cholangitis, causing false-positive findings (54). F-18 FDG PET caused a change in the therapeutic management in about 30% of the patients. Therefore, F-18 FDG PET may have a gaining role for staging of patients with CCC (Fig. 6). Further studies indicate sensitivity values from 61% up to 90%, respectively (54, 56, 57). False-positive findings have been reported due to biliary stent-associated inflammatory reactions. In the study by Anderson et al., a high sensitivity of F-18 FDG PET regarding detection of distant metastases has been described, resulting in a change in the therapeutic management in a significant number of patients (54).

F-18 FDG PET(-CT) is not routinely performed in gallbladder cancer since the majority of tumors are diagnosed accidentally after cholecystectomy. Reports indicate that PET may be useful to identify residual tumor tissue with a sensitivity of 78% and a specificity of 80% (54). Dual time-point imaging may further increase the capability of F-18 FDG PET for differentiating benign from malignant tumors. Nishiyama et al. reported an increase in sensitivity from 83% to 96% when delayed PET imaging is used for interpretation and to a value of 100% if combined early and delayed imaging are evaluated, using cut-off values of F-18 FDG SUV = 4.5 (early PET scan) and 2.9 (delayed PET scan), respectively. However, this approach was associated with a reduced specificity of 44% compared to 56% using standard PET imaging (58, 59).

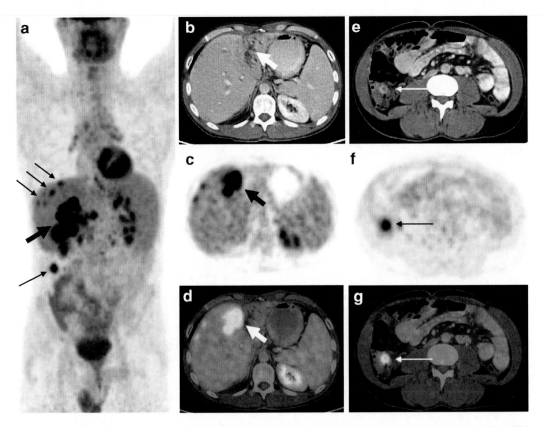

Fig. 6. Initial staging of a 61-year-old patient with cholangiocellular carcinoma (CCC). (a) whole-body view of F-18 FDG PET indicating the primary tumor (*large arrow*), metastatic sites in the liver (*small arrows*), and an additional extrahepatic metastasis in the abdomen (*small arrow*). Appearance of the malignant primary and metastatic liver lesions of CCC at CT (b), F-18 FDG PET (c), and F-18 FDG PET-CT (d). (e, f, g) Demonstration of the metastatic site in the abdomen at helical CT (e), F- 18 FDG PET (f), and F-18 FDG PET-CT (g).

9. Liver Metastases

9.1. Imaging

Ultrasound and MRI have displaced conventional scintigraphic modalities for the detection of liver metastases. Functional liver scintigraphy and colloid scintigraphy play only a marginal role for the differential diagnosis of hepatic tumors (60). The sensitivity in noncurrent clinical studies is reported to be as high as 60–90% (60). Due to an increased glucose metabolism, liver metastases usually present with increased focal F-18 FDG uptake. In colorectal cancer, F-18 FDG PET has a high sensitivity and specificity (91% and 95%) for detecting liver metastases (61). However, for detection of smaller metastases with a size <10 mm, the sensitivity is markedly reduced (62). In a meta-analysis from 2002, F-18 FDG PET had the highest median sensitivity compared to that of CT and MRI (63). It can be expected that multi-slice CT and contrast-enhanced MRI have a higher sensitivity, especially for the detection of metastases markedly smaller than 10 mm. There is an advantage for F-18 FDG PET regarding a higher specificity and the option to detect extrahepatic metastases and local recurrence of the primary tumor. Recently, Ruers et al. reported a PET-based change of the therapeutic management in 10 of 51 patients (20%) (64). This was made possible by the detection or exclusion of liver metastases or extrahepatic tumor deposits. In patients with increasing tumor markers, F-18 FDG PET has been demonstrated to have a high sensitivity of 93% and a high specificity of 98% to detect or exclude local recurrence or hepatic metastases with high accuracy (65).

9.2. PET(-CT) for Response Monitoring in Liver Metastases

The more frequently performed imaging modalities such as CT, MRI, or US do not always allow a reliable estimation of therapy response. Especially, the clinically relevant demonstration of response to treatment at an early time point after initiation of a specific treatment protocol using morphometric criteria is relatively difficult. Also, at the end of therapy, residual vital tumor tissue cannot be reliably excluded and differentiated from therapy-related fibrosis. F-18 FDG PET has been demonstrated to be superior compared to morphology-based imaging modalities regarding therapy monitoring in primary tumors (e.g., colorectal cancer) and liver metastases. The progression of liver metastases could be detected significantly earlier with PET (5 vs. 8.4 months) compared to that with CT (8.5 vs. 9.8 months) (66). F-18 FDG PET is now increasingly used for monitoring response to selective internal radiotherapy with ^{90}Y microspheres (SIRT). However, only case reports are published in the literature. The clinical evaluation of new PET tracers such as Ga-68 DOTATOC, F-18 galacto-RGD, or F-18 FLT will increase the possibilities of response monitoring with PET(-CT).

10. Conventional Nuclear Medical Imaging Modalities for Imaging Hepatobiliary Cancers

Recently, the importance of conventional imaging modalities for the clinical work-up of liver lesions has decreased. However, with the availability of hybrid scanners (SPECT-CT), these techniques may become more important in the future and are, therefore, briefly summarized.

10.1. Blood Pool Scintigraphy

Blood pool scintigraphy relies on the infusion of Tc-99m-labeled erythrocytes for the visualization of blood flow in the liver or the blood pool. The major indication for blood pool scintigraphy is the detection of liver hemangioma. Because of the cavernous structure, the tracer accumulation is low at the beginning of the examination and increases over time. Liver metastases usually present with intense focal uptake of the radiotracer.

10.2. Colloid Scintigraphy of the Liver

In the liver, there are approximately 15% Kupffer cells which have the potential to accomplish phagocytosis. Depending on the size of the particles, the integrity of phagocytosis can be assessed with Tc-99m-labeled colloid particles (particle size 200–1,000 nm). Diseases leading to destruction of the reticuloendothelial system (RES) of the liver usually present as an area of decreased or missing uptake of the radiotracer. However, the specificity of this modality is low (67). At colloid scintigraphy, HCC usually presents with a photopenic defect; however, it remains difficult to differentiate malignoma-associated lesions and areas of decreased uptake caused by liver cirrhosis.

10.3. Hepatobiliary Functional Scintigraphy

Tc-99m-labeled iminodiacetate derivatives (e.g., Tc-99m IDA) have been established which are actively taken up by hepatocytes and excreted consecutively by the biliary system. Reabsorption in the intestines does not occur. The maximum uptake in the liver parenchyma can be observed about 10 ± 3 min post-injury; after 10 ± 4 min, the ductus choledochus becomes visible and the gall-bladder can be detected after 15 ± 5 min. Diseases that are associated with destruction and loss of function of the liver parenchyma usually present as a photopenic defect (e.g., metastases). At functional liver scintigraphy, a reduced or missing tracer uptake in the parenchymal phase can be observed. The mode of tracer uptake, however, shows an overlap to that of focal nodular hyperplasia (FNH) (68). The intensity of the tracer uptake is also affected by tumor grading. Therefore, different uptake patterns from a photopenic defect to intense focal uptake can be observed in the parenchymal phase. Therefore, reliable criteria for the diagnosis of HCC are missing, similar to morphologic imaging modalities.

10.4. Octreotide Scintigraphy

Neuroendocrine tumors usually present with increased expression levels of somatostatin receptors (SSTR). Radiolabeled ligands such as In-111 DTPA-DPhe-octreotide have the ability to detect SSTR-positive liver metastases or primary liver or pancreatic tumors specifically (69). Besides detection of metastases, octreotide scintigraphy can also be used to evaluate a potential therapeutic option with somatostatin analogs and to monitor response to treatment.

10.5. Less Frequently Performed Imaging Modalities

Liver metastases from malignant tumors of the chromoaffine tissue (e.g., pheochromocytoma) can be specifically detected with I-123/131 MIBG (70). Radiolabeled antibodies that specifically bind to cell surface molecules of neutrophil granulocytes (anti-NCA95) can be used for specific detection of intrahepatic abscesses. For the same purpose, leukocyte scintigraphy can be used utilizing autologous leukocytes labeled with In-111 oxine or with Tc-99m HMPAO. The detection of malignant liver tumors or abscesses can also be performed using Ga-67 citrate scintigraphy (71).

References

1. Kuehl, H., Veit, P., Rosenbaum, S.J., Bockisch, A., Antoch, G. (2007) Can PET-CT replace separate diagnostic CT for cancer imaging? Optimizing CT protocols for imaging cancers of the chest and abdomen *J Nucl Med* **48(1)**, 45S–57S.

2. Reubi, J.C., Schar, J.C., Waser, B., et al. (2000) Affinity profiles for human somatostatin receptor subtypes SST1–SST5 of somatostatin radiotracers selected for scintigraphic and radiotherapeutic use *Eur J Nucl Med* **27(3)**, 273–82.

3. Hofmann, M., Maecke, H., Borner, R., et al. (2001) Biokinetics and imaging with the somatostatin receptor PET radioligand (68) Ga-DOTATOC: preliminary data *Eur J Nucl Med* **28(12)**:1751–7.

4. Francis, D.L., Visvikis, D., Costa, D.C., et al. (2003)Potential impact of [18F]3'-deoxy-3'-fluorothymidine versus [18F]fluoro-2-deoxy-D-glucose in positron emission tomography for colorectal cancer *Eur J Nucl Med Mol Imaging* **30(7)**, 988–94.

5. Herrmann, K., Eckel, F., Schmidt, S., et al. (2008) In vivo characterization of proliferation for discriminating cancer from pancreatic pseudotumors *J Nucl Med* **49(9)**, 1437–44.

6. Beer, A.J., Haubner, R., Sarbia, M., et al. (2006) Positron emission tomography using [18F]Galacto-RGD identifies the level of integrin alpha(v)beta3 expression in man *Clin Cancer Res* **12(13)**, 3942–9.

7. Santo, E. (2004) Pancreatic cancer imaging: which method *Jop* **5(4)**, 253–7.

8. Sohn, T.A., Yeo, C.J., Cameron, J.L., et al. (2000) Resected adenocarcinoma of the pancreas-616 patients: results, outcomes, and prognostic indicators. *J Gastrointest Surg* **4(6)**, 567–79.

9. Yeo, C.J., Abrams, R.A., Grochow, L.B., et al. (1997) Pancreaticoduodenectomy for pancreatic adenocarcinoma: postoperative adjuvant chemoradiation improves survival. A prospective, single-institution experience *Ann Surg* **225(5)**, 621–33; discussion 633–6

10. Cardenes, H.R., Chiorean, E.G., Dewitt, J., Schmidt, M., Loehrer, P. (2006) Locally advanced pancreatic cancer: current therapeutic approach *Oncologist* **11(6)**, 612–23.

11. Bipat, S., Phoa, S.S., van Delden, O.M., et al. (2005) Ultrasonography, computed tomography and magnetic resonance imaging for diagnosis and determining resectability of pancreatic adenocarcinoma: a meta-analysis *J Comput Assist Tomogr* **29(4)**, 438–45.

12. Megibow, A.J., Zhou, X.H., Rotterdam, H., et al. (1995) Pancreatic adenocarcinoma: CT versus MR imaging in the evaluation of resectability--report of the Radiology Diagnostic Oncology Group *Radiology* **195(2)**, 327–32.

13. Borbath, I., Van Beers, B.E., Lonneux, M., et al. (2005) Preoperative assessment of pancreatic tumors using magnetic resonance imaging, endoscopic ultrasonography, positron emission tomography and laparoscopy *Pancreatology* **5(6)**, 553–61.

14. DeWitt, J., Devereaux, B., Chriswell, M., et al. (2004) Comparison of endoscopic ultrasonography and multidetector computed tomography for detecting and staging pancreatic cancer *Ann Int Med* **141(10)**, 753–63.

15. Mertz, H.R., Sechopoulos, P., Delbeke, D., Leach, S.D. (2000) EUS, PET, and CT scanning for evaluation of pancreatic adenocarcinoma *Gastrointest Endosc* **52(3)**, 367–71.

16. Soriano, A., Castells, A., Ayuso, C., et al. (2004) Preoperative staging and tumor resectability assessment of pancreatic cancer: prospective study comparing endoscopic ultrasonography, helical computed tomography, magnetic resonance imaging, and angiography *Am J Gastroenterol* **99(3)**, 492–501.

17. Bares, R., Dohmen, B.M., Cremerius, U., Fass, J., Teusch, M., Bull, U. (1996) Results of positron emission tomography with fluorine-18 labeled fluorodeoxyglucose in differential diagnosis and staging of pancreatic carcinoma *Radiologe* **36**, 435–40.

18. Bares, R., Klever, P., Hauptmann, S., et al. (1994) F-18 fluorodeoxyglucose PET in vivo evaluation of pancreatic glucose metabolism for detection of pancreatic cancer *Radiology* **192(1)**, 79–86.

19. Delbeke, D., Rose, D.M., Chapman, W.C., et al. (1999) Optimal interpretation of FDG PET in the diagnosis, staging and management of pancreatic carcinoma *J Nucl Med* **40(11)**, 1784–91.

20. Diederichs, C.G., Staib, L., Glatting, G., Beger, H.G., Reske, S.N. (1998) FDG PET: elevated plasma glucose reduces both uptake and detection rate of pancreatic malignancies *J Nucl Med* **39(6)**, 1030–1033.

21. Friess, H., Langhans, J., Ebert, M., et al. (1995) Diagnosis of pancreatic cancer by 2[18F]-fluoro-2-deoxy-D-glucose positron emission tomography *Gut* **36(5)**, 771–7.

22. Heinrich, S., Goerres, G.W., Schafer, M., et al. (2005) Positron emission tomography/computed tomography influences on the

management of resectable pancreatic cancer and its cost-effectiveness *Ann Surg* **242(2)**, 235–43.

23. Inokuma, T., Tamaki, N., Torizuka, T., et al. (1995) Evaluation of pancreatic tumors with positron emission tomography and F-18 fluorodeoxyglucose: comparison with CT and US *Radiology* **195(2)**, 345–52.

24. Kato, T., Fukatsu, H., Ito, K., et al. (1995) Fluorodeoxyglucose positron emission tomography in pancreatic cancer: an unsolved problem *Eur J Nucl Med* **22(1)**, 32–9.

25. Koyama, K., Okamura, T., Kawabe, J., et al. (2001) Diagnostic usefulness of FDG PET for pancreatic mass lesions *Ann Nucl Med* **15(3)**, 217–24.

26. Lemke, A.J., Niehues, S.M., Hosten, N., et al. (2004) Retrospective digital image fusion of multidetector CT and 18F-FDG PET: clinical value in pancreatic lesions – a prospective study with 104 patients *J Nucl Med* **45(8)**, 1279–86.

27. Nakamoto, Y., Higashi, T., Sakahara, H., et al. (2000) Delayed (18)F-fluoro-2-deoxy-D-glucose positron emission tomography scan for differentiation between malignant and benign lesions in the pancreas *Cancer* **89(12)**, 2547–54.

28. Nishiyama, Y., Yamamoto, Y., Monden, T., et al. (2005) Evaluation of delayed additional FDG PET imaging in patients with pancreatic tumour *Nucl Med Commun* **26(10)**, 895–901.

29. Sendler, A., Avril, N., Helmberger, H., et al. (2000) Preoperative evaluation of pancreatic masses with positron emission tomography using 18F-fluorodeoxyglucose: diagnostic limitations *World J Surg* **24(9)**, 1121–9.

30. Valinas, R., Barrier, A., Montravers, F., Houry, S., Talbot, J.N., Huguier, M. (2002) 18 F-fluorodeoxyglucose positron emission tomography for characterization and initial staging of pancreatic tumors *Gastroenterol Clin Biol* **26(10)**, 888–92.

31. van Kouwen, M.C., Jansen, J.B., van Goor, H., de Castro, S., Oyen, W.J., Drenth, J.P. (2005) FDG-PET is able to detect pancreatic carcinoma in chronic pancreatitis *Eur J Nucl Med Mol Imaging* **32(4)**, 399–404.

32. Zimny, M., Bares, R., Fass, J., et al. (1997) Fluorine-18 fluorodeoxyglucose positron emission tomography in the differential diagnosis of pancreatic carcinoma: a report of 106 cases *Eur J Nucl Med* **24(6)**, 678–82.

33. Delbeke, D., Coleman, R.E., Guiberteau, M.J., et al. (2006) Procedure guideline for tumor imaging with 18F-FDG PET-CT 1.0 *J Nucl Med* **47(5)**, 885–95.

34. Diederichs, C.G., Staib, L., Vogel, J., et al. (2000) Values and limitations of 18F-fluorodeoxyglucose-positron-emission tomography with preoperative evaluation of patients with pancreatic masses *Pancreas* **20(2)**, 109–116.

35. Ruf, J., Lopez Hanninen, E., Oettle, H., Plotkin, M., Pelzer, U., Stroszczynski, C, et al. (2005) Detection of recurrent pancreatic cancer: comparison of FDG-PET with CT/MRI. *Pancreatology* **5(2–3)**, 266–272.

36. Zimny, M., Fass, J., Bares, R., et al. (2000) Fluorodeoxyglucose positron emission tomography and the prognosis of pancreatic carcinoma *Scand J Gastroenterol* **35(8)**, 883–8.

37. Lyshchik, A., Higashi, T., Nakamoto, Y., et al. (2005) Dual-phase 18F-fluoro-2-deoxy-D-glucose positron emission tomography as a prognostic parameter in patients with pancreatic cancer *Eur J Nucl Med Mol Imaging* **32(4)**, 389–97.

38. Higashi, T., Sakahara, H., Torizuka, T., et al. (1999) Evaluation of intraoperative radiation therapy for unresectable pancreatic cancer with FDG PET *J Nucl Med* **40(9)**, 1424–33.

39. Maisey, N.R., Webb, A., Flux, G.D., et al. (2000) FDG-PET in the prediction of survival of patients with cancer of the pancreas: a pilot study *Br J Cancer* **83(3)**, 287–93.

40. Adams, S., Baum, R., Rink, T., Schumm-Drager, P.M., Usadel, K.H., Hor, G. (1998) Limited value of fluorine-18 fluorodeoxyglucose positron emission tomography for the imaging of neuroendocrine tumours *Eur J Nucl Med* **25(1)**, 79–83.

41. Murakami, T., Mochizuki, K., Nakamura, H. (2001) Imaging evaluation of the cirrhotic liver *Semin LiverDis* **21(2)**, 213–24.

42. Fung, K.T., Li, F.T., Raimondo, M.L., et al. (2004) Systematic review of radiological imaging for hepatocellular carcinoma in cirrhotic patients *Br J Radiol* **77(920)**, 633–40.

43. Park, M.S., Kim, T.K., Kim, K.W., et al. (2004) Differentiation of extrahepatic bile duct cholangiocarcinoma from benign stricture: findings at MRCP versus ERCP *Radiology* **233(1)**, 234–40.

44. Delbeke, D., Martin, W.H., Sandler, M.P., Chapman, W.C., Wright, J.K., Jr., Pinson, C.W. (1998) Evaluation of benign vs malignant hepatic lesions with positron emission tomography *Arch Surg* **133(5)**, 510-5; discussion 515–6.

45. Gambhir, S.S., Czernin, J., Schwimmer, J., Silverman, D.H., Coleman, R.E., Phelps, M.E. (2001) A tabulated summary of the FDG PET literature *J Nucl Med* **42(5)**, 1S–93S.

46. Okazumi, S., Isono, K., Enomoto, K., et al. (1992) Evaluation of liver tumors using fluorine-18-fluorodeoxyglucose PET: characterization of

tumor and assessment of effect of treatment *J Nucl Med* **33(3)**, 333–9.

47. Lin, W.Y., Tsai, S.C., Hung, G.U. (2005) Value of delayed 18F-FDG-PET imaging in the detection of hepatocellular carcinoma *Nucl Med Commun* **26(4)**, 315–21.

48. Sugiyama, M., Sakahara, H., Torizuka, T., et al. (2004) 18F-FDG PET in the detection of extrahepatic metastases from hepatocellular carcinoma *J Gastroenterol* **39(10)**, 961–8.

49. Ho, C.L., Yu, S.C., Yeung, D.W. (2003) 11C-acetate PET imaging in hepatocellular carcinoma and other liver masses *J Nucl Med* **44(2)**, 213–21.

50. Ho, C.L., Chen, S., Yeung, D.W., Cheng, T.K. (2007) Dual-tracer PET-CT imaging in evaluation of metastatic hepatocellular carcinoma *J Nucl Med* **48(6)**, 902–9.

51. Yamamoto, Y., Nishiyama, Y., Kameyama, R., et al. (2008) Detection of hepatocellular carcinoma using 11C-choline PET: comparison with 18F-FDG PET *J Nucl Med* **49(8)**, 1245–8.

52. Kubota, K., Hisa, N., Nishikawa, T., et al. (2001) Evaluation of hepatocellular carcinoma after treatment with transcatheter arterial chemoembolization: comparison of Lipiodol-CT, power Doppler sonography, and dynamic MRI *Abdom Imaging* **26(2)**, 184–90.

53. Chen, Y.K., Hsieh, D.S., Liao, C.S., et al. (2005) Utility of FDG-PET for investigating unexplained serum AFP elevation in patients with suspected hepatocellular carcinoma recurrence *Anticancer Res* **25(6C)**, 4719–25.

54. Anderson, C.D., Rice, M.H., Pinson, C.W., Chapman, W.C., Chari, R.S., Delbeke, D. (2004) Fluorodeoxyglucose PET imaging in the evaluation of gallbladder carcinoma and cholangiocarcinoma *J Gastrointest Surg* **8(1)**, 90–7.

55. Lee, J.D., Yang, W.I., Park, Y.N., et al. (2005) Different glucose uptake and glycolytic mechanisms between hepatocellular carcinoma and intrahepatic mass-forming cholangiocarcinoma with increased (18)F-FDG uptake *J Nucl Med* **46(10)**, 1753–9.

56. Prytz, H., Keiding, S., Bjornsson, E., et al. (2006) Dynamic FDG-PET is useful for detection of cholangiocarcinoma in patients with PSC listed for liver transplantation *Hepatology* **44(6)**, 1572–80.

57. Widjaja, A., Mix, H., Wagner, S., et al. (1993) Positron emission tomography and cholangiocarcinoma in primary sclerosing cholangitis *Z Gastroenterol* **37(8)**, 731–3.

58. Nishiyama, Y., Yamamoto, Y., Kimura, N., et al. (2007) Comparison of early and delayed FDG PET for evaluation of biliary stricture *Nucl Med Commun* **28(12)**, 914–9.

59. Nishiyama, Y., Yamamoto, Y., Fukunaga, K., et al. (2006) Dual-time-point 18F-FDG PET for the evaluation of gallbladder carcinoma. *J Nucl Med* **47(4)**, 633–8.

60. Lunia, S., Parthasarathy, K.L., Bakshi, S., Bender, M.A. (1975) An evaluation of 99mTc-sulfur colloid liver scintiscans and their usefulness in metastatic workup: a review of 1,424 studies *J Nucl Med* **16(1)**, 62–5.

61. Delbeke, D., Vitola, J.V., Sandler, M.P., et al. (1997) Staging recurrent metastatic colorectal carcinoma with PET *J Nucl Med* **38(8)**, 1196–1201.

62. Fong, Y., Saldinger, P.F., Akhurst, T., et al. (1999) Utility of 18F-FDG positron emission tomography scanning on selection of patients for resection of hepatic colorectal metastases. *Am J Surg* **178(4)**, 282–7.

63. Kinkel, K., Lu, Y., Both, M., Warren, R.S., Thoeni, R.F. (2002) Detection of hepatic metastases from cancers of the gastrointestinal tract by using noninvasive imaging methods (US, CT, MR imaging, PET): a meta-analysis *Radiology* **224(3)**, 748–56.

64. Ruers, T.J., Langenhoff, B.S., Neeleman, N., et al. (2002) Value of positron emission tomography with [F-18]fluorodeoxyglucose in patients with colorectal liver metastases: a prospective study. *J Clin Oncol* **20(2)**, 388–95.

65. Valk, P.E., Abella-Columna, E., Haseman, M.K., et al. (1999) Whole-body PET imaging with [18F]fluorodeoxyglucose in management of recurrent colorectal cancer *Arch Surg* **134(5)**, 503–11; discussion 511–13.

66. Langenhoff, B.S., Oyen, W.J., Jager, G.J., et al. (2002) Efficacy of fluorine-18-deoxyglucose positron emission tomography in detecting tumor recurrence after local ablative therapy for liver metastases: a prospective study. *J Clin Oncol* **20(22)**, 4453–8.

67. Sciuk, J., Schober, O. (1997) Nuclear medicine diagnosis of space-occupying lesions of the liver *Der Internist* **38(10)**, 917–23.

68. Rubin, R.A., Lichtenstein, G.R. (1993) Hepatic scintigraphy in the evaluation of solitary solid liver masses *J Nucl Med* **34(4)**, 697–705.

69. Olsen, J.O., Pozderac, R.V., Hinkle, G., et al. (1995) Somatostatin receptor imaging of neuroendocrine tumors with indium-111 pentetreotide (Octreoscan) *Semin Nucl Med* **25(3)**, 251–61.

70. Khafagi, F.A., Shapiro, B., Fischer, M., Sisson, J.C., Hutchinson, R., Beierwaltes, W.H. (1991) Phaeochromocytoma and functioning paraganglioma in childhood and adolescence: role of iodine 131 metaiodobenzylguanidine *Eur J Nucl Med* **18(3)**, qw191–8.

71. Sostre, S., Villagra, D., Morales, N.E., Rivera, J.V. (1988) Dual-tracer scintigraphy and

subtraction studies in the diagnosis of hepato-cellular carcinoma *Cancer* **61(4)**, 667–72.

72. Eckel, F., Herrmann, K., Schmidt, S., Hillerer, C., Wieder, H.A., Krause, B.J, et al. Imaging of proliferation in hepatocellular carcinoma with the in vivo marker 18F-fluorothymidine. *J Nucl Med* 2009 Sep; **50(9)**, 1441–1447.

73. Mansour, J.C., Schwartz, L., Pandit-Taskar, N., D'Angelica, M., Fong, Y., Larson, S.M, et al. (2006) The utility of F-18 fluorodeoxyglu-cose whole body PET imaging for determin-ing malignancy in cystic lesions of the pancreas. *J Gastrointest Surg* **10(10)**, 1354–1360.

74. Sahani, D.V., Kalva, S.P., Fischman, A.J., Kadavigere, R., Blake, M., Hahn, P.F, et al. (2005) Detection of liver metastases from adenocarcinoma of the colon and pancreas: comparison of mangafodipir trisodium-enhanced liver MRI and whole-body FDG PET. *AJR Am J Roentgenol* **185(1)**, 239–246.

75. Frohlich, A., Diederichs, C.G., Staib, L., Vogel, J., Beger, H.G., Reske, S.N. (1999) Detection of liver metastases from pancreatic cancer using FDG PET. *J Nucl Med* **40(2)**, 250–255.

Chapter 15

Prostate Cancer

Hossein Jadvar

Abstract

Prostate cancer is biologically and clinically a heterogeneous disease and its imaging evaluation will need to be tailored to the specific phases of the disease in a patient-specific, risk-adapted manner. We first present a brief overview of the natural history of prostate cancer before discussing the role of various imaging tools, including opportunities and challenges, for different clinical phases of this common disease in men. We then review the preclinical and clinical evidence on the potential and emerging role of positron emission tomography with various radiotracers in the imaging evaluation of men with prostate cancer.

Key words: Prostate, Cancer, PET

1. Natural History and Biology of Prostate Cancer

Prostate cancer is the most common cancer and the second leading cause of cancer death affecting men in USA. In 2009, the estimated incidence of and deaths from this disease were 192,280 cases and 27,360 cases, respectively (1). As life expectancy increases, so will the incidence of this disease, creating what will become an epidemic male health problem. Prostate cancer is a heterogeneous disease characterized by an overall long natural history in comparison to the other solid tumors, with a wide spectrum of biological behavior that ranges between indolent and aggressive states (2, 3).

Prostate-specific antigen (PSA), a 34-kD androgen-regulated exocrine serine protease that cleaves the prostate-derived protein "seminogelin" in the seminal fluid for the liquefaction of the semen, is produced by both the normal and the diseased prostate cells and can be measured in the serum as an "organ-specific marker" in two major isoforms: PSA complexed to α1-antichymotrypsin and uncomplexed free PSA (4). Various PSA parameters

Malik E. Juweid and Otto S. Hoekstra (eds.), *Positron Emission Tomography*, Methods in Molecular Biology, vol. 727,
DOI 10.1007/978-1-61779-062-1_15, © Springer Science+Business Media, LLC 2011

employed for monitoring include PSA density, PSA velocity, PSA half-life, PSA nadir, PSA doubling time, time to PSA elevation, age-specific PSA reference ranges, and free to total PSA ratio (5–8). After radical prostatectomy, PSA should be undetectable with hypersensitive tests (detection threshold <0.1 ng/mL) 6 weeks after the operation (9).

In the post-PSA era, most patients (about 92%) present with locoregional disease, while metastatic disease is the initial presentation in about 5% of patients, with the remaining 3% classified as unknown (1). Despite highly successful treatments for localized prostate cancer, approximately 40% of men will eventually (most within 10 years from primary treatment) experience a detectable rise in the serum PSA level (biochemical failure), suggesting that prostate cancer can metastasize relatively early in the course of the disease, probably as a result of genetic instability including loss of metastasis-suppressor genes (10). A portion of men with increasing serum PSA level will develop locally recurrent disease and as many as two-thirds will have evidence of osseous metastatic involvement (11–14). Patients at highest risk for bone metastases include men aged older than 65 years, those with high-grade high-stage neoplasms, those who fail primary curative therapies (radical prostatectomy and radiation therapy), and those who develop biochemical recurrence after hormonal therapy (15–17). Patient's age may have additional independent influence on the natural history of disease such that in men younger than 35 years of age, the tumor is invariably poorly differentiated, rapidly growing with bulky soft tissue metastases, and is associated with negative tumor markers (18). Moreover, it appears that racial differences in the biology of androgen-independent carcinoma do not contribute to the inferior survival of black men compared to that of white men with metastatic prostate cancer (19).

Pound et al. in their landmark article documented the natural history of progression to metastatic disease and death after PSA elevation following radical prostatectomy and no adjuvant hormonal therapy (20). A detectable serum PSA level of at least 0.2 ng/mL was considered as an evidence for biochemical recurrence. The actuarial metastasis-free survival for all men was 82% at 15 years after surgery. The median actuarial time to metastases was 8 years from the time of PSA relapse. Once men developed metastatic disease, the median survival time to death was 5 years. The time to biochemical progression, PSA doubling time, and Gleason score were predictive of the probability and time to development of metastatic disease. The time interval from surgery to the appearance of metastatic disease was predictive of time until death (20). Once men develop hormone refractory metastatic disease, the 1-year survival is about 24% with a median survival of only 8–18 months (21).

Androgens are essential for the development, growth, and maintenance of the prostate. The effects of androgens are exerted via the nuclear androgen receptor (AR), which is a ligand-dependent (either testosterone or α-dihydrotestosterone) transcription activator involved in cellular proliferation and differentiation, and is present in all histologic types of prostate tumors, in recurrent carcinoma, and in tumor metastases (22–25). Almost all patients respond favorably to androgen ablation, but virtually all patients will relapse to an androgen-independent clinical state. The hormone-refractory state is believed to occur via bypassing or sensitizing the AR pathway. The factor involved may be AR mutation such that the receptor is activated either promiscuously or in a ligand-independent manner. Other factors include amplification of coactivators, activation of oncogenes, and autocrine growth factor stimulation (25).

Prediction of prognosis is an important objective in the clinical decision-making process, patient counseling, and assessing treatment outcomes (26). To this end, Partin tables and nomograms have been developed. Partin tables use the clinical stage, Gleason score, age, and nuclear morphometry to predict disease-free survival among patients with clinically localized prostate cancer after surgery (27). Nomograms utilize pretreatment clinical variables to predict clinical outcomes (28, 29). However, such clinically derived models cannot directly guide a specific therapy or provide accurate objective means for early prediction of treatment response and comparison of clinical trials for either the current conventional therapies or the potentially new treatments.

The role of PSA changes in predicting prognosis in patients with metastatic prostate cancer who are treated with androgen withdrawal therapy has also been investigated. It appears that patients with high initial PSA level have a worse cause-specific survival and that serial PSA measurements can distinguish nonfavorable responders early in the course of treatment and assist in monitoring disease progression (30–34). This is in fact what is done nowadays clinically. PSA doubling time has been found to be useful in predicting systemic progression-free survival (defined as time to evidence of metastatic disease on bone scintigraphy) in patients with biochemical failure (defined as PSA level ≥ 0.4 ng/mL) following radical prostatectomy (35). In patients with metastatic cancer who are treated with androgen ablation therapy, PSA changes in combination with the initial Gleason grade may be useful in determining the time to androgen-independent progression (36, 37). In patients with hormone-refractory metastatic cancer who are treated with chemotherapy, PSA can predict pain end points as well as progression-free survival and overall survival (38).

However, despite the utility of PSA as an "organ-specific marker," it is not ideal due to its nonspecificity and low sensitivity.

PSA should not be considered as a direct measure of tumor growth since the serum level is influenced by the volume of the benign epithelium, grade of carcinoma, inflammation, androgen levels, growth factors, and the extracellular matrix (39). PSA may be undetectable or low in view of disseminated prostate cancer (40–42) and there is emerging data to suggest that various therapies may affect PSA expression in a manner unrelated to the impact on tumor growth (43–45). Additionally, PSA is frequently a source of great anxiety and overstated diagnostic expectations for the patient, designated by the term "PSA-itis" (46).

2. Diagnostic Imaging Evaluation of Prostate Cancer

As oncology departures from nonspecific diagnosis and treatment toward patient-specific approach to therapy, accurate knowledge of the presence and extent of disease becomes even more crucial in order to tailor the treatment plan appropriately (47). This information in combination with the physiologic, histologic, antigenic, molecular, and genetic markers of the disease will provide unprecedented opportunities for the new era of imaging-based cancer diagnosis and therapy (48).

Imaging evaluation of prostate cancer remains challenging (49). Initial imaging differential diagnosis may be made when suspected (e.g., high serum PSA level and abnormal digital rectal examination) with ultrasound and/or magnetic resonance imaging (MRI) using endorectal probes and image-guided biopsies. Imaging also provides important information on local extent of disease and examines for potential regional and distant metastatic disease in high-risk patients. Determination of the most optimal method for imaging evaluation of men with PSA relapse (biochemical failure) remains unsettled, but the goal of imaging is to determine if there is recurrence in the treated prostate bed or if distant disease is present (or both). Current imaging tests, including ultrasound, CT, MRI, bone scintigraphy, and In-111 capromab pendetide (*Prostascint*, Cytogen, Princeton, NJ), are not sufficiently accurate to detect local recurrence or metastatic disease in prostate cancer (50–52). Such determination, however, is critical since it impacts therapeutic management, including consideration for salvage therapy for local recurrence and systemic treatment for metastatic disease.

Prostascint is a radiolabeled antibody targeted at the prostate-specific membrane antigen (PSMA), which is a glycoprotein expressed in both the benign and the neoplastic prostatic epithelial cells. It is upregulated in hormone-resistant states and in metastatic disease (53, 54). Despite the relevance of PSMA in prostate cancer, Prostascint has limited predictive value in imaging the prostate fossa, particularly following radiation therapy, has low sensitivity for detecting osseous metastases, is technically demanding, and requires interpretation at sites with experience and expertise (52).

Although bone scintigraphy can be useful in detecting osseous metastases, the false-positive rate is high (55), and it cannot detect soft tissue or lymph node involvement, which is quite prevalent with metastatic spread of this disease. Bone scintigraphy has limited sensitivity in detecting metastases when the serum PSA level is below 2 ng/mL and only best correlates at high PSA levels of >16 ng/mL (56–58). Additionally, a "flare" phenomenon may be observed with the initiation of hormonal ablation and even chemotherapy in the setting of clinical and serologic improvement, but worsening scan pattern (59). However, in patients who do not fit into this clinical scenario, bone scan progression may be considered when there are larger lesions, new lesions, or a combination of both (60). There have been some efforts in developing methods for quantification of bone scintigraphy in order to facilitate quantitative determination of the extent of osseous metastatic disease and changes associated with response to treatment (61–63). Quantitative bone scintigraphy may also have prognostic utility, with the percentage of positive area of bone metastases as an independent predictor of disease death in patients with prostate cancer (64, 65). Moreover, CT has been shown to be useful for additional evaluation of suspected skeletal metastases following bone scintigraphy by characterizing the radiographic appearance of the lesions (66).

Newer imaging methods using lymphotropic superparamagnetic nanoparticles in conjunction with high-resolution MRI may also allow the detection of small and otherwise undetectable lymph-node metastases in patients with prostate cancer (67). However, the exact clinical utility of such diagnostic imaging approach in a diverse group of patients will still need to be determined.

3. Role of PET in Prostate Cancer

The clinical experience with PET(-CT) in uroradiology and, in particular, prostate cancer is expanding (68, 69). Here, we briefly discuss the use of various PET radiotracers in prostate cancer with an emphasis on F-18 FDG (the most common radiotracer used in oncologic PET) as well as radiolabeled acetate and choline, which are the two other most studied radiotracers in prostate cancer.

3.1. Fluorodeoxyglucose (F-18 FDG)

PET with F-18 FDG has become an important diagnostic imaging tool for the identification of a diverse group of common and rare malignancies (70–73). With the current availability of hybrid PET-CT imaging systems, it is possible to localize metabolic abnormalities and characterize the metabolic activity of normal and abnormal structures precisely, thereby increasing diagnostic confidence and reducing equivocal image interpretations. Clinical utility of F-18 FDG PET has included initial diagnosis, staging and restaging of cancer, detection of metastases, prediction and evaluation of therapy response, differentiation of post-therapy changes from residual or recurrent tumor, and prognostication. The ability of F-18 FDG PET to detect cancer is based upon elevated glucose metabolism in the malignant tissue in comparison to that in the normal tissue, as a result of increased expression of cellular membrane glucose transporters (mainly GLUT-1) and enhanced hexokinase (HK-II) enzymatic activity in tumors (74, 75).

It has generally been presumed that PET with F-18 FDG may not be useful in prostate cancer (76). This notion is probably based on the observed heterogeneity of tumor metabolic activity that can overlap with normal tissue, and benign prostatic hyperplasia (BPH) (77–81). F-18 FDG PET may not be useful in the diagnosis and staging of clinically organ-confined disease and in the detection of locally recurrent disease due to the overlap of tumor uptake with scar tissue and also because of the intense urine activity in the adjacent urinary bladder (82). F-18 FDG is also not specific for cancer, and false positives may occur with prostatitis (83).

Although the exact etiology for the observed variability of glucose metabolism in prostate cancer remains unclear, this observation probably reflects the biological range of the disease and other biologic modulatory factors including tumor hypoxia (84, 85). Technical and image-processing factors may also play an important role in the observed heterogeneity of F-18 FDG accumulation in prostate cancer. For example, significantly lower tissue F-18 FDG accumulation, with ensuing false-negative results, has been noted when filtered-back projection is employed instead of iterative reconstruction with segmented attenuation, irrespective of the biological heterogeneity (86, 87). In particular, it has been demonstrated that in selected patients, iterative reconstruction can contribute significantly to the detection of prostate cancer with F-18 FDG PET (87).

Despite the above notions and the overall heterogeneity of published studies in relatively small number of subjects, several animal-based translational and human-based clinical studies have demonstrated that F-18 FDG PET can be useful in certain clinical circumstances in prostate cancer. The general clinical themes in which F-18 FDG PET may have significant diagnostic utility include the following (88–110):

- Imaging evaluation of patients with high Gleason score primary tumors (90)

- Patients with high serum PSA and PSA velocity after initial primary treatment – detection rate of about 31% at a sensitivity of 80% and specificity of 73% with a PSA threshold of 2.4 ng/mL, and sensitivity of 71% and specificity of 77% with a PSA velocity threshold of 1.3 ng/mL/y (95); sensitivity of 75% and specificity of 100% in men with PSA relapse after treatment of localized prostate cancer (94)

- Assessment of the extent of disease in men with advanced androgen-independent disease

- Detection of metabolically active osseous and soft tissue metastases (97) (Fig. 1)

- Assessment of response to treatment – F-18 FDG accumulation in the primary prostate cancer and metastatic sites decreased 1–5 months after initiation of androgen deprivation therapy (91); >33% increase in average SUVmax of up to 5 lesions or appearance of new lesions could dichotomize castrate metastatic prostate cancer patients treated with anti-microtubule chemotherapy as progressors or nonprogressors (98) (Fig. 2)

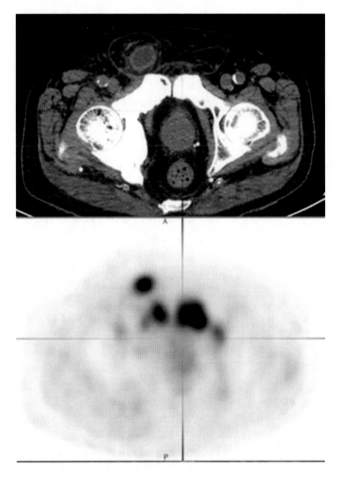

Fig. 1. Metastatic prostate cancer in bone (symphysis) and an enlarged right inguinal lymph node.

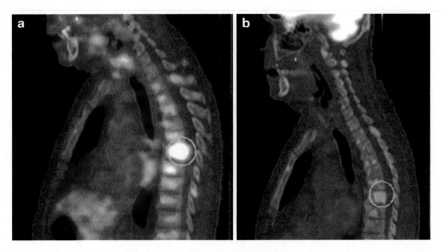

Fig. 2. A 69-year-old man with metastatic prostate cancer, (**a**) hypermetabolic upper thoracic vertebra with a SUVmax of 5.0 prior to androgen ablation therapy, PSA = 98 ng/ml (**b**) SUVmax of 2.7 for the same lesion after androgen ablation, PSA = 21 ng/ml, demonstrating decline in the lesion metabolic activity in response to therapy.

- Prognostication – patients with primary prostate tumors with high SUV had a poorer prognosis in comparison to those with low SUV (93)

Since F-18 FDG uptake in the prostate tumor appears to be directly dependent on the androgen presence and stimulation, F-18 FDG PET may also be useful in the prediction of the time to androgen-refractory state (e.g., early increase in castrate tumor F-18 FDG uptake) that may allow earlier therapeutic modification to be made for the purpose of averting or delaying this clinical state in order to improve overall outcome (91, 111). Moreover, F-18 FDG PET may be more useful than In-111 Prostascint in the detection of metastatic disease in patients with high PSA or PSA velocity (112).

However, more experience would be needed to determine the exact clinical utility of F-18 FDG PET in the above and other clinical circumstances during the natural history of prostate cancer. For example, a prospective clinical trial is currently underway to help define the role of F-18 FDG PET-CT in therapy assessment and in outcome prediction (time to hormone-refractory state and survival) in men with androgen-naïve and androgen-refractory metastatic prostate cancer (113).

3.2. C-11 Acetate

Acetate participates in cytoplasmic lipid synthesis, which is believed to be increased in tumors. The cellular retention of radiolabeled acetate in prostate cancer cell lines is primarily due to the incorporation of the radiocarbon into phosphatidylcholine and neutral lipids of the cells (114, 115). It has been suggested that fatty acid metabolism rather than glycolysis may be dominant in prostate cancer in view of alteration in several enzymes involved in the metabolism of fatty acids and enhanced beta-oxidation pathway (116). Very recent in vitro and animal model in vivo studies by the group at Washington University in St. Louis confirmed the extensive involvement of the fatty acid synthesis pathway in C-11 acetate uptake in prostate tumors as an imaging marker for fatty acid synthase expression (117). Fatty acid synthase is the major enzyme required for converting carbohydrates to fatty acids, and its upregulation plays a role in tumorigenesis of the prostate in the transgenic adenocarcinoma of mouse prostate (TRAMP) model (118).

The lack of accumulation of acetate in urine is also advantageous to imaging prostate cancer in particular, because the prostate bed remains unobstructed by the adjacent high levels of radioactivity in the urinary bladder, commonly a problem with F-18 FDG (119). Although there can be a considerable overlap between the uptake level in primary cancer and in normal prostate gland, the uptake generally appears to be greater in the tumor than in the normal tissue (120). C-11 acetate may also be useful in the detection of tumor recurrence in some patients who had been treated previously with prostatectomy or radiation, with lesion detectability of 75% and false-positive rate that can be up to 15% (121–129). In a comparative study with F-18 FDG, the median C-11 acetate uptake was higher than that with F-18 FDG for local recurrence and regional lymph node metastases, while the reverse was noted with distant metastases (130). In another similar study, C-11 acetate identified disease in 30% of patients in comparison to 9% with F-18 FDG, when the analysis was limited to findings confirmed by other correlative imaging studies that were likely considered to represent tumor activity (125) (Fig. 3). In this same report, the success rate of lesion detection by C-11 acetate was dependent on PSA level, with 59% positive rate in patients with serum PSA >3 ng/mL that declined significantly to 4% in patients with serum PSA levels ≤3 ng/mL.

When compared to F-18 fluorocholine (F-18 FCH) in patients with very low prostate-specific antigen values (<1 ng/mL), both C-11 acetate and F-18 FCH could detect local residual/recurrent disease in about half of the patients, while endorectal probe MRI could detect the disease in about 83% of the patients (131). In another relatively similar study, it was found that fusion of C-11 acetate PET and MRI was able to localize recurrent tumor precisely in 73% of abnormal uptake sites that influenced clinical management in 28% of patients (132). In an animal model of prostate cancer, it has also been shown that androgen deprivation may decrease acetate uptake in the tumor, similar to what has been noted with F-18 FDG (92, 111). A suitable 3-compartment, 3-parameter model for C-11 acetate uptake kinetics in prostate cancer has recently been reported (133).

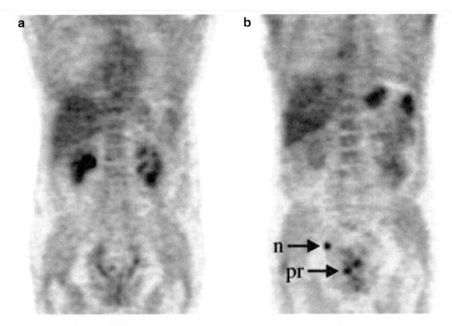

Fig. 3. A 71-year-old male with PSA relapse (PSA = 3.7 ng/mL at 8 years after definitive prostate radiation therapy, Gleason score 10). (**a**) FDG PET scan is normal, (**b**) C-11 acetate PET shows tracer accumulation, a right pelvic metastatic node, and local recurrence in the prostate bed (used with permission from Ref. (125)).

Moreover, the radiation dosimetry for C-11 acetate in humans has been reported (134).

A fluorine-18-labeled formulation of acetate (that allows commercial regional distribution similar to F-18 FDG) has also been reported with potential use in prostate cancer (135). A comparative animal study of C-11 acetate and F-18 fluoroacetate showed that for most organs (except for blood, muscle, and fat), the tumor-to-organ uptake ratios at 30 min after tracer administration were higher with F-18 fluoroacetate, whereas the tumor-to-heart and tumor-to-prostate ratios were similar (136).

3.3. Choline

Radiolabeled choline accumulates in prostate tumor (137). Therefore, choline PET has been found to be useful in the imaging of prostate cancer (138–149) (Fig. 4). The biological basis for radiolabeled choline uptake in tumors is the malignancy-induced upregulation of choline kinase, which leads to the incorporation and trapping of choline in the form of phosphatidylcholine (lecithin) in the tumor cell membrane. Choline uptake in prostate tumor appears to be uncorrelated to cellular proliferation (as depicted by Ki-67), but may be affected by hypoxia (84, 150). It has been demonstrated that under aerobic conditions, both androgen-sensitive and androgen-independent prostate tumors show higher choline uptake than that with radiolabeled acetate or with F-18 FDG. However, during hypoxia, the tumor uptake

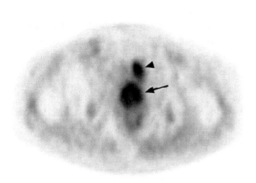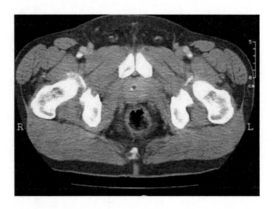

Fig. 4. A 63-year-old man with moderately differentiated prostate cancer and osseous metastasis in left pubis on C-11 choline PET-CT (used with permission from Ref. (156)).

with F-18 FDG and acetate is higher than that with choline (84). Both C-11- and F-18-labeled choline have been synthesized and investigated (151–155). C-11 has a shorter half-life (20 min) that requires an onsite cyclotron facility and generally displays no or little bladder urine activity (156).

A recent retrospective study compared the diagnostic performance of MRI, 3D MRS, combined MRI-MRS, and C-11 choline PET-CT for intraprostatic tumor sextant localization with histology as the standard of reference (157). The sensitivity and specificity were 55 and 86%, respectively, for PET-CT; 54 and 75%, respectively, for MRI; and 81% and 67%, respectively, for MRS. Therefore, in this study, C-11 choline PET-CT demonstrated a lower sensitivity relative to that of MRS alone or combined with MRI. Opposite findings have been reported by Japanese investigators, in that C-11 choline PET was more sensitive than MRI and MRS for the detection of primary prostate lesions (PET: 100% vs. MRI: 60% vs. MRS: 65%, respectively) (158). These conflicting results may be due to differing methodology in data collection or analysis, and in patient population. Research is underway to provide more sophisticated image fusion software for accurate registration of anatomic MRI, diffusion MRI, C-11 choline PET, and histologic sections of the prostate gland (159). German investigators compared C-11 choline PET-CT with whole-body MRI retrospectively for staging of prostate cancer (160). Diagnostic validation was by histology, follow-up, or consensus reading. Overall sensitivity and specificity were 97 and 77%, respectively, for C-11 choline PET and 79 and 94%, respectively, for whole-body MRI. Therefore, the two imaging modalities were found to be complementary.

A study rather similar to the MRI reports that compared transrectal ultrasonography (TRUS) and C-11 choline PET-CT in patients with clinically localized prostate cancer showed that both

PET and TRUS tended to understage prostate cancer. Therefore, the authors suggested that reliable clinical decision making (e.g., with regard to decision for nerve-sparing radical prostatectomy) might not be possible based on the findings on these imaging modalities (161). Despite the above reports, other investigations have found a relatively good diagnostic performance for C-11 choline PET(-CT) in the detection of primary prostate cancer. For example, Scher et al. reported a sensitivity of 87% and specificity of 62% for the detection primary prostate cancer with histopathological examination of resection specimen or biopsy as the reference standard (162). Interestingly, the group from Italy reported nearly the reverse values, with sensitivity of 66% and specificity of 81% for localization of primary prostate cancer on a sextant histopathologic analysis (163). Martorana et al. assessed the diagnostic performance of C-11 choline PET-CT for nodules ≥5 mm in 43 patients with known prostate cancer before the initial 12-core transrectal biopsy (164). PET demonstrated a sensitivity of 83% in this setting but had very low sensitivity for the assessment of extraprostatic extension in comparison to MRI (22 vs. 63%, respectively, $P < 0.001$). Therefore, although C-11 choline PET may be helpful in detecting primary prostate cancer, the sensitivity may depend on several factors that will need to be defined (e.g., tumor grade, size, and location).

C-11 choline PET has been evaluated for detecting local, regional, and metastatic prostate cancer (165). The tracer uptake was noted to decrease both in the primary tumor and in the metastases after hormonal therapy, although this has been disputed in other studies (166, 167). In another study, C-11 choline was determined to localize recurrence in higher percentage of men after primary radiation therapy than after radical prostatectomy (78 vs. 38%, respectively) (144). The reason for such difference based on the type of primary therapy remains unclear. The potential utility of C-11 choline PET-CT for the detection of local recurrence after radical prostatectomy has also been demonstrated with a sensitivity of 73% and specificity of 88% (149).

Italian researchers reported a sensitivity and specificity of 64 and 90% for the detection of nodal metastases in men with PSA failure after radical retropubic prostatectomy (168) that was somewhat similar to the reported sensitivity of 80% and specificity of 96% for staging lymph nodes preoperatively at the time of initial diagnosis (143). In a comparative study with F-18 FDG, C-11 choline was found to be generally superior to F-18 FDG for restaging prostate cancer, although statistical testing of the observed differences between F-18 FDG and C-11 choline diagnostic performance measures was not reported (145).

A German group showed that PET-CT significantly improves the lesion localization and characterization with C-11 choline (169). In a similar study from Italy, C-11 acetate PET-CT demonstrated sensitivity and specificity of 60 and 98%, respectively, on a patient basis, and 41 and 99%, respectively, on a nodal basis, for the detection of pelvic lymph node metastasis in patients who underwent radical prostatectomy with extended pelvic lymph node dissection (170). Therefore, although this study suggested a low sensitivity for nodal staging in patients with intermediate to high risk for prostate cancer, it still performed better than clinical staging nomograms with regard to improved specificity.

A F-18-labeled formulation of choline has also been developed and preliminarily tested in men with prostate cancer. Price et al. showed that murine xenograft of prostate cancer accumulated higher F-18 FDG than F-18 FCH (F-18 fluorocholine), while interestingly in human studies, the FCH uptake in lesions was higher than that with F-18 FDG (171). The exact reason for such observation remains unclear but may be due to the biological differences between an implanted tumor and a native tumor. F-18-FCH uptake overlaps among normal, benign, and malignant tissue (similar to C-11 acetate and C-11 choline) (172, 173). In one recent report, disease was missed in a significant number of patients (up to 75%) with elevated PSA (172), although in another report the results were more encouraging (174). A dual-phase study (7 min and 1 h after F-18 FCH administration) has also been evaluated, which showed that it may be helpful in distinguishing malignant from benign tissue in view of the observation that malignant tissue displays stable or increasing tracer accumulation, whereas benign tissue shows decreasing uptake (175). A similar observation has also been reported with F-18 FDG for improving the differential diagnosis of malignant from benign (e.g., inflammation) conditions.

Italian investigators showed that the detection rate of F-18 FCH PET-CT in patients with biochemical relapse is dependent on the serum PSA level (176). In this study, F-18 FCH PET demonstrated a detection rate of 20% for PSA ≤1 ng/mL, 44% for $1 < PSA \leq 5$ ng/mL, and 82% for PSA >5 ng/mL. In the study by Karuse and colleagues from Germany, the detection rate of C-11 choline PET-CT was 36% for PSA <1 ng/mL, 43% for $1 \leq PSA < 2$ ng/mL, 62% for $2 \leq PSA < 3$ ng/mL, and 73% for PSA ≥3 ng/mL. Androgen deprivation therapy also did not show a significant effect on the detection rate of C-11 choline PET-CT ($P=0.37$) (167). Similar positive dependence of C-11 choline PET-CT lesion detection rate on PSA level has been reported by other investigators (177–179), although there are also reports of no significant correlation (patient-based analysis) between lesion maximum SUV, PSA level, Gleason score, or pathological stage at the time of initial diagnosis (147, 180). Whereas few investigations have reported that C-11 choline may be useless in detecting disease when PSA is less than 5 ng/mL (144) or less than 4 ng/mL with Gleason sum score of less than 8 (181), another study with

F-18 FCH showed up to 41% true positive findings in restaging patients with PSA <5 ng/mL (182). Therefore, despite some mixed results, it appears that in general terms, the sensitivity of PET with either of the two choline tracers may directly depend on the serum PSA level with the expectation that at higher PSA levels, the probability of lesion localization increases.

Although both acetate and choline appear to be more or less equally useful in imaging prostate cancer in individual patients (183) and are probably more advantageous than F-18 FDG in some clinical circumstances, such as detection of the locally recurrent disease (130, 145), large clinical studies in well-defined clinical situations will be needed to determine their exact diagnostic role in prostate cancer.

3.4. F-18 Fluoride

F-18 fluoride is highly sensitive for the detection of osseous metastases from prostate cancer (184, 185). A recent animal model PET-CT study compared F-18 FDG and F-18 fluoride in the characterization of osteolytic, osteoblastic, and mixed lesions of prostate cancer (186). F-18 fluoride accumulation in lesions correlated with bone volume measured on histomorphometric analysis, while F-18 FDG accumulation strongly correlated with soft tissue measurements. Interestingly, mixed lesions demonstrated minimal uptake of both tracers. Another recent study compared F-18 FCH and F-18 fluoride PET-CT in 17 men preoperatively and 21 men postoperatively for suspected recurrence and/or metastatic disease (187). The sensitivity and specificity for the detection of osseous metastases were 81 and 93%, respectively, for F-18 fluoride and 74 and 99%, respectively, for F-18 FCH. F-18 FCH appeared to be more useful for early detection of marrow involvement. It was also noted that F-18 fluoride could be negative in highly dense sclerotic lesions, presumably reflecting treated disease.

Even-Sapir and colleagues from Israel performed a prospective comparative study of Tc-99m MDP planar and SPECT bone scintigraphy with F-18 fluoride PET(-CT) in 44 patients with high-risk prostate cancer (188). The sensitivity and specificity for the detection of osseous metastases were 70 and 57%, respectively, for planar bone scintigraphy; 92 and 82%, respectively, for SPECT; 100 and 62%, respectively, for F-18 fluoride PET; and 100 and 90%, respectively, for F-18 fluoride PET-CT. F-18 fluoride PET-CT was statistically more sensitive and specific than planar and SPECT bone scintigraphy, and more specific than F-18 fluoride PET.

3.5. Other PET Radiotracers

Several other radiotracers have also been investigated in the evaluation of prostate cancer, including radiolabeled methionine, carbon monoxide, water, hydroxytryptophan, putrescine, penciclovir (in association with ex vivo transduced mutant herpes simplex virus type 1 thymidine kinase reporter gene), thymidine, ethanolamine, integrins, and androgens (189–203). All these radiotracers are not readily available and their diagnostic roles remain unclear. Future studies may establish well-defined diagnostic utility for these and the other novel PET radiotracers in the assessment of prostate cancer. Here, we briefly discuss the available data on some of the promising tracers.

3.6. C-11 Methionine

Another positron-emitting radiotracer that has been used to image tumors is the radiolabeled amino acid carbon-11 methionine (C-11 Met). Uptake of this radiotracer reflects the presence of transmethylation pathways in some tumors. C-11 Met, because of the relatively short 20-min half-life of the C-11 label, must be produced locally for administration and is currently not commercially available. An early study of the use of PET with C-11 Met in prostate cancer showed higher tumor-to-blood ratio and more rapid and uniform tumor uptake than F-18 FDG (194). Another comparative study of F-18 FDG and C-11 Met in 12 patients with progressive metastatic prostate cancer (based on increasing PSA level and increasing disease burden on conventional imaging) demonstrated a sensitivity of 48% for F-18 FDG that was substantially lower that for C-11 Met at 72% (198). However, specificities were not reported. A more recent report on 20 men with increased serum PSA level (range 3.5–28.6 ng/mL) and negative repeat biopsies showed a positive tumor detection rate of 35%, suggesting that C-11 Met PET guidance can enhance biopsy yield (204).

3.7. F-18 FDHT

16β-18F-fluoro-5α-dihydrotestosterone (F-18 FDHT) is a PET tracer suitable for imaging androgen receptors. Larson et al. showed a tumor localization rate of 78% with a lesion SUVmax of 5.3 using F-18 FDHT (vs. F-18 FDG detection rate of 97% and lesion SUVmax of 5.2) (205) (Fig. 5). Metabolism of F-18 FDHT was rapid with 80% conversion within 10 min to radiolabeled metabolites bound to plasma proteins. In another study, it was demonstrated that FDHT uptake in prostate cancer lesions decreases significantly after administration of androgen receptor antagonist (flutamide), supporting the receptor-mediated process of FDHT uptake, and that the uptake is positively correlated with PSA level (206). Radiation dosimetry of FDHT has also been reported (207).

3.8. Anti-FACBC

1-Amino-3-18F-fluorocyclobutane-1-carboxylic acid (F-18 FACBC) is a synthetic l-leucine analog that shows initial high uptake in pancreas and liver (critical organ) followed by rapid clearance and low urinary excretion (208). Animal studies have shown that prostate cancer has higher tracer uptake than inflammation and BPH. Schuster et al. studied 15 patients with newly

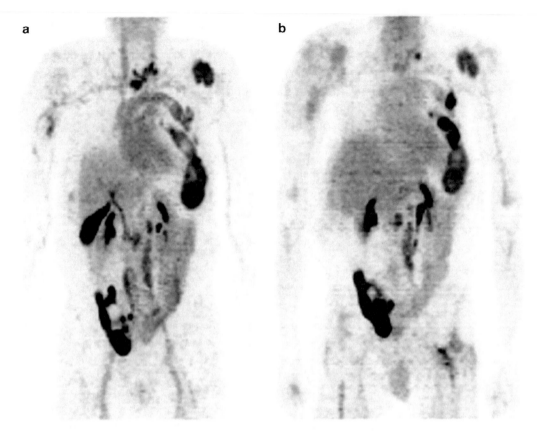

Fig. 5. (*Right panel*) 16ß-18F-fluoro-5-dihydrotestosterone (F-18 FDHT) and (*left panel*) F-18 FDG PET scans in the same patient show different levels and extent of uptake of the two tracers in the metastatic prostate cancer lesions (neck, left shoulder, and left chest) (used with permission from Ref. (205)).

diagnosed and recurrent prostate carcinoma. Presence or absence of disease was correctly identified in 40 of 48 prostate sextants; pelvic nodal status correlated in 7 of 9 patients, with higher malignant lymph node uptake of tracer seen in both the staging and restaging of patients compared with benign nodal uptake (209).

3.9. F-18 FLT and F-18 FMAU

F-18 fluorothymidine (F-18 FLT) is a PET radiotracer for monitoring cellular proliferation (DNA synthesis) that relies upon thymidine kinase 1 (TK1) enzymatic activity. Studies have shown that FLT can be a useful tracer for monitoring antitumor response to treatment, although the DNA salvage pathway may be a complicating factor in quantitative image interpretation (210, 211). It has been demonstrated in animal models of human prostate cancer that F-18 FLT may be useful for monitoring androgen ablation therapy that results in marked reduction of F-18 FLT accumulation in the tumor (202). However, the high physiologic uptake in the bone marrow can hinder the detection of osseous metastatic lesions.

Another cellular proliferation tracer, 1-(2′-deoxy-2′-fluoro-beta-D-arabinofuranosyl)thymine (FMAU), may also be useful in the imaging of prostate cancer. This thymidine analog tracer is preferably phosphorylated by mitochondrial thymidine kinase 2 (TK2) and incorporated into the DNA (212–217). It has the advantages of low urinary excretion and bone marrow localization, two factors important in the imaging evaluation of prostate cancer. In a recent study of F-18 FMAU in a number of patients with diverse tumors, a SUV of 3.0 was noted in prostate cancer, with the highest physiologic uptake seen in the liver and kidneys (218, 219).

Acknowledgment

This work was supported by grants from the National Institutes of Health – National Cancer Institute Grant No. R01-CA111613 and R21- CA142426.

References

1. SEER: The Surveillance, Epidemiology, and End Results Program (http://seer.cancer.gov) – based within the Surveillance Research Program (SRP) at the National Cancer Institute (NCI).

2. Frank, I.N., Graham, S., Jr., Nabors, W.L. (1991) Urologic and Male Genital Cancers. In: Holleb AI, Fink DJ, Murphy GP, editors. Clinical Oncology. Atlanta: American Cancer Society; pp. 280–283.

3. Kessler, B., Albertsen, P. (2003) The natural history of prostate cancer *Urol Clin North Am* **30**, 219–26.

4. Lin, D.W., Noteboom, J.L., Blumenstein, B.A., et al. (1998) Serum percent free prostate-specific antigen in metastatic prostate cancer *Urology* **52**, 366–71.

5. Ploch, N.R., Brawer, M.K. (1994) How to use prostate-specific antigen *Urology* **43(2)**, 27–35.

6. Fowler, J.E., Jr., Pandey, P., Seaver, L.E., et al. (1995) Prostate specific antigen regression and progression after androgen deprivation for localized and metastatic prostate cancer *J Urol* **153**, 1860–5.

7. Small, E.J. (1998) Prostate cancer: incidence, management and outcomes. *Drugs Aging* **13**, 71–81.

8. Lukes, M., Urban, M., Zalesky, M., et al. (2001) Prostate-specific antigen: current status *Folio Biol* (Praha) **47**, 41–9.

9. Boccon-Gibod, L. (1995) Prostate-specific antigen or PSA. Facts and probabilities *Presse Med* **24**, 1471–2.

10. Dong, J.T., Rinker-Schaeffer, C.W., Ichikawa, T., et al. (1996) Prostate cancer – biology of metastasis and its clinical implications. *World J Urol* **14**, 182–9.

11. Yu, K.K., Hawkins, R.A. (2000) The prostate: diagnostic evaluation of metastatic disease. *Radiol Clin North Am* **38**, 139–57.

12. Carroll, P. (2001) Rising PSA after a radical treatment *Eur Urol* **40(2)**, 9–16.

13. McMurtry, C.T., McMurtry, J.M. (2003) Metastatic prostate cancer: complications and treatment *J Am Geriatr Soc* **51**, 1136–42.

14. Timme, T.L., Satoh, T., Tahir, S.A., et al. (2003) Therapeutic targets for metastatic prostate cancer *Curr Drug Targets* **4(3)**, 251–61.

15. De la Taille, A., Vancherot, F., Salomon, L., et al. (2001) Hormone-refractory prostate cancer: a multi-step and multi-event process *Prostate Cancer Prostatic Dis* **4**, 204–12.

16. Carlin, B.I., Andriole, G.L. (2000) The natural history, skeletal complications, and management of bone metastases in patients with prostate carcinoma. *Cancer* **88(12)**, 2989–94.

17. Herold, D.M., Hanlon, A.L., Movsas, B., et al. (1998) Age-related prostate cancer metastases *Urology* **51**, 985–90.

18. Sandhu, D.P., Munson, K.W., Benghiat, A., et al. (1992) Natural history and prognosis of prostate carcinoma in adolescents and men under 35 years of age. *Br J Urol* **69**, 525–9.

19. Fowler, J.E., Bigler, S.A., Renfroe, D.L., et al. (1997) Prostate specific antigen in black and white men after hormonal therapies for prostate cancer *J Urol* **158**, 150–4.

20. Pound, C.R., Partin, A.W., Eisenberger, M.A., et al. (1999) Natural history of progression after PSA elevation following radical prostatectomy *JAMA* **281**, 1591–7.

21. Fossa, S.D., Dearnaley, D.P., Law, M., et al. (1992) Prognostic factors in hormone-resistant progressing cancer of the prostate *Ann Oncol* **3**, 331–5.

22. Trapman, J., Brinkmann, A.O. (1996) The androgen receptor in prostate cancer *Pathol Res Pract* **192**, 752–60.

23. Culig, Z., Hobisch, A., Hittmair, A., et al. (1997) Androgen receptor gene mutations in prostate cancer. Implications for disease progression and therapy *Drugs Aging* **10**, 50–8.

24. Culig, Z., Klocker, H., Bartsch, G., et al. (2002) Androgen receptors in prostate cancer *Endocr Relat Cancer* **9**, 155–70.

25. Jenster, G. (1999) The role of the androgen receptor in the development and progression of prostate cancer *Semin Oncol* **26**, 407–21.

26. Smaletz, O., Scher, H.I. (2002) Outcome predictions for patients with metastatic prostate cancer *Semin Urol Oncol* **20**, 155–63.

27. Partin, A.W., Steinberg, G.D., Pitcock, R.V., et al. (1992) Use of nuclear morphometry, Gleason histologic scoring, clinical stage, and age to predict disease-free survival among patients with prostate cancer *Cancer* **70**(1), 161–8.

28. Smaletz, O., Scher, H.J., Small, E.J., et al. (2002) Nomogram for overall survival of patients with progressive metastatic prostate cancer after castration *J Clin Oncol* **20**, 3972–82.

29. Cho, D., Di Blasio, C.J., Rhee, A.C., et al. (2003) Prognostic factors for survival in patients with hormone-refractory prostate cancer (HRPC) after initial androgen deprivation therapy (ADT). *Urol Oncol* **21**, 282–91.

30. Miller, J.I., Ahmann, F.R., Drach, G.W., et al. (1992) The clinical usefulness of serum prostate specific antigen after hormonal therapy of metastatic prostate cancer *J Urol* **147**, 956–61.

31. Kelly, W.K., Scher, H.I., Mazumdar, M., et al. (1993) Prostate-specific antigen as a measure of disease outcome in metastatic hormone refractory prostate cancer *J Clin Oncol* **11**, 596–7.

32. Matzkin, H., Perito, P.E., Soloway, M.S. (1993) Prognostic factors in metastatic prostate cancer *Cancer* **72**(12), 3788–92.

33. Spencer, J.A., Chug, W.J., Hudson, E., et al. (1998) Prostate specific antigen level and Gleason score in predicting the stage of newly diagnosed prostate cancer *Br J Radiol* **71**, 1130–5.

34. Furuya, Y., Akakura, K., Tobe, T., et al. (2001) Prognostic significance of changes in prostate-specific antigen in patients with metastatic prostate cancer after endocrine treatment *Int Urol Nephrol* **32**, 659–63.

35. Roberts, S.G., Blute, M.L., Bergstralh, E.J., et al. (2001) PSA doubling time as a predictor of clinical progression after biochemical failure following radical prostatectomy for prostate cancer *Mayo Clin Proc* **76**, 576–81.

36. Oosterlinck, W., Mattelaer, J., Casselman, J., et al. (1997) PSA evolution: a prognostic factor in treatment of advanced prostatic carcinoma with total androgen blockade. Data from a Belgian multicentric study of 546 patients *Acta Urol Belg* **65**, 63–71.

37. Benaim, E.A., Pace, C.M., Lam, P.M., et al. (2002) Nadir prostate-specific antigen as a predictor of progression to androgen-independent prostate cancer *Urology* **59**, 73–8.

38. Small, E.J., McMillan, A., Meyer, M., et al. (2001) Serum prostate-specific antigen decline as a marker of clinical outcome in hormone-refractory prostate cancer patients: association with progression-free survival, pain end points, and survival *J Clin Oncol* **19**, 1304–11.

39. Crawford, E.D., DeAntoni, E.P., Ross, C.A. (1996) The role of prostate-specific antigen in the chemoprevention of prostate cancer *J Cell Biochem* **25**, 149–55.

40. Safa, A.A., Reese, D.M., Carter, D.M., et al. (1998) Undetectable serum prostate-specific antigen associated with metastatic prostate cancer: a case report and review of the literature *Am J Clin Oncol* **21**, 323–6.

41. Sella, A., Konichezky, M., Flex, D., et al. (2000) Low PSA metastatic androgen-independent prostate cancer *Eur Urol* **38**, 250–4.

42. Beardo, P., Fernandez, P.L., Corral, J.M., et al. (2001) Undetectable prostate specific antigen in disseminated prostate cancer *J Urol* **166**, 993.

43. Dreicer, R. (1997) Metastatic prostate cancer: assessment of response to systemic therapy *Semin Urol Oncol* **15**, 28–32.

44. Bauer, K.S., Figg, W.D., Hamilton, J.M., et al. (1999) A pharmacokinetically guided Phase II study of carboxyamido-triazole in androgen-independent prostate cancer. *Clin Cancer Res* **5(9)**, 2324–9.

45. Horti, J., Dixon, S.C., Logothetis, C., et al. (1999) Increased transcriptional activity of PSA in the presence of TNP-470, an angiogenesis inhibitor. *Br J Cancer* **79**, 1588–93.

46. Lofters, A., Juffs, H.G., Pond, G.R., et al. (2002) "PSA-itis": knowledge of serum prostate specific antigen and other causes of anxiety in men with metastatic prostate cancer. *J Urol* **168(6)**, 2516–20.

47. Hricak, H., Schoder, H., Pucar, D., et al. (2003) Advances in imaging in the postoperative patient with a rising prostate-specific antigen level *Semin Oncol* **30**, 616–34.

48. Benaron, D.A. (2002) The future of cancer imaging *Cancer Metastasis Rev* **21**, 45–78.

49. Yu, K.K., Hricak, H. (2000) Imaging prostate cancer *Radiol Clin North Am* **38**, 59–85.

50. Engelbrecht, M.R., Barentsz, J.O., Jager, G.J., et al. (2000) Prostate cancer staging with imaging *BJU Int* **86(1)**, 123–34.

51. Haseman, M.K., Reed, N.L., Rosenthal, S.A. (1996) Monoclonal antibody imaging of occult prostate cancer in patients with elevated prostate-specific antigen. Positron emission tomography and biopsy correlation *Clin Nucl Med* **21(9)**, 704–13.

52. Haseman, M.K., Rosenthal, S.A., Polascik, T.J. (2000) Capromab pendetide imaging of prostate cancer *Cancer Biother Radiopharm* **15(2)**:131–40.

53. Fair, W.R., Israeli, R.S., Heston, W.D. (1997) Prostate-specific membrane antigen *Prostate* **32**, 140–8.

54. Elgamal, A.A., Holmes, E.H., Su, S.L., et al. (2000) Prostate-specific membrane antigen (PSMA): current benefits and future value. *Semin Surg Oncol* **18**, 10–16.

55. Roudier, M.P., Vesselle, H., True, L.D., et al. (2003) Bone histology at autopsy and matched bone scintigraphy findings in patients with hormone refractory prostate cancer: the effect of biphosphonate therapy on bone scintigraphy results *Clin Exp Metastasis* **20**, 171–80.

56. Lee, C.T., Oesterling, J.E. (1997) Using prostate-specific antigen to eliminate the staging radionuclide bone scan *Urol Clin North Am* **24**, 389–94.

57. Modoni, S., Calo, E., Nardella, G., et al. (1997) PSA and bone scintigraphy *Int J Biol Markers* **12**, 158–61.

58. Murphy, G.P., Troychak, M.J., Cobb, O.E., et al. (1997) Evaluation of PSA, free PSA, PSMA, and total and bone alkaline phosphatase levels compared to bone scans in the management of patients with metastatic prostate cancer *Prostate* **33**, 141–6.

59. Coleman, R.E., Mashiter, G., Whitaker, K.B., et al. (1988) Bone scan flare predicts successful systemic therapy for bone metastases *J Nucl Med* **29**, 1354–9.

60. Bubley, G.J., Carducci, M., Dahut, W., et al. (1999) Eligibility and response guidelines for phase II clinical trials in androgen-independent prostate cancer: recommendations from the prostate-specific antigen working group *J Clin Oncol* **17**, 3461–7.

61. DeLuca, S.A., Castronovo, F.P., Rhea, J.T. (1983) The effects of chemotherapy on bony metastases as measured by quantitative skeletal imaging *Clin Nucl Med* **8**, 11–13.

62. Drelichman, A., Decker, D.A., Al-Sarraf, M., et al. (1984) Computerized bone scan. A potentially useful technique to measure response in prostate carcinoma *Cancer* **53**, 1061–5.

63. Imbriaco, M., Larson, S.M., Yeung, H.W., et al. (1998) A new parameter for measuring metastatic bone involvement by prostate cancer: the bone scan index *Clin Cancer Res* **4**, 1765–72.

64. Noguchi, M., Kikuchi, H., Ishibashi, M., et al. (2003) Percentage of the positive area of bone metastasis is an independent predictor of disease death in advanced prostate cancer *Br J Cancer* **88(2)**, 195–201.

65. Yahara, J., Noghuchi, M., Noda, S. (2003) Quantitative evaluation of bone metastases in patients with advanced prostate cancer during systemic treatment *BJU Int* **92**, 379–84.

66. Rafii, M., Firooznia, H., Kramer, E., et al. (1988) The role of computed tomography in evaluation of skeletal metastases *J Comput Tomogr* **12**, 19–24.

67. Harisinghani, M.G., Barentsz, J.O., Hahn, P.F., et al. (2003) Noninvasive detection of clinically occult lymph-node metastases in prostate cancer *N Eng J Med* **348(25)**, 2491–9.

68. Bouchelouche, K., Oehr, P. (2008) Recent developments in urologic oncology: positron emission tomography molecular imaging *Curr Opin Oncol* **20**, 321–6.

69. Sanz, G., Rioja, J., Zudaire, J.J., et al. (2004) PET and prostate cancer *World J Urol* **22**, 351–2.

70. Conti, P.S., Lilien, D.L., Hawley, K., et al. (1996) PET and [F-18]-FDG in oncology: a clinical update. *Nucl Med Biol* **23**, 717–35.

71. Fischman, A.J. (1996) Positron emission tomography in the clinical evaluation of metastatic cancer *J Clin Oncol* **14**(3), 691–6.

72. Jadvar, H., Fischman, A.J. (1999) Evaluation of rare tumors with [F-18]fluorodeoxyglucose positron emission tomography. *Clin Positron Imaging* **2**, 153–8.

73. Kostakoglu, L., Agress, H., Jr., Goldsmith, S.J. (2003) Clinical role of FDG PET in evaluation of cancer patients *Radiographics* **23**, 315–40.

74. Macheda, M.L., Rogers, S., Bets, J.D. (2005) Molecular and cellular regulation of glucose transport (GLUT) proteins in cancer. *J Cell Physiol* **202**, 654–62.

75. Smith, T.A. (2000) Mammalian hexokinases and their abnormal expression in cancer *Br J Biomed Sci* **57**, 170–8.

76. Takahashi, N., Inoue, T., Lee, J., Yamaguchi, T., Shizukuishi, K. (2007) The roles of PET and PET/CT in the diagnosis and management of prostate cancer *Oncology* **72**, 226–33.

77. Effert, P.J., Bares, R., Handt, S., et al. (1996) Metabolic imaging of untreated prostate cancer by positron emission tomography with 18fluorine-labeled deoxyglucose. *J Urol* **155**, 994–8.

78. Hofer, C., Laubenbacher, C., Block, T., et al. (1999) Fluorine-18-fluorodeoxyglucose positron emission tomography is useless for the detection of local recurrence after radical prostatectomy. *Eur Urol* **36**, 31–5.

79. Patel, P., Cohade, C., DeWeese, T., et al. (2002) Evaluation of metabolic activity of prostate gland with PET-CT. *J Nucl Med* **43**(5), 119P.

80. Salminen, E., Hogg, A., Binns, D., et al. (2002) Investigations with FDG-PET scanning in prostate cancer show limited value for clinical practice *Acta Oncol* **41**(5), 425–9.

81. von Mallek, D., Backhaus, B., Muller, S.C., et al. (2006) Technical limits of PET/CT with 18FDG in prostate cancer. *Aktuelle Urol* **37**, 218–21.

82. Liu, I.J., Zafar, M.B., Lai, Y.H., et al. (2001) Fluorodeoxyglucose positron emission tomography studies in diagnosis and staging of clinically organ-confined prostate cancer *Urology* **57**, 108–11.

83. Kao, P.F., Chou, Y.H., Lai, C.W. (2008) Diffuse FDG uptake in acute prostatitis *Clin Nucl Med* **33**, 308–10.

84. Hara, T., Bansal, A., DeGrado, T.R. (2006) Effect of hypoxia on the uptake of [methyl-3H]choline, [1–14C]acetate and [18F]FDG in cultured prostate cancer cells. *Nucl Med Biol* **33**, 977–84.

85. Pugachev, A., Ruan, S., Carlin, S., et al. (2005) Dependence of FDG uptake on tumor microenvironment *Int J Radiat Oncol Biol Phys* **62**, 545–53.

86. Etchebehere, E.C., Macapinlac, H.A., Gonen, M., Humm, K., Yeung, H.W., Akhurst, T., et al. (2002) Qualitative and quantitative comparison between images obtained with filtered back projection and iterative reconstruction in prostate cancer lesions of 18F-FDG PET. *Q J Nucl Med* **46**, 122–30.

87. Turlakow, A., Larson, S.M., Coakley, F., Akhurst, T., Gonen, M., Macapinlac, H.A., et al. (2001) Local detection of prostate cancer by positron emission tomography with 2-fluorodeoxyglucose: comparison of filtered back projection and iterative reconstruction with segmented attenuation correction. *Q J Nucl Med* **45**, 235–44.

88. Shreve, P.D., Grossman, H.B., Gross, M.D., et al. (1996) Metastatic prostate cancer: initial findings of PET with FDG *Radiology* **199**, 751–6.

89. Oyama, N., Akino, H., Kanamaru, H., et al. (1998) Fluorodeoxyglucose positron emission tomography in diagnosis of untreated prostate cancer *Nippon Rinsho* **56**, 2052–5.

90. Oyama, N., Akino, H., Suzuki, Y., et al. (1999) The increased accumulation of [18F] fluorodeoxyglucose in untreated prostate cancer. *Jpn J Clin Oncol* **29**, 623–9.

91. Oyama, N., Akino, H., Suzuki, Y., et al. (2001) FDG PET for evaluating the change of glucose metabolism in prostate cancer after androgen ablation *Nucl Med Commun* **22**, 963–9.

92. Oyama, N., Kim, J., Jones, L.A., et al. (2002) MicroPET assessment of androgenic control of glucose and acetate uptake in the rat prostate and a prostate cancer tumor model *Nucl Med Biol* **29**, 783–90.

93. Oyama, N., Akino, H., Suzuki, Y., et al. (2002) Prognostic value of 2-deoxy-2-[F-18] fluoro-D-glucose positron emission tomography imaging for patients with prostate cancer. *Mol Imaging Biol* **4**, 99–104.

94. Chang, C.H., Wu, H.C., Tsai, J.J., et al. (2003) Detecting metastatic pelvic lymph nodes by (18)f-2-deoxyglucose positron emission tomography in patients with prostate-specific antigen relapse after treatment for localized prostate cancer. *Urol Int* **70**(4), 311–5.

95. Schoder, H., Herrmann, K., Gonen, M., Hricak, H., Eberhard, S., Scardino, P., et al.

(2005) 2-[18F]fluoro-2-deoxyglucose positron emission tomography for detection of disease in patients with prostate-specific antigen relapse after radical prostatectomy. *Clin Cancer Res* 11, 4761–9.

96. Jadvar, H., Pinski, J.K., Conti, P.S. (2003) FDG PET in suspected recurrent and metastatic prostate cancer *Oncol Rep* 10(5), 1485–8.

97. Morris, N.J., Akhurst, T., Osman, I., et al. (2002) Fluorinated deoxyglucose positron emission tomography imaging in progressive metastatic prostate cancer *Urology* 59, 913–8.

98. Morris, M.J., Akhurst, T., Larson, S.M., Ditullio, M., Chu, E., Siedlecki, K., et al. (2005) Fluorodeoxyglucose positron emission tomography as an outcome measure for castrate metastatic prostate cancer treated with antimicrotubule chemotherapy *Clin Cancer Res* 11, 3210–6.

99. Bucerius, J., Ahamadzadehfar, H., Hortling, N., Joe, A.Y., Palmedo, H., Biersack, H.J. (2007) Incidental diagnosis of a PSA-negative cancer by (18)FDG PET/CT in a patient with hypopharyngeal cancer. *Prostate Cancer Prostatic Dis* 10, 307–10.

100. Agus, D.B., Golde, D.W., Squouros, G., Ballanqrud, A., Cordon-Cardo, C., Scher, H.I. (1998) Positron emission tomography of a human prostate cancer xenograft: association of changes in deoxyglucose accumulation with other measures of outcome following androgen withdrawal *Cancer Res* 58, 3009–14.

101. Sung, J., Espiritu, J.I., Segall, G.M., Terris, M.K. (2003) Fluorodeoxyglucose positron emission tomography studies in the diagnosis and staging of clinically advanced prostate cancer *BJU Int* 92, 24–7.

102. Ludwig, V., Hopper, O.W., Martin, W.H., Kikkawa, R., Delbeke, D. (2003) [18F] fluoro- deoxyglucose positron emission tomography surveillance of hepatic metastases from prostate cancer following radiofrequency ablation: a case report. *Am Surg* 69, 593–8.

103. Yeh, S.D., Imbriaco, M., Larson, S.M., et al. (1996) Detection of bony metastases of androgen-independent prostate cancer by PET-FDG *Nucl Med Biol* 23, 693–7.

104. Haberkorn, U., Bellemann, M.E., Altmann, A., et al. (1997) PET 2-fluoro-2-deoxyglucose uptake in rat prostate adenocarcinoma during chemotherapy with gemcitabine. *J Nucl Med* 38, 1215–21.

105. Heicappell, R., Muller-Mattheis, V., Reinhardt, M., et al. (1999) Staging of pelvic lymph nodes in neoplasms of the bladder and prostate by positron emission tomography with 2-[(18)F]-2-deoxy-D-glucose. *Eur Urol* 36, 582–7.

106. Sanz, G., Robles, J.E., Gimenez, M., et al. (1999) Positron emission tomography with 18fluorine-labelled deoxyglucose: utility in localized and advanced prostate cancer. *BJU Int* 84, 1028–31.

107. Shimizu, N., Masuda, H., Yamanaka, H., et al. (1999) Fluorodeoxyglucose positron emission tomography scan of prostate cancer bone metastases with flare reaction after endocrine therapy *J Urol* 161, 608–9.

108. Kotzerke, J., Gschwend, J.E., Neumaier, B. (2002) PET for prostate cancer imaging: still a quandary or the ultimate solution *J Nucl Med* 43(2), 200–2.

109. Zhang, Y., Saylor, M., Wen, S., et al. (2006) Longitudinally quantitative 2-deoxy-2-[18F] fluoro-D-glucose micro positron emission tomography imaging for efficacy of new anticancer drugs: a case study with bortezomib in prostate cancer murine model. *Mol Imaging Biol* 8, 300–8.

110. Mullerad, M., Eisenberg, D.P., Akhurst, T.J., et al. (2006) Use of positron emission tomography to target prostate cancer gene therapy by oncolytic herpes simplex virus *Mol Imaging Biol* 8, 30–5.

111. Jadvar, H., Li, X., Shahinian, A., et al. (2005) Glucose metabolism of human prostate cancer mouse xenografts *Mol Imaging* 4, 91–7.

112. Seltzer, M.A., Barbaric, Z., Belldegrun, A., et al. (1999) Comparison of helical computerized tomography, positron emission tomography and monoclonal antibody scans for evaluation of lymph node metastases in patients with prostate specific antigen relapse after treatment for localized prostate cancer *J Urol* 162, 1322–8.

113. Jadvar, H. (2008) [F-18]-Fluorodeoxyglucose (FDG) positron emission tomography and computed tomography (PET-CT) in metastatic prostate cancer. USC Norris Comprehensive Cancer Center. ClinicalTrials. gov Identifier: NCT00282906. Accessed August 20, 2008.

114. Yoshimoto, M., Waki, A., Yonekura, Y., et al. (2001) Characterization of acetate metabolism in tumor cells in relation to cell proliferation: acetate metabolism in tumor cells *Nucl Med Biol* 28, 117–22.

115. Shreve, P.D., Lannone, P., Weinhold, P. (2002) Cellular metabolism of [1-C14]-acetate in prostate cancer cells in vitro. *J Nucl Med* 43(5), 272P.

116. Liu, Y. (2006) Fatty acid oxidation is a dominant bioenergetic pathway in prostate cancer *Prostate Cancer Prostatic Dis* 9, 230–4.

117. Vavere, A.L., Kridel, S.J., Wheeler, F.B., et al. (2008) 1–11C-acetate as a PET radiopharmaceutical for imaging fatty acid synthase expression in prostate cancer. *J Nucl Med* **49**, 327–34.

118. Pflug, B.R., Pecher, S.M., Brink, A.W., et al. (2003) Increased fatty acid synthase expression and activity during progression of prostate cancer in the TRAMP model *Prostate* **57**, 245–54.

119. Seltzer, M.A., Jahan, S.A., Dahlbom, M., et al. (2003) Combined metabolic imaging using C-11 acetate and FDG PET for the evaluation of patients with suspected recurrent prostate cancer. *J Nucl Med* **44(5)**, 132P.

120. Kato, T., Tsukamoto, E., Kuge, Y., et al. (2002) Accumulation of [(11)C]acetate in normal prostate and benign prostatic hyperplasia: comparison with prostate cancer. *Eur J Nucl Med Mol Imaging* **29(11)**, 1492–5.

121. Hautzel, H., Muller-Mattheis, V., Herzog, H., et al. (2002) The (11C) acetate positron emission tomography in prostatic carcinoma. New prospects in metabolic imaging *Urologe A* **41**, 569–76.

122. Kotzerke, J., Volkmer, B.G., Neumaier, B., et al. (2002) Carbon-11 acetate positron emission tomography can detect local recurrence of prostate cancer. *Eur J Nucl Med Mol Imaging* **29(10)**, 1380–4.

123. Oyama, N., Akino, H., Kanamaru, H., et al. (2002) 11C-acetate PET imaging of prostate cancer. *J Nucl Med* **43(2)**, 181–6.

124. Seltzer, M.A., Jahan, S., Dahlbom, M., et al. (2002) C-11 acetate PET imaging of primary and locally recurrent prostate cancer: comparison to normal controls. *J Nucl Med* **43(5)**, 117P.

125. Oyama, N., Miller, T.R., Dehdashti, F., et al. (2003) 11C-acetate PET imaging of prostate cancer: detection of recurrent disease at PSA relapse. *J Nucl Med* **44(4)**, 549–55.

126. Dimitrakopoulou-Strauss, A., Strauss, L.G. (2003) PET imaging of prostate cancer with 11C-acetate. *J Nucl Med* **44(4)**, 556–8.

127. Sandblom, G., Sorensen, J., Lundin, N., et al. (2006) Positron emission tomography with C11-acetate for tumor detection and localization in patients with prostate specific antigen relapse after radical prostatectomy. *Urology* **67**, 996–1000.

128. Jadvar, H., Li, X., Park, R., Shahinian, A., et al. (2008) Quantitative autoradiography of radiolabeled acetate in mouse xenografts of human prostate cancer *J Nucl Med* **47(1)**, 421P- 422P.

129. Albrecht, S., Buchegger, F., Soloviev, D., et al. (2007) 11C-acetate PET in the early evaluation of prostate cancer recurrence. *Eur J Nucl Med Mol Imaging* **34**, 185–96.

130. Fricke, E., Machtens, S., Hofmann, M., et al. (2003) Positron emission tomography with (11)C- acetate and (18)F-FDG in prostate cancer patients. *Eur J Nucl Med Mol Imaging* **30(4)**, 607–11.

131. Vees, H., Buchegger, F., Albrecht, S., et al. (2007) 18F-choline and/or 11C-acetae positron emission tomography: detection of residual or progressive subclinical disease at very low prostate-specific antigen values (<1 ng/mL) after radical prostatectomy. *BJU Int* **99**, 1415–20.

132. Watchter, S., Tomek, S., Kurtaran, A., et al. (2006) 11C-acetate positron emission tomography imaging and image fusion with computed tomography and magnetic resonance imaging in patients with recurrent prostate cancer. *J Clin Oncol* **24**, 2513–9.

133. Schiepers, C., Hoh, C.K., Nuyts, J., et al. (2008) 1–11C-acetate kinetics of prostate cancer. *J Nucl Med* **49**, 206–15.

134. Seltzer, M.A., Jahan, S.A., Sparks, R., et al. (2004) Radiation dose estimates in humans for (11)C-acetate whole-body. PET *J Nucl Med* **45(7)**, 1233–6.

135. Matthies, A., Ezziddin, S., Ulrich, E.M., et al. (2004) Imaging of prostate cancer metastases with 18F-fluoroacetate using PET/CT. *Eur J Nucl Med Mol Imaging* **31**, 797.

136. Ponde, D.E., Dence, C.S., Oyama, N., et al. (2007) 18F-fluoroacetate: a potential acetate analog for prostate tumors imaging – in vivo evaluation of 18F-fluoroacetate versus 11C-acetate. *J Nucl Med* **48**, 420–8.

137. Zheng, Q.H., Gradner, T.A., Raikwar, S., et al. (2004) [11C]choline as a PET biomarker for assessment of prostate cancer tumor models. *Bioorg Med Chem* **12**, 2887–93.

138. Hara, T., Kosaka, N., Kishi, H. (1998) PET imaging of prostate cancer using carbon-11-choline. *J Nucl Med* **39(6)**, 990–5.

139. Kotzerke, J., Prang, J., Neumaier, B., et al. (2000) Experience with carbon-11 choline positron emission tomography in prostate carcinoma. *Eur J Nucl Med* **27(9)**, 1415–9.

140. Picchio, M., Landoni, C., Messa, C., et al. (2002) Positive [11C]choline and negative [18F]FDG with PET in recurrence of prostate cancer. *Am J Roentgenol AJR* **179**, 482–4.

141. de Jong, I.J., Pruim, J., Elsinga, P.H., et al. (2002) Visualization of prostate cancer with 11C- choline positron emission tomography. *Eur Urol* **42(1)**, 18–23.

142. Blumstein, N.M., Wollenweber, F., Wahl, A., et al. (2003) [11C]choline PET/CT a therapy

optimizing tool for prostatectomised patients with increasing PSA level. J Nucl Med 44(5), 133P.

143. de Jong, I.J., Pruim, J., Elsinga, P.H., et al. (2003) Preoperative staging of pelvic lymph nodes in prostate cancer by 11C-choline PET. *J Nucl Med* **44(3)**, 331–5.

144. de Jong, I.J., Pruim, J., Elsinqa, P.H., et al. (2003) 11C-choline positron emission tomography for the evaluation after treatment of localized prostate cancer. *Eur Urol* **44**, 38–9.

145. Picchio, M., Messa, C., Landoni, C., et al. (2003) Value of [11C]choline-positron emission tomography for re-staging prostate cancer: a comparison with [18F]fluorodeoxy-glucose- positron emission tomography. *J Urol* **169(4)**, 1337–40.

146. Kanda, T., Nakagomi, K., Goto, S., et al. (2008) Visualization of prostate cancer with 11C- choline positron emission tomography (PET): localization of primary and recurrent prostate cancer. *Hinyokika Kiyo* **54**, 325–32.

147. Reske, S.N., Blumstein, N.M., Neumaier, B., et al. (2006) Imaging prostate cancer with 11C- choline PET/CT. *J Nucl Med* **47**, 1249–54.

148. Reske, S.N. (2008) [(11C)Choline uptake with PET/CT for the initial diagnosis of prostate cancer: relation to PSA levels, tumor stage and anti-androgenic therapy. *Eur J Nucl Med Mol Imaging* **35(9)**, 1740–1.

149. Reske, S.N., Blumstein, N.M., Glatting, G. (2008) [(11C)]choline PET/CT imaging in occult local relapse of prostate cancer after radical prostatectomy. *Eur J Nucl Med Mol Imaging* **35**, 9–17.

150. Breeuwsma, A.J., Pruim, J., Jongen, M.M., et al. (2005) In vivo uptake of [11C]choline does not correlate with cell proliferation in human prostate cancer. *Eur J Nucl Med Mol Imaging* **32**, 668–73.

151. Reischl, G., Bieg, C., Schmiedl, O., et al. (2004) Highly efficient automated synthesis of [(11)C]choline for multi dose utilization. *Appl Radiat Isot* **60**, 835–8.

152. DeGrado, T.R., Baldwin, S.W., Wang, S., et al. (2001) Synthesis and evaluation of (18) F-labeled choline analogs as oncologic PET tracers. *J Nucl Med* **42**, 1805–14.

153. DeGrado, T.R., Coleman, R.E., Wang, S., et al. (2001) Synthesis and evaluation of 18F-labeled choline as an oncologic tracer for positron emission tomography: initial findings in prostate cancer. *Cancer Res* **61(1)**, 110–117.

154. DeGrado, T.R., Reiman, R.E., Price, D.T., et al. (2002) Pharmacokinetics and radiation dosimetry of 18F-fluorocholine. *J Nucl Med* **43**, 92–6.

155. Hara, T., Kosaka, N., Kishi, H. (2002) Development of F-18 fluoroethylcholine for cancer imaging with PET: synthesis, biochemistry, and prostate cancer imaging. *J Nucl Med* **43**, 187–99.

156. Sutinen, E., Nurmi, M., Roivainen, A., et al. (2004) Kinetics of [(11C)]choline uptake in prostate cancer: a PET study. *Eur J Nucl Med Mol Imaging* **31**, 317–24.

157. Testa, C., Schiavina, R., Lodi, R., et al. (2007) Prostate cancer: sextant localization with MR imaging, MR spectroscopy, and 11C-choline PET-CT. *Radiology* **244**, 797–806.

158. Yamaguchi, T., Lee, J., Uemura, H., et al. (2005) Prostate cancer: a comparative study of 11C-choline PET and MR imaging combined with proton MR spectroscopy. *Eur J Nucl Med Mol Imaging* **32**, 742–8.

159. Park, H., Piert, M.R., Khan, A., et al. (2008) Registration methodology for histological sections and in vivo imaging of human prostate *Acad Radiol* **15**, 1027–39.

160. Eschmann, S.M., Pfannenberg, A.C., Rieger, A., et al. (2007) Comparison of 11C-choline PET-CT and whole body MRI for staging of prostate cancer. *Nuklearmedizin* **46**, 161–8.

161. Rinnab, L., Blumstein, N.M., Mottaghy, F.M., et al. (2007) 11C-choline positron emission tomography/computed tomography and transrectal ultrasonography for staging localized prostate cancer. *BJU Int* **99**, 1421–6.

162. Scher, B., Seitz, M., Albinger, W., et al. (2007) Value of 11C-choline PET and PET-CT in patients with suspected prostate cancer. *Eur J Nucl Med Mol Imaging* **34**, 45–53.

163. Farsad, M., Schiavina, R., Castellucci, P., et al. (2005) Detection and localization of prostate cancer: correlation of (11C) C-choline PET/CTPET-CT with histo-pathologic step-section analysis. *J Nucl Med* **46**:1642–9.

164. Martorana, G., Schiavina, R., Cort, B., et al. (2006) 11C-choline positron emission tomography/computed tomography for tumor localization of primary prostate cancer in comparison with 12-core biopsy. *J Urol* **176**, 954–60.

165. Kishi, H., Minowada, S., Kosaka, N., et al. (2002) C-11 choline PET helps determine the outcome of hormonal therapy of prostate cancer. *J Nucl Med* **43(5)**, 117P.

166. Jadvar, H., Gurbuz, A., Li, X., et al. (2008) Choline autoradiography of human prostate

cancer xenograft: effect of castration *Mol Imaging* 7(**3**), 147–52.

167. Krause, B.J., Souvatzpglou, M., Tuncel, M., et al. (2008) The detection rate of [(11)C]Choline-PET/CT depends on the serum PSA-value in patients with biochemical recurrence of prostate cancer. *Eur J Nucl Med Mol Imaging* **35**, 18–23.

168. Scattoni, V., Picchio, M., Suardi, N., et al. (2007) Detection of lymph-node metastases with integrated [11C]choline in patients with PSA failure after radical retropubic prostatectomy: results confirmed by open pelvic-retroperitoneal lymphadenectomy. *Eur Radiol* **52**, 423–9.

169. Tuneel, M., Souvatzoglou, M., Herrmann, K., et al. (2008) (11C)Choline positron emission tomography/computed tomography for staging and restaging of patients with advanced prostate cancer. *Nucl Med Biol* **35**, 689–95.

170. Schiavina, R., Scattoni, V., Castellucci, P., et al. (2008) (11C)-choline positron emission tomography/computerized tomography for preoperative lymph-node staging in intermediate-risk and high-risk prostate cancer: comparison with clinical staging nomograms. *Eur Urol* **54**, 392–401.

171. Price, D.T., Coleman, R.E., Liao, R.P., et al. (2002) Comparison of [18 F]fluorocholine and [18F]fluorodeoxyglucose for positron emission tomography of androgen dependent and androgen independent prostate cancer. *J Urol* **168**, 273–80.

172. Igerc, I., Kohlfurst, S., Gallowitsch, H.J., et al. (2008) The value of 18F-choline PET/CT in patients with elevated PSA-level and negative prostate needle biopsy for localization of prostate cancer. *Eur J Nucl Med Mol Imaging* **35**, 976–83.

173. Yoshida, S., Nakagomi, K., Goto, S., et al. (2005) 11C-choline positron emission tomography in prostate cancer: primary staging and recurrent site staging. *Urol Int* **74**, 214–20.

174. Kwee, S.A., Coel, M.N., Lim, J., et al. (2005) Prostate cancer localization with 18fluorine fluorocholine positron emission tomography. *J Urol* **173**, 252–5.

175. Kwee, S.A., Wei, H., Sesterhenn, I., et al. (2006) Localization of primary prostate cancer with dual-phase 18F-fluorocholine PET. *J Nucl Med* **47**, 262–9.

176. Pelosi, E., Arena, V., Skanjeti, A., et al. (2008) Role of whole-body (18F)-choline PET/CT in disease detection in patients with biochemical relapse after radical treatment for prostate cancer. *Radiol Med* **113**(6), 895–904.

177. Schilling, D., Schlemmer, H.P., Wagner, P.H., et al. (2008) Histological verification of 11C- choline-positron emission tomography/computed tomography positive lymph nodes in patients with biochemical failure after treatment for localized prostate cancer. *BJU Int* **102**, 446–51.

178. Husarik, D.B., Miralbell, R., Dubs, M., et al. (2008) Evaluation of [(18)F]-choline PET/CT for staging and restaging of prostate cancer. *Eur J Nucl Med Mol Imaging* **35**, 253–63.

179. Rinnab, L., Mottaghy, F.M., Blumstein, N.M., et al. (2007) Evaluation of [11C]choline positron emission tomography in patients with increasing prostate-specific antigen levels after primary treatment for prostate cancer. *BJU Int* **100**, 786–93.

180. Cimitan, M., Bortolus, R., Morassut, S., et al. (2006) 18F-fluorocholine PET/CT imaging for the detection of recurrent prostate cancer at PSA relapse: experience in 100 consecutive patients. *Eur J Nucl Med Mol Imaging* **33**, 1387–98.

181. Giovacchini, G., Picchio, M., Coradesschi, E., et al. (2008) [(11C)C]choline uptake with PET/CT for the initial diagnosis of prostate cancer: relation to PSA levels, tumor stage and anti-androgenic therapy. *Eur J Nucl Med Mol Imaging* **35**, 1065–73.

182. Heinisch, M., Dirisamer, A., Loidl, W., et al. (2006) Positron emission tomography/computed tomography with F-18 fluorocholine for restaging of prostate cancer patients: meaningful at PSA <5 ng/mL. *Mol Imaging Biol* **8**, 43–8.

183. Kotzerke, J., Volkmer, B.G., Glatting, G., et al. (2003) Intra-individual comparison of [11C]acetate and [11C]choline PET for detection of metastases of prostate cancer. *Nuklearmedizin* **42**, 25–30.

184. Dotan, Z.A. (2008) Bone imaging in prostate cancer *Nat Clin Prac Urol* **5**, 434–44.

185. Langsteger, W., Heinisch, M., Fogelman, I. (2006) The role of fluorodexoyglucose, 18F-dihydroxyphenylalanine, 18F-choline, and 18F-fluoride in bone imaging with emphasis on prostate and breast. *Semin Nucl Med* **36**, 73–92.

186. Hsu, W.K., Virk, M.S., Feeley, B.T., et al. (2008) Characterization of osteolytic, osteoblastic, and mixed lesions in a prostate cancer mouse model using 18F-FDG and 18F-fluoride PET/CT. *J Nucl Med* **49**, 414–21.

187. Beheshti, M., Vali, R., Waldenberger, P., et al. (2008) Detection of bone metastases in patients with prostate cancer by F-18 fluorocholine and F-18 fluoride PET-CT:

a comparative study. *Eur J Nucl Med Mol Imaging* **35(10)**, 1766–74.

188. Even-Sapir, E., Metser, U., Mishani, E., et al. (2006) The detection of bone metastases in patients with high risk prostate cancer: 99mTc-MDP planar bone scintigraphy, single- and multi-filed-of-view SPECT, 18F-fluoride PET, and 18F-fluoride PET/CT. *J Nucl Med* **47**, 287–97.

189. Yang, H., Berger, F., Tran, C., et al. (2003) MicroPET imaging of prostate cancer in LNCAP-SR39TK-GFP mouse xenografts. *Prostate* **55**, 39–47.

190. Hwang, D.R., Mathias, C.J., Welch, M.J., et al. (1990) Imaging prostate derived tumors with PET and N-(3-[18F]fluoropropyl) putrescine. *Int J Rad Appl Instrum B* **17**, 525–32.

191. Inaba, T. (1992) Quantitative measurements of prostatic blood flow and blood volume by positron emission tomography *J Urol* **148**, 1457–60.

192. Liu, A., Carlson, K.E., Katzenllenbogen, J.A. (1992) Synthesis of high affinity fluorine-substituted ligands for the androgen receptor. Potential agents for imaging prostatic cancer by positron emission tomography *J Med Chem* **35**, 2113–29.

193. Wang, G.J., Volkow, N.D., Wolf, A.P., et al. (1994) Positron emission tomography study of human prostatic adenocarcinoma using carbon-11 putrescine. *Nucl Med Biol* **21(1)**, 77–82.

194. Macapinlac, H.A., Humm, J.L., Akhurst, T., et al. (1999) Differential metabolism and pharmacokinetics of L-[1-(11)C]-methionine and 2-[(18)F]fluoror-2-deoxy-D-glucose (FDG) in androgen independent prostate cancer. *Clin Positron Imaging* **2**, 173–81.

195. Kalkner, K.M., Ginman, C., Nilsson, S., et al. (1997) Positron emission tomography (PET) with 11C-5-hydroxytryptophan (5-HTP) in patients with metastatic hormone-refractory prostatic adenocarcinoma. *Nucl Med Biol* **24**, 319–25.

196. Kalkner, K.M., Nilsson, S., Bergstrom, M., et al. (1997) PET with hydroxytryptophan as tracer in hormone-refractory prostatic adenocarcinoma: evaluation of decarboxylation in vivo *In Vivo* **11**, 377–81.

197. Kurdziel, K., Bacharach, S., Carrasquillo, J., et al. (2000) Using PET 18F-FDG, 11CO, and 15O-water for monitoring prostate cancer during a phase II anti-angiogenic drug trial with thalidomide. *Clin Positron Imaging* **3**, 144.

198. Nunez, R., Macapinlac, H.A., Yeung, H., et al. (2002) Combined 18F-FDG and C-11 methionine PET scans in patients with newly progressive metastatic prostate cancer. *J Nucl Med* **43**, 46–55.

199. Chen, X., Jadvar, H., Pinski, J.K., et al. (2003) PET imaging of prostate cancer xenografts in bone *Mol Imaging* #110.

200. Dehdashti, F., Picus, J., Michalski, J.M., et al. (2003) Positron emission tomographic assessment of androgen receptors in prostate carcinoma. *J Nucl Med* **44(5)**, 131P.

201. Kurdziel, K.A., Figg, W.D., Carrasquillo, J.A., et al. (2003) Using positron emission tomography 2-deoxy-2-[18F]fluoro-D-glucose, 11CO, and 15O-water for monitoring androgen independent prostate cancer. *Mol Imaging Biol* **5**, 86–93.

202. Oyama, N., Ponde, D.E., Dence, C., et al. (2004) Monitoring of therapy in androgen-dependent prostate tumor model by measuring tumor proliferation *J Nucl Med* **45**, 519–25.

203. Mintz, A., Wang, L., Ponde, D.E. (2008) Comparison of radiolabeled choline and ethanolamine as a probe for cancer detection *Cancer Biol Ther* **7(5)**, 742–7.

204. Toth, G., Lengyel, Z., Balkay, L., et al. (2005) Detection of cancer with 11C-methionine positron emission tomography. *J Urol* **173**, 66–9.

205. Larson, S.M., Morris, M., Gunther, I., et al. (2004) Tumor localization of 16-beta-18F-fluoro-5-alpha-dihydrotestosterone versus 18F-FDG in patients with progressive, metastatic prostate cancer. *J Nucl Med* **45**, 366–73.

206. Dehdashti, F., Picus, J., Michalski, J.M., et al. (2005) Positron tomographic assessment of androgen receptors in prostate carcinoma *Eur J Nucl Med Mol Imaging* **32**, 344–50.

207. Zanzonico, P.B., Finn, R., Pentlow, K.S., et al. (2004) PET-based radiation dosimetry in man of 18F-fluorodihydrotestosterone, a new radiotracer for imaging prostate cancer. *J Nucl Med* **45**, 1966–71.

208. Oka, S., Hattori, R., Kurosaki, F., et al. (2007) A preliminary study of anti-1-amino-3-18F-fluorocyclobuyl-1-carboxylic acid for the detection of prostate cancer. *J Nucl Med* **48**, 46–55.

209. Schuster, D.M., Votaw, J.R., Nieh, P.T., et al. (2007) Initial experience with radiotracer anti-1-amino-3–18F-fluorocyclobutane-1-carboxylic acid with PET/CT in prostate carcinoma. *J Nucl Med* **48**, 56–63.

210. Shields, A.F. (2006) Positron emission tomography measurement of tumor metabolism and growth: its expanding role in oncology *Mol Imaging Biol* **8**, 141–50.

211. Couturier, O., Leost, F., Campone, M., et al. (2005) Is 3'-deoxy-[18F]fluorothymidine ([18F])-FLT) the next tracer for routine clinical PET after [18]-FDG. *Bull Cancer* **92**, 789–98.

212. Conti, P.S., Alauddin, M.M., Fissekis, J.R., et al. (1995) Synthesis of 2'-fluoro-5-[11C]-methyl-1-beta-D-arabinofurasyluracil ([11C]-FMAU): a potential nucleoside analog for in vivo study of cellular proliferation with PET. *Nucl Med Biol* **22**, 783–9.

213. Nishii, R., Volgia, A.Y., Mawlawi, O., et al. (2008) Evaluation of 2'-deoxy-2'-[(18)F]fluoro-5-methyl-1-beta-L:-arabinofuranosyluracil ([(18)F]-L:-FMAU) as a PET imaging agent for cellular proliferation: comparison with [(18)F]-D:-FMAU and [(18)F]FLT. *Eur J Nucl Med Mol Imaging* **35**, 990–8.

214. Bading, J.R., Shahinian, A.H., Bathija, P., et al. (2000) Pharmacokinetics of the thymidine analog 2'-fluoro-5-[(14)C]-methyl-1-beta-D-arabinofuranosyluracil [(14)C] FMAU in rat prostate tumor cell. *Nucl Med Biol* **27**, 361–8.

215. Bading, J.R., Shahinian, A.H., Vail, A., et al. (2004) Pharmacokinetics of the thymidine analog 2'-fluoro-5-methyl-1-beta-D-arabinofuranosyluracil (FMAU) in tumor-bearing rats. *Nucl Med Biol* **31**, 407–18.

216. Tehrani, O.S., Douglas, K.A., Lawhorn-Cres, J.M., et al. (2008) Tracking cellular stress with labeled FMAU reflects changes in mitochondrial TK2. *Eur J Nucl Med Mol Imaging* **35**, 1480–8.

217. Tehrani, O.S., Muzik, O., Heilbrun, L.K., et al. (2007) Tumor imaging using 1-(2'-deoxy-18F-fluoro-beta-D-arabinofuranosyl)thymine and PET. *J Nucl Med* **48**, 1436–41.

218. Sun, H., Mangner, T.J., Collins, J.M., et al. (2005) Imaging DNA synthesis in vivo with 18F-FMAU and PET. *J Nucl Med* **46(2)**, 292–6.

219. Sun, H., Sloan, A., Mangner, T.J., et al. (2005) Imaging DNA synthesis with [18F] FMAU and positron emission tomography in patients with cancer. *Eur J Nucl Med Mol Imaging* **32**, 15–22.

Chapter 16

Brain Tumors

Serge Goldman and Benoit J.M. Pirotte

Abstract

For most cancers, PET is essentially a diagnostic tool. For brain tumors, PET has got its main contribution at the level of the therapeutic management. Indeed, specific reasons render the therapeutic management of brain tumors, especially gliomas, a real challenge. Although some gliomas may appear well-delineated on conventional neuroimaging such as CT and MRI, they are by nature infiltrating neoplasms and the interface between tumor and normal brain tissue may not be accurately defined. Moreover, gliomas may present as ill-defined lesions for which various MRI sequences combination does not provide a unique contour for tumor delineation. Also, gliomas are often histologically heterogeneous with anaplastic areas evolving within a low-grade tumor, and contrast-enhancement on CT or MRI does not represent a good marker for anaplastic tissue detection. Finally, assessment of tumor residue, recurrence, or progression, may be altered by different signals related to inflammation or adjuvant therapies, and contrast enhancement on CT and MRI is not an appropriate marker at the postoperative or posttherapeutic stage. These limitations of conventional neuroimaging in detecting tumor tissue, delineating tumor extent and evidencing anaplastic changes, lead to potential inaccuracy in lesion targeting at different steps of the management (diagnostic, surgical, postoperative, and posttherapeutic stages). Molecular information provided by PET has proved helpful to supplement morphological imaging data in this context. F-18 FDG and amino-acid tracers such as C-11 methionine (C-11 MET) provide complementary metabolic data that are independent from the anatomical MR information. These tracers help in the definition of glioma extension, detection of anaplastic areas, and postoperative follow-up. Additionally, PET data have a prognostic value independently of histology. To take advantage of PET data in glioma treatment, PET might be integrated in the planning of image-guided biopsy, resection, and radiosurgery.

Key words: Brain neoplasms, Pathology, Radionuclide, Imaging/surgery, Carbon radioisotopes/diagnostic use, Diagnosis, Differential, Fluorodeoxyglucose F18/diagnostic use, Glioma, Humans, Image processing, Computer-assisted methionine/analogs, Computer-assisted derivatives/diagnostic use, Neuronavigation, Positron-emission tomography, Stereotaxic techniques

1. PET and Brain Tumor Specificities

In the early 1990s, PET emerged as an innovative diagnostic method in oncology, but the first demonstration that PET imaging of cancer might be of clinical benefit was made a decade

Malik E. Juweid and Otto S. Hoekstra (eds.), *Positron Emission Tomography*, Methods in Molecular Biology, vol. 727,
DOI 10.1007/978-1-61779-062-1_16, © Springer Science+Business Media, LLC 2011

earlier, particularly in case of brain tumors. PET was at that time dedicated to brain and heart studies, and brain tumors were just one among other neurological diseases for which functional imaging was proposed. Apart from this historical point, brain tumors hold a particular place in clinical PET because of the features that differentiate brain tumors from most cancers studied with PET. The first feature conferring a prominent place to molecular imaging in neuro-oncology is brain inaccessibility, in contrast with most organs that may be sampled by non- or minimally invasive procedures. So, there is a powerful drive to develop molecular imaging that would probe brain tumors with such an accuracy that sampling for histological analysis would be unnecessary in situations that do not require therapeutic surgical access. The second feature is related to the organ that hosts these tumors. Functions in the brain are distributed; in other words, consequences of malignant lesions are extremely variable in function of the site of implantation. Also, function distribution in the brain is such that some regions ensure vital or major functions with no possible vicariance in case of injury: when compared to the main organs where cancer develops (lung, intestine, breast, prostate, liver, etc.), the brain is unique in the sense that loss of a few grams of tissue might lead to death or major handicap. Thus again functional imaging plays a crucial role in the management of brain tumors: defining the precise anatomical relationship of a lesion with highly functional brain areas is indeed essential, as is the meticulous tailoring of ablative treatments. The third characteristic of brain tumors is the extreme regional heterogeneity of some primitive neoplasms that arise in the brain. As a consequence of this heterogeneity, each part of the lesion might have a different biological behavior. Aggressiveness of a tumor, which is defined on the basis of its most aggressive component, is not evenly distributed in the lesion. Therefore, molecular imaging has a role to play in targeting lesion areas that will set the right diagnosis and that will require selective attention during ablative procedure planning. This introduction set the scene for PET use in neuro-oncology that will not be limited to what we expect from PET in other oncological situations: high diagnostic value easily summarized by the cardinal specificity, sensitivity, positive and negative predictive values.

As for tumors of other organs, malignant lesions in the brain might arise from the different cellular components of the brain. The classification of brain tumors proposed by the World Health Organization is actually based on a differentiation by cellular types (1). In adults, metastasis from somatic cancers is the most frequent neoplastic lesion in supratentorial localization, with the most frequent sites of origin being the lung, breast, melanoma, kidney and gastrointestinal tumors. Glioblastoma is the most common tumor arising from glial cells, and it is the most aggressive form of these gliomas. Astrocytomas, either low-grade (grade II) or anaplastic (grade III), are more frequent than the tumors arising from the oligodendrogial cells, i.e. grade II and grade III oligodendrogliomas that are most infiltrating tumors. Grading of gliomas is based on the presence of histological signs of anaplasia (mitosis, nuclear atypia, endothelial proliferation, and necrosis) that set local progression potential of the tumor. Metastatic dissemination of malignant brain tumors is indeed rare, except for ependymomas that may disseminate through the cerebrospinal fluid. Primary cerebral lymphomas represent a particular category of tumors that has become more frequent with the increased number of immunodeficient patients. Pituitary adenomas are not neuroectodermal in origin, but their localization often imposes a neurosurgical approach in their management and their endocrine nature renders their metabolic investigation appealing. Tumors of the meninges or those originating in the nerves are most frequently benign and will not be considered in this chapter. In contrast to adults, a majority of brain tumors in children are infratentorial (in the cerebellum and brainstem).

2. Challenges in Brain Tumor Management

2.1. At the Diagnostic Stage

A growing brain lesion is usually revealed and diagnosed after the occurrence of neurological symptoms. At that stage, surgery plays an important role in the treatment of brain tumors by reducing tumor cell volume and mass effect, and also by providing histological diagnosis and grading. In some situations, however, context and lesion's appearance may seriously challenge this recommended management.

2.1.1. Incidental Brain Lesions

When a brain lesion is diagnosed incidentally, the neoplastic nature or the evolving potential of the lesion is not manifest and the necessity of biopsy or resection can be questioned. Such situations are not rare, either in children explored for epilepsy, or in patients in whom a brain lesion has been diagnosed on a CT or MRI scan prescribed for independent reasons (i.e. sinusitis, trauma, and viral meningitis). Lesion's appearance on MRI is not always sufficient to accurately define management option for incidental brain lesions. Incidental brain lesions often present on MRI as well-delineated, with neither edema nor enhancement. These features may suggest non-evolving or indolent tumors (e.g. dysembryoplastic neuroepithelial tumors) or non-tumor lesions (e.g. dysplasia), so that, although the lesions seem accessible to resection, MRI follow-up may appear safer than surgery. Then, clinicians are facing a difficult choice between two risks: that of recommending unnecessary surgery and that of affording the risk of leaving in place a potentially aggressive lesion in a conservative setting. Therefore, at the diagnostic stage, clinicians might need more data about the evolving potential of unclear incidental brain lesions in order to better define, justify, and sustain the therapeutic choice.

2.1.2. Infiltrative Unresectable Brain Lesions

In other cases, the tumor may appear so infiltrative or located so close to eloquent gray matter, such as brainstem or primary sensory–motor cortical areas, that it might be estimated unresectable. Although allowing direct and precise visualization of brain tumors and structures, MR imaging cannot predict tumor diagnosis or grading and therefore cannot be used as sole basis for therapy. Indeed, in neuro-oncology, no adjuvant therapy can be reasonably applied without histological diagnosis and grading. In unresectable brain lesions, a surgical biopsy is then required and the technique of stereotactic biopsy represents the most adapted diagnostic procedure for this purpose. CT and MR images combining T1-weighted sequences with or without gadolinium injection (T1 ± Gd-DTPA), T2-weigthed, fluid-attenuated inversion-recovery (FLAIR) and diffusion sequences can be acquired in stereotactic conditions, allowing target selection in contrast-enhanced areas or in T2/FLAIR highly hypersignal areas for defining biopsy trajectories. Multiple trajectories harvesting staged samples represent the technique of choice to increase the diagnostic yield of the procedure and to reduce the risk of harvesting non-diagnostic or nonrepresentative samples. Increasing the sampling, however, also increases the risk of morbidity related to the procedure.

Diagnostic yield and risk of stereotactic biopsy represent major concerns in neurosurgery that reach their paroxysm in the management of brainstem lesions. Indeed, in the past decade, the utility, risk, and indication of a stereotactic biopsy in intrinsic infiltrative lesions of the brainstem have been widely questioned, especially in children. The management of these lesions requires careful consideration of the risk related to serial biopsy trajectories but also of the level of radiological diagnostic certainty (2). Indeed, the preoperative radiological diagnosis may be inaccurate for tumor type in about 25% of the cases and up to 13% of such lesions are non-neoplastic lesions. Therefore, the consequences of empiric therapy should not be underestimated before making appropriate treatment recommendations.

2.2. At the Therapeutic Stage

Surgical resection plays a major role in the treatment of brain gliomas. Indeed, it has been shown that the quality of the surgical resection played an important role on the patient's outcome in many glial tumor subtypes.

2.2.1. Prognostic Value of Surgical Resection in Brain Tumors

In adults, a longer survival after a surgical resection than after a stereotactic biopsy has been largely demonstrated in brain gliomas, particularly in low-grade gliomas (3–5). Moreover, routine application of image-guided neurosurgery has improved the accuracy and safety of neurosurgical interventions.

In high-grade gliomas such as anaplastic astrocytomas and glioblastomas, a similar benefit of resection has also been reported (6–8). The clinical benefit of radical resection remains debated (9), but a retrospective multivariate statistical analysis of 285 consecutive patients suffering from a high-grade gliomas has demonstrated that patients in whom maximal resection was performed lived longer than those who have received a partial surgery (10). A multivariate analysis of 416 patients with a glioblastoma has demonstrated a significant survival advantage ($p < 0.0001$) when the resection included more than 98% of the tumor volume (using MR volumetric quantification method), as compared to those in which the resection included less than 98% (median survival 13 months and 8.8 months, respectively) (11). Recently, the use of fluorescence-labeled markers to detect brain tumor tissue during surgical resection has improved the amount of tumor tissue removed and increased the survival in high-grade gliomas (12, 13).

In children, the benefit of a maximal tumor resection has also been demonstrated in low-grade gliomas and is probably more significant than in adults. Indeed, maximal surgical resection remains the main therapeutic step for many pediatric tumor types, including ependymomas, craniopharyngiomas, astrocytomas, and even medulloblastomas (14–19). Moreover, failure to achieve complete resection often results in tumor progression requiring further therapies in patients with pilocytic astrocytomas, the supposedly most indolent form of glioma. Similarly, in most children with ependymomas, this failure is ultimately fatal. Therefore, a maximal tumor resection increases children's survival in the majority of cases.

2.2.2. Radiosurgery in Brain Tumors

Radiosurgery is a stereotactic treatment defined as the delivery of a single, high dose of radiation allowing the precise and complete destruction of chosen target structures containing pathologic and healthy cells, without significant concomitant or late radiation damage to adjacent tissues. Radiosurgery is proposed in the multimodality management of brain tumors, including gliomas (20). High rate of successful treatment is attained for brain lesions, such as metastases, that do not extensively infiltrate the surrounding tissue. Since this closed-head intervention fully relies on the information provided by imaging procedures, accuracy of lesion delineation on the chosen imaging modality is of upmost importance in radiosurgery.

2.3. At the Postoperative Stage

At different steps of the postoperative stage, clinicians need an accurate method to assess either the completeness of the surgical resection or the efficacy of the adjuvant therapy on tumor growth.

2.3.1. Assessing Surgical Resection and Second-Look Surgery

Since the completeness of the resection may represent a curative factor in many brain tumors, especially in children, immediate postoperative (within 48 h after surgery) MR imaging (included T1 ± Gd-DTPA, T2 and FLAIR images) is mandatory, even in tumors considered by the surgeon as totally resected. A residual abnormal signal on immediate postoperative MR images is considered as a tumor fragment left in place. That is of major importance, especially because second-look surgery – defined as the resection of residual tumor before progression on follow-up imaging – has been promoted with acceptable morbidity in order to improve the outcome in many tumor types (15, 21). Moreover, early second-look surgery presents significant advantages. It avoids delay in applying adjuvant therapy and therapeutic escalation, and it reduces the risks related to surgical dissections of a tissue with late postoperative reactions (scar and arachnoiditis).

2.3.2. Assessing Response to Adjuvant Therapy and Early Detection of Recurrence

MR follow-up along and after application of adjuvant therapy (radiation therapy, chemotherapy, immunotherapy) is largely used to assess tumor response; it relies on changes in tumor characteristics such as size (reflected by different MR signals), peri-tumor edema, mass effect, and intensity of contrast enhancement. The accurate assessment of tumor response to therapy and also the accurate early detection of tumor recurrence are of major importance in order to promptly adapt and target therapeutic strategy.

3. Morphological Imaging Limitations

3.1. Detection of Tumor Tissue

Studies correlating the diagnostic yield of stereotactic biopsy with MR imaging illustrated the limitations of MR imaging in defining tumor tissue (22, 23). When multiple serial biopsies are performed, the success rate and the pertinence of the established diagnosis are high but failures occur due to inadequate targeting (24–26). Samples may consist in specimens irrelevant to the identification of brain tumors, such as non-tumor parenchyma, gliosis, and necrosis. In brainstem tumors, for example, the diagnostic yield of MR-guided stereotactic biopsy ranges between 83 and 96% (2).

MRI accuracy is also limited for the detection of tumor residue immediately after operation (even when T1, T2, FLAIR sequences are performed within 3 days), for the delineation of abnormal residual signals and for the differentiation between residue signals and inflammatory reactions even on FLAIR imaging sequences (21). Therefore, MRI alone cannot reliably set the decision for a complementary surgical approach.

During and after adjuvant therapy application, MR images are not always reflecting tumor response since abnormal signals may falsely increase or decrease during and after therapy application, within and around the tumor. Moreover, the occurrence of clinical deterioration is not always documented by tumor regrowth on imaging. Finally, MR imaging may not always reveal tumor recurrence early enough to allow prompt therapy escalation.

3.2. Detection of Anaplastic Tissue

Regional variation in the level of malignancy of brain gliomas cannot be unequivocally distinguished on MR imaging, even with contrast injection or multiple sequences. Therefore, MR-guided stereotactic biopsy might harvest tissue samples that are non-diagnostic (necrotic tissue in tumors) or unrepresentative leading to underestimated grading (low-grade tissue in high-grade tumors). Also, partial tumor removal under MR-guided neurosurgery may not target the tumor portions that present the highest potential of evolution (27, 28).

3.3. Accurate Tumor Delineation

CT- or MR-guided navigation for volumetric resection of brain tumors may be of limited help in some situations. Indeed, although providing a direct and multiplanar visualization of brain tumors, sensitivity and specificity of MR imaging in detecting tumor tissue are not high enough to ensure accurate tumor delineation. In high-grade gliomas, the contrast-enhanced area provided by T1-Gd-DTPA-weighted images usually represents the volume that neurosurgeons plan to remove. This is particularly true when tumor limits are not well defined and when neighboring eloquent areas are displaced by mass effect and edema. Low-grade gliomas, for example, oligodendrogliomas, fibrillar astrocytomas (more rarely pilocytic astrocytomas and gangliogliomas) may present as particularly infiltrative and ill-defined lesions on conventional MR imaging, especially on T1 $\pm$ Gd-DTPA (10). Tumor enhancement may be discrete or heterogeneous and does not always allow precise delineation for complete image-guided resection. Moreover, the abnormal signal on T2-weighted or FLAIR MR sequences is often not sharply delineated, and it may be much more extended than the tumor itself. The combined analysis of all MR sequences (T1 $\pm$ Gd-DTPA, T2-weighted and FLAIR) provides neither a more reliable nor a more accurate contour for image-guided resection in high-grade gliomas, and therefore does not improve tumor delineation. Lack of accuracy of MR for tumor boundaries definition in low-grade and high-grade gliomas, in adults and in children, is reflected in the literature (sensitivity and specificity to detect tumor tissue: 96% and 53% and to detect tumor grade: 72% and 65%) (19, 25, 29–34).

4. Specific Challenges in Pediatric Brain Tumors

In a majority of children, the accurate management of a newly diagnosed brain mass on MRI does not raise much discussion. However, in some cases, MRI may present many limitations that can make the choice of the accurate surgical option a real challenge. The surgical management of pediatric brain tumors, basically performed with MR imaging, needs to be improved. Indeed, there are challenges specific to the tumor types found in children compared to adults. Briefly: (1) some low-grade (pilocytic astrocytomas, ependymomas, teratomas) and high-grade (PNET, germinomas) tumors are specific of the pediatric population, and the tendency of some of them (PNET, ependymomas, pilocytic astrocytomas, germinomas) to disseminate in the cerebro-spinal fluid represents a crucial challenge in their management; (2) pediatric brain tumors have a higher proportion of low-grade tumors, of tumors with mixed (glioneuronal) or atypical (xanthoastrocytoma) cell population and of lesions with very low or questionable evolving potential (hamartoma, dysplasia, dysembryoplastic neuroepithelial) tumors; (3) moreover, many types of supratentorial pediatric tumors (pilocytic astrocytomas, gangliogliomas, and ependymomas) are rather well-delineated, displace more than infiltrate the functional tissue, making them usually accessible to a total removal; (4) indications and place of stereotactic biopsy are subsequently less frequent than in adults and the issue of the histological heterogeneity, observed in adult gliomas, has never been demonstrated by histological correlations in pediatric gliomas or even studied in other tumor types; (5) a complete tumor removal is much more frequently feasible and crucial for the outcome in children than in adults (15).

Because of these specificities, some MR imaging limitations have a particular impact in the pediatric population. Not detecting the tumor nature of a lesion, for instance in the context of focal epilepsy, might delay an adequate surgical management. Also, limitation in the quality of tumor delineation might have particularly deleterious consequences in children.

5. General Applications of PET for Brain Tumors

5.1. Methodology (Tracers, Acquisition, and Analysis)

PET provides independent and complementary information on level and distribution of brain tumors metabolism (23, 35–39), especially with two types of tracers: F-18 fluorodeoxyglucose (F-18 FDG), which assess glucose metabolism, and amino acid tracers. Other tracers used are tracking changes in blood volume and perfusion, and nucleic acid and lipid syntheses. In particular, the thymidine analog 3'-deoxy-3'-F-18 fluorothymidine (F-18 FLT) has been proposed to directly assess DNA synthesis for tumor cell proliferation estimation.

Data acquisition for F-18 FDG PET slightly differs from what is recommended in other PET applications. In order to get data in a standardized way, in particular when follow-up studies are planned, it is important to maintain the patient in a controlled state of rest in order to avoid variations in brain metabolism. Indeed, most data analysis will rely on visual or calculated comparison between tumor and normal brain metabolism. Again, in order to aim at standardization, it is also recommend maintaining a fasting state even if increased contrast between tumor and background has been reported after glucose administration (40). Considering the high uptake of F-18 FDG in the brain, F-18 FDG is generally administered at about half the doses administered for a whole body scan. PET acquisition is done, as for other neurological indications, starting 40 min postinjection for a duration that varies in function of the system used. Late images, acquired several hours postinjection, might lead to higher contrast between the tumor and the surrounding brain due to a slow but significant dephosphorylation of the metabolized F-18 FDG that occurs preferentially in the normal brain (41). For practical reasons, these late images are rarely acquired. If using a PET-CT system, CT acquisition is not essential except for transmission correction purpose. Attenuation maps may be calculated using ellipses drawn on the various slices and considering a homogenous attenuation coefficient. 2-D PET acquisition and filtered back projection reconstructions are acceptable for brain tumor imaging. Visual data analysis is greatly improved by coregistration of the PET images with various MRI sequences. This is particularly important for lesions located within the cortical or subcortical gray matter. PET-MR fusion is essential to evaluate tracer uptake within a lesion area detected on MRI. Lesion uptake is compared to that in normal white matter since gray matter uptake is often higher than the uptake in the tumor, even in the highly malignant glioblastoma.

Labeled amino acid tracers developed so far for PET imaging are distributed in two categories. There are tracers actively incorporated into the proteins, such as [^{11}C]methyl-L-methionine (C-11 MET) or 2-F-18-fluoro-L-tyrosine and 4-F-18-fluoro-L-phenylalanine, potentially allowing studies of protein synthesis rate, while others, such as 2-F-18-fluoro-$\propto$-methyl-L-tyrosine (F-18 FMT), 3,4-dihydroxy-6-18F-fluoro-L-phenylalanine (FDOPA) and O-(2-F-18-fluoroethyl)-L-tyrosine (F-18 FET) are not integrated into proteins and are therefore valuable tools to specifically evaluate the transport process.

The amino acid tracer that has been extensively studied for use in brain tumor evaluation is C-11 MET. More recently, aromatic amino acid tracers have been investigated, principally to take profit of their chemical structure that allows high-yield fluor-18 labeling, the necessary step toward a large-scale use. The main tracers of this type are FET and F-18-FDOPA.

Uptake of amino acid tracers in brain tumors is essentially related to the rate of the active transport processes, even for the tracers that are also incorporated into proteins. Therefore, differences in brain tumor uptake distribution of the various tracers are limited, in particular for what concerns C-11 MET, F-18 FET, and F-18 FDOPA (42, 43). Still, differences in uptake kinetics exist between nonnatural amino acids, such as FET, and natural amino acids, due to differences in transport systems affinity. Also, influence of the extra- and intracellular amino acid content might differ for different amino acid tracers because of differences in the transport and exchange systems involved (44, 45). Due to the potential influence of amino acid load on the tracer uptake, it is recommended to perform PET with amino acid tracers in the fasting state. Most of the pertinent information on the tracer uptake is obtained in the very early phase postinjection, but visual and semiquantitative analyses of the images are usually done on images acquired starting from 20 to 30 min postinjection for a duration ranging between 15 and 30 min, depending on doses and PET system sensitivity. Even more than for PET-F-18 FDG, coregistration with MRI is essential for lesion localization with amino acid tracers since these tracers provide less anatomical landmarks than F-18 FDG.

Relation between amino acid tracer uptake and histological and biological changes within brain tumors has been principally investigated with C-11 MET. Since the transport system present in the vasculature plays an important role in the whole transport process, it is not surprising that, in stereotactic comparisons, C-11 MET uptake is regionally correlated to cerebral blood volume measured with MR and with histological index of endothelial proliferation (46). C-11 MET uptake is also correlated to mitotic activity within the tumors and, more globally, its level relates to the local presence of histological signs of anaplasia (46, 47).

The thymidine analog 3'-deoxy-3'-^{18}F-fluorothymidine (F-18 FLT) has also been proposed to directly assess DNA synthesis to estimate tumor cell proliferation. As for extra-cranial cancer applications, this tracer has been essentially proposed for therapy monitoring, based on the concept that change in DNA synthesis should be the most direct index of therapeutic effects on tumor proliferation (48). F-18 FLT uptake in gliomas seems to be more tightly correlated to the Ki-67 histological proliferation index than C-11 MET uptake, but sensitivity of this tracer for the detection of anaplastic gliomas might be lower than required for clinical application, and dependence of F-18 FLT uptake on blood-brain barrier disruption raises the question of its specificity (49, 50).

F-18 Fluorocholine has been proposed as a tracer of phospholipid metabolism, but its use has been very limited and pathophysiological significance of its higher uptake in malignant lesions remains undefined (51). Blood volume and perfusion imaging of gliomas provide information on vascular tumor changes that reflect oncogenic processes related to angiogenesis. Data on these vascular aspects might be accessed by PET imaging with traditional tracers (52, 53), but MRI might appear more suitable than PET in this matter (46, 54). Considering the role of various forms of radiation therapy in the management of brain tumors, it is attractive to have access to regional information on local hypoxia within the lesion. Data on F-18 fluoromisonidazole (F-18 FMISO) metabolite retention, a marker of cellular hypoxia, remain scarce in gliomas but larger access to such tracers might boost research in this field (55–57).

A methodological issue that is common to PET studies with the different tracers relates to data analysis. The two main aspects to consider are the type of quantification and the delineation of the lesion for quantitative analysis. The type of quantification obviously depends of the biological process under analysis. Some general modelizations are applicable for brain tumor studies that give access to specific or global kinetic parameters. For instance, the metabolic rate calculated using such a model to quantify F-18 FLT uptake is correlated to the proliferation index obtained in vitro (58). In most cases, however, and in particular for F-18 FDG and amino acid tracers, tumor-over-background ratio are used because they do not require dynamic image acquisitions and complex quantifications have not been biologically validated. It is preferable to calculate ratios to a background that is representative of a relatively constant normal brain metabolism; using mirror regions of interest is therefore not recommended since the relative amount of gray and white matters will vary in the reference region, depending on tumor localization. For the analysis of tumor response to therapeutic agents, in absence of surgical resection, it may be interesting to evaluate the changes in the global tumor load. Indices that integrate intensity of the signal and extension of the lesion have been proposed for that purpose (59). Delineation of the lesion is another issue that has implication for the quantification of the signal and for the definition of the tumor area when PET data are used to plan therapeutic procedures. Methods that rely on MRI data to delineate regions of interest for tracer uptake quantification suffer from the difficulty to define what MRI sequences might reliably reflect tumor extension, as already discussed. Gliomas should be considered as lesions that have variable bulk and infiltrative components (60, 61). Methods of tumor delineation that are validated histologically are rare and based on a quite limited number of points of stereotactic comparison between image and histological data (61, 62). Recently, a 3-D

Gaussian model to define tumor limits has been validated for PET-C-11 MET in brain metastases, but this approach only considers the bulk component of the lesion since brain metastases usually have a limited propensity to infiltrate the normal brain (63).

5.2. Value of PET in Neuro-Oncology: General Applications

The largest PET experience in neuro-oncology has been acquired with F-18 FDG (35, 37, 39, 64). Highly malignant tumors are characterized by an increased F-18 FDG uptake, and the clinical value of adding F-18 FDG PET to morphological information has been established for various clinical situations: differential diagnosis of brain lesion, anticipation of malignancy level, prognosis, detection of anaplastic components, persistence or recurrence of malignant tissue and effect of adjuvant therapy. In particular, F-18 FDG uptake is a more accurate reflection of tumor grade than contrast enhancement. Various studies in adult gliomas have shown that F-18 FDG uptake is anatomically heterogeneous within the tumor and correlates with the degree of local histological anaplasia (38, 47). F-18 FDG uptake in primary central nervous system lymphoma is usually extremely high, except in rare cases with predominant necrosis (65–68).

C-11 MET has also been largely validated in neuro-oncology (28, 69, 70). The clinical value of C-11 MET PET comes from the high contrast between uptake in tumor and in surrounding brain tissue. Such a contrast is not found for F-18 FDG uptake due to the high glucose consumption in the normal gray matter. Therefore, C-11 MET PET is characterized by a high sensitivity for the detection of tumor cells, a quality of interest when limits between the infiltrative peripheral component of the tumor and the intact brain are to be defined. Not surprisingly, the value of C-11 MET PET, compared to other imaging modalities, has been highlighted for the definition of tumor boundaries (28, 46, 71).

Brain tumors are among the rare cancers for which pediatric applications of PET are quite frequent. Still, very few studies have been published on PET in pediatric neuro-oncology. The first F-18 FDG PET studies of isolated cases showed a relationship between F-18 FDG uptake and degree of tumor malignancy, and these studies highlighted the heterogeneity of F-18 FDG uptake in pediatric brain tumors (15). A study focused on functional brain mapping using F-18 FDG-, C-11 MET- and O-15 H_2O-PET correlated with MR images for preoperative neurosurgical planning in pediatric brain tumors, in order to characterize the relationship between potentially resectable tumors and functionally eloquent brain areas (72). Another study with F-18 FDG PET and C-11 MET PET in 27 untreated primary pediatric brain tumors found that both F-18 FDG and C-11 MET uptakes were associated with the grade of malignancy and provided valuable additional information on clinical tumor aggressiveness (73). Also, a study of F-18 FDG PET and O-15 H_2O-PET, coregistrated to MRI has confirmed the correlation between F-18 FDG uptake and histological grade in high-grade pediatric brain tumors, just as it has been shown earlier in adults (74).

Our experience illustrates the high specificity of PET in the management of unclear incidental lesions. We recently reviewed the impact of PET results in the management of incidental brain lesions in 55 children seen in our center. Surgery was proposed to all 17 patients who had a significantly increased tracer uptake in the lesion. A tumor diagnosis was obtained in all these operated cases. A low or absent PET tracer uptake was estimated to correspond to an indolent low-grade tumor or a non-tumor tissue, and sustained a conservative option. Follow-up showed a stable condition in all 38 patients with low tracer uptake and in those patients who had been operated on, histology yielded non-tumor lesions or indolent tumors that were dysembryoplastic neuroepithelial tumors, and low-grade astrocytomas (75). Sasaki et al. have reported high C-11 MET uptake in focal cortical dysplasias that would need to be regarded as "false positive" in terms of tumor detection (76). Nevertheless, cortical dysplasias are mainly found in children evaluated for focal epilepsy, and detection of C-11 MET uptake, focally and moderately enhanced within the cortical band, actually helps in the therapeutic decision when epilepsy is drug-resistant. From our experience, the main role of PET-C-11 MET in pediatric incidental brain lesion remains to support conservative decision when low tracer uptake is found, since this metabolic finding reasonably excludes aggressive lesion that would progress and render delayed surgery more hazardous.

Prognostic value of F-18 FDG PET and C-11 MET -PET in brain gliomas is a matter of interest because classical histology does not strictly determine the prognosis. Since histology is available for most lesions and is obviously a major prognostic factor, it is important to evaluate the prognostic value of PET within a histological category or with a multivariate approach that includes histological data in the analysis. Studies have shown that the level of C-11 MET uptake is a prognostic index of survival, separately in glioblastoma and in grade II and grade III gliomas (4, 5, 77, 78). At least part of this prognostic value resides in the correlation between C-11 MET uptake and proliferative indices (105). A multivariate analysis conducted in patients with gliomas of different grades confirmed this independent prognostic value of C-11 MET PET (79). Prognostic value of other amino acid tracers, such as F-18 FET, has also been established, in particular for low-grade gliomas (80).

PET value for the *immediate postoperative assessment* has also been investigated. Early experience with F-18 FDG PET showed that the main advantage of F-18 FDG PET, as compared to the imaging methods relying on contrast enhancement, is that F-18 FDG uptake is not much influenced by the postoperative changes and steroid treatment (81). Experience in adults as well as in children showed that early postoperative PET (performed within 8 days after surgery), especially using C-11 MET, improves the diagnostic accuracy of tumor residue detection, as compared with that obtained with MRI (performed within 48 h after surgery and including T1 ± Gd-DTPA, T2-weighted and FLAIR sequences). Early postoperative PET, performed to assess the completeness of tumor resection, illustrates the high specificity and sensitivity of C-11 MET PET, as confirmed by early reoperations (Fig. 1). Indeed, a study has shown that tumor residue is always found at reoperation in cases presenting residual C-11 MET uptake, while MR signals lead to false-positive results (21). In that study, there were no false-negative results since the long-term follow-up showed no tumor progression in cases with no postoperative PET tracer uptake, whatever the MR signals were. This impact of PET data on early postoperative evaluation is of particular value in glial tumors such as ependymomas, low-grade astrocytomas, and hemangiopericytomas, in which radical surgery is a key factor of prognosis.

After the early postoperative period, the first clinical question that requires imaging evaluation is the *detection of recurrence*. The differential diagnosis between brain tumor recurrence and radionecrosis has been among the first oncological application proposed for F-18 FDG PET (82). It appears that the value of F-18 FDG PET in this application exists but sensitivity and specificity are not as high as hoped, reaching 75% and 81%, respectively, in a study that shows how the sensitivity of the method is improved

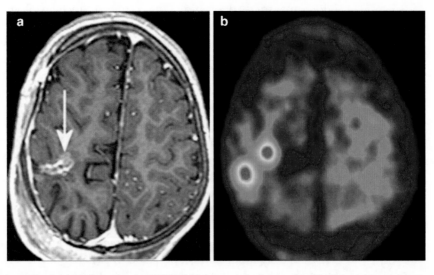

Fig. 1. Postoperative Axial MR (**a**) and C-11 MET PET (**b**) images of a 4-year-old girl with a right parietal ependymoma, showing residual C-11 MET uptake at sites where MR signals were unconclusive. Sites of C-11 MET uptake corresponded to residual tumor at reoperation.

by coregistration with MRI (83). Despite the high sensitivity of PET amino acid tracers, their global accuracy in this differentiation might be quite similar to the one of F-18 FDG (84, 85). Still, data indicate that amino acid tracers are more effective than F-18 FDG for the sensitive detection of recurrent high-grade gliomas, since patients with recurrent lesions with no increased F-18 FDG uptake were detected with 89% sensitivity with C-11 MET PET in an analysis of 42 patients with histological confirmation (86). Pituitary adenoma is a particular type of intracranial tumor for which metabolic imaging is of high value in recurrence and active residue detection. Metabolic investigation of pituitary adenomas has been proposed 20 years ago, but this application remained rarely investigated in the literature (87, 88). Its value at the postoperative stage is related to the difficulties in MRI interpretation after surgery. PET with amino-acid tracers is a sensitive method to detect adenoma residue producing peptidic hormones, and it may be used to orient further surgical or radiosurgical treatments (89). Even the so-called non-secreting adenomas present with high uptake of amino-acid tracers and this may be used in the follow-up of residues that have no manifestation in hormonal blood testing (89).

Another major issue in patients' follow-up is the *detection of anaplastic transformation* within low-grade gliomas. F-18 FDG PET has also been proposed for this purpose. Again, the value of F-18 FDG PET in this matter has been demonstrated in early studies (90), but here the sensitivity of various amino acid tracers is the most beneficial (91, 92). The demonstration that F-18 FDG and C-11 MET uptake are higher in tumor areas with anaplastic changes backs the use of PET in the follow-up of low-grade tumors (38, 46, 47), and early treatment of local sites that develop increased uptake of these tracers might reasonably be proposed.

A role of PET imaging that is extremely promising, in general, is the metabolic assessment of nonsurgical therapies (93). Considering the limitations of morphological imaging in the evaluation of brain tumors after therapeutic interventions, it seems attractive to make use of metabolic correlates of tumor cell activity to evaluate therapeutic response to nonablative interventions. Advantages of this approach are shown for brachytherapy (94, 95). Metabolic changes induced by the chemotherapeutic agents used in the treatment of glioblastoma have been demonstrated. A study showed the superiority of F-18 FET-PET imaging over MRI in predicting stable disease after paclitaxel in recurrent glioblastoma (96). A study in patients with oligodendroglioma demonstrated that metabolic changes on C-11 MET PET were far more pronounced than the volumetric changes calculated on MRI FLAIR sequences, after chemotherapy with procarbazine, CCNU, and vincristine (PCV) (59). In glioblastoma, the very early metabolic change found in patients responsive to nitrosourea compounds is actually an increase in glucose metabolism manifested on F-18 FDG PET, a finding that is interpreted as reflecting cellular processes kindled by an efficient therapeutic aggression of the cancer tissue (97, 98).

6. Specific Applications of PET for Brain Tumor Management: PET Guidance of Therapy

The increasing availability and routine application of image-guided neurosurgery – or neuronavigation – improve the accuracy and safety of neurosurgical interventions. First application of image-guided neurosurgery was the sampling of brain lesions by stereotaxic biopsies, avoiding direct open access to the brain. Technological advances that ensure real-time image-guidance have paved the way to a more recent application, the optimization of tumor resection by using contours representing tumor limits and brain structures defined on anatomical imaging. Limitation of MRI for both applications, i.e. defining the most representative area of a brain tumor for adequate histological diagnosis and defining the external limits of a tumor in order to plan its optimal ablation, has urged the addition of metabolic information for the planning of image-guided neurosurgical procedures. Demonstration of a local relationship between histological features and PET data is the theoretical basis of PET image use in neuronavigation planning. This demonstration has been made by correlative studies on stereotactic procedures that allow parallel analysis of PET and histological data in restricted tumor sites (38, 46, 47, 54).

We introduced PET-guidance of stereotactic biopsy in our center in 1992 (Fig. 2) (22). In our experience, the diagnostic yield of stereotactic biopsy is increased by the metabolic targeting, essentially by reducing the number of non-diagnostic and nonrepresentative samples (23, 99, 100). The value of the method has been particularly highlighted for the evaluation of brainstem lesions (101). A study compared the contributions of C-11 MET and F-18 FDG for PET-guided stereotactic biopsy of brain gliomas. In 32 patients with glioma, stereotactic C-11 MET and F-18 FDG PET were integrated in the MR planning of stereotactic brain biopsy. Non-diagnostic samples were never collected from areas of increased C-11 MET or F-18 FDG uptake, while nine non-diagnostic trajectories were targeted toward abnormal MR signals (99). In all patients with increased uptake of both tracers, the focus of highest C-11 MET uptake corresponded to the focus of highest F-18 FDG uptake, but the extent of uptake of both tracers was variable. Because C-11 MET provided a more sensitive signal, it was judged that amino-acid tracers are the molecules of choice for single-tracer PET-guided neurosurgical procedures in gliomas (99).

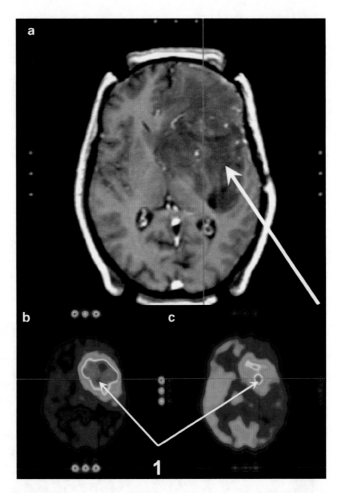

Fig. 2. Comparison in stereotactic conditions of MR imaging (**a**), C-11 MET PET (**b**), and F-18 FDG PET (**c**) of a right frontal WHO grade III anaplastic astrocytoma in which a biopsy was preferred to a resection because the lesion was very infiltrative (**a**). C-11 MET-PET (**b**) and F-18 FDG PET (**c**) showed heterogeneous tracer uptake. The focus of highest metabolic activity was used as a target for biopsy (*thin arrows* on **b** and **c**). This F-18 FDG PET-guided biopsy sampled the anaplastic tissue contrary to the biopsy performed in an area of abnormal MR signal but lower F-18 FDG uptake, which yielded a sample with histological characteristics of a low-grade tumor (*large arrow* on **a**).

In order to use PET information preoperatively, it is necessary to integrate PET images in the set of images used for planning of the surgical procedures. To allow perfect coregistration of PET and MR images, the technique has initially consisted in acquiring PET and CT/MR images in the same stereotactic conditions on the same day. This required adaptation of the stereotaxic system designed for CT or MR imaging. In particular, it is necessary to perfectly secure the base ring of this system on the PET couch using a specific clamp. In order to create a fiducial reference system for PET, it is convenient to modify commercial MR localizers to accommodate tubings filled with F-18 fluoride solution (22, 23).

More recently, improvements in automatic voxel-based registration algorithms have allowed the validation of frameless acquisition techniques, particularly convenient for navigation planning of volumetric resections. The criterion of choice between frame-based or frameless approaches is the trade-off between accuracy and reliability against minimal invasiveness and clinical routine feasibility. All the navigation data planned on the workstation are displayed in the eyepiece of the surgical microscope and visible in the operative field, including the PET contours of the tumor. The neurosurgical resection primarily aims at the total removal of the tumor defined by these contours (28). The surgical planning established preoperatively is followed in order to achieve a total resection of the tumor as defined by PET and MR (Fig. 3). Alternatively, at least the resection of the tumor limits based on the PET tracer is aimed at, or a partial resection focused on the area of the highest tracer uptake being located outside the infiltrated functional structure is performed. An analysis of

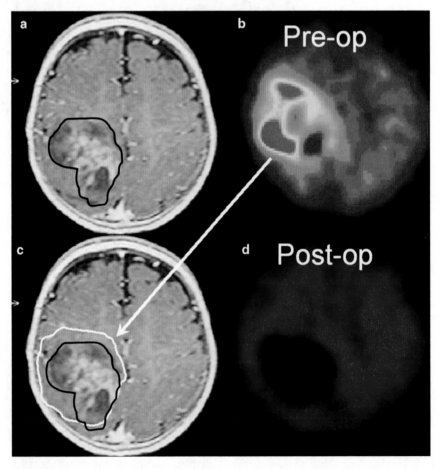

Fig. 3. Axial MR (**a** and **c**) and C-11 MET PET (**b**) images of a 1-year-old with a right parietal WHO grade I ganglioglioma showing the PET contour (*white line*) projected on MR imaging and larger than the MR contour (*black line*). Postoperative C-11 MET PET (**d**) shows no residual C-11 MET uptake.

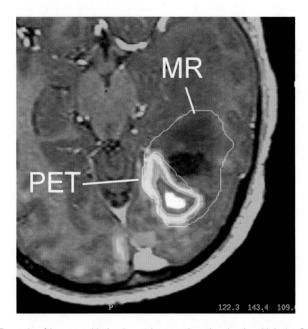

Fig. 4. Example of image-guided volumetric resection planning in which the C-11 MET PET-defined contour (PET, rainbow-colored) of a left posterior temporal anaplastic oligoastrocytoma projects within the MR-defined contour (MR, contour in *blue*). The MR contour, defined with a fusion of the T1 ± Gd-DTPA (no contrast enhancement), T2 and FLAIR sequences, is much larger than the PET contour.

103 image-guided resections of brain tumors shows that in 83 procedures (80%), PET improved tumor delineation and contributed to define a final target contour different from that obtained with MR alone (Fig. 4). Total resection of the increased PET tracer uptake was achieved in 54 procedures (52%) and provided a longer survival ($p = 0.007$) compared to patients with postoperative residual PET tracer uptake.

Radiosurgery is another therapeutic domain in which local metabolic information might improve the local treatment of a brain tumor. We recently reported on the experience acquired with PET-guidance of Leksell Gamma Knife® radiosurgery. The integration of stereotactic PET in radiosurgery allowed us to treat 130 patients (including 10 children) with the combination of MR/CT and PET guidance. Abnormal PET uptake was found in 88% of the 149 target volumes defined, and information provided by PET altered significantly the MR-based definition of the tumor in 73% of the cases (102–104).

Acknowledgment

FRS-FNRS and National Lottery – Belgium.

References

1. Louis, D.N., Ohgaki, H., Wiestler, O.D., Cavenee, W.K., Burger, P.C., Jouvet, A., et al. (2007) The 2007 WHO classification of tumours of the central nervous system. *Acta Neuropathol* **114**, 97–109.

2. Pirotte, B.J., Lubansu, A., Massager, N., Wikler, D., Goldman, S., Levivier, M. (2007) Results of positron emission tomography guidance and reassessment of the utility of and indications for stereotactic biopsy in children with infiltrative brainstem tumors. *J Neurosurg* **107**, 392–9.

3. Mariani, L., Siegenthaler, P., Guzman, R., Friedrich, D., Fathi, A.R., Ozdoba, C., et al. (2004) The impact of tumour volume and surgery on the outcome of adults with supratentorial WHO grade II astrocytomas and oligoastrocytomas. *Acta Neurochir (Wien)* **146**, 441–8.

4. De Witte, O., Levivier, M., Violon, P., Salmon, I., Damhaut, P., Wikler, D., Jr., et al. (1996) Prognostic value positron emission tomography with [18F]fluoro-2-deoxy-D-glucose in the low-grade glioma. *Neurosurgery* **39**, 470–6; discussion 476–7.

5. De Witte, O., Goldberg, I., Wikler, D., Rorive, S., Damhaut, P., Monclus, M., et al. (2001) Positron emission tomography with injection of methionine as a prognostic factor in glioma. *J Neurosurg* **95**, 746–50.

6. Daneyemez, M., Gezen, F., Canakci, Z., Kahraman, S. (1998) Radical surgery and reoperation in supratentorial malignant glial tumors. *Minim Invasive Neurosurg* **41**, 209–13.

7. Kowalczuk, A., Macdonald, R.L., Amidei, C., Dohrmann, G., 3rd, Erickson, R.K., Hekmatpanah, J., et al. (1997) Quantitative imaging study of extent of surgical resection and prognosis of malignant astrocytomas. *Neurosurgery* **41**, 1028–36; discussion 1036–8.

8. Yokoyama, J., Ikawa, H., Endow, M., Fuchimoto, Y., Watanabe, K., Hosoya, R., et al. (1995) The role of surgery in advanced neuroblastoma. *Eur J Pediatr Surg* **5**, 23–6.

9. Hess, K.R. (1999) Extent of resection as a prognostic variable in the treatment of gliomas. *J Neurooncol* **42**, 227–31.

10. Pirotte, B., Levivier, M., Goldman, S., Massager, N., Wikler, D., De Witte, O., et al. (2009) PET-guided volumetric resection of supratentorial high grade gliomas: A survival analysis in 66 consecutive patients. *Neurosurgery* **64**(3), 471–81; discussion 481.

11. Lacroix, M., Abi-Said, D., Fourney, D.R., Gokaslan, Z.L., Shi, W., DeMonte, F., et al. (2001) A multivariate analysis of 416 patients with glioblastoma multiforme: prognosis, extent of resection, and survival. *J Neurosurg* **95**, 190–8.

12. Stummer, W., Reulen, H.J., Meinel, T., Pichlmeier, U., Schumacher, W., Tonn, J.C., et al. (2008) Extent of resection and survival in glioblastoma multiforme: identification of and adjustment for bias. *Neurosurgery* **62**, 564–76; discussion 564–76.

13. Sanai, N., Berger, M.S. (2008) Glioma extent of resection and its impact on patient outcome. *Neurosurgery* **62**, 753–64; discussion 264–6.

14. Pollack, I.F. (1999) The role of surgery in pediatric gliomas. *J Neurooncol* **42**, 271–88.

15. Pirotte, B., Acerbi, F., Lubansu, A., Goldman, S., Brotchi, J., Levivier, M. (2007) PET imaging in the surgical management of pediatric brain tumors. *Childs Nerv Syst* **23**, 739–51.

16. Black, P.M. (1991) Brain tumor. Part 2. *N Engl J Med* **324**, 1555–64.

17. Black, P.M. (1991) Brain tumors. Part 1. *N Engl J Med* **324**, 1471–6.

18. Albright, A.L. (1993) Pediatric brain tumors. *CA Cancer J Clin* **43**, 272–88.

19. Foreman, N.K., Love, S., Gill, S.S., Coakham, H.B. (1997) Second-look surgery for incompletely resected fourth ventricle ependymomas: technical case report. *Neurosurgery* **40**, 856–60; discussion 860.

20. Larson, D.A., Gutin, P.H., McDermott, M., Lamborn, K., Sneed, P.K., Wara, W.M., et al. (1996) Gamma knife for glioma: selection factors and survival. *Int J Radiat Oncol Biol Phys* **36**, 1045–53.

21. Pirotte, B., Levivier, M., Morelli, D., Van Bogaert, P., Detemmerman, D., David, P., et al. (2005) Positron emission tomography for the early postsurgical evaluation of pediatric brain tumors. *Childs Nerv Syst* **21**, 294–300.

22. Levivier, M., Goldman, S., Bidaut, L.M., Luxen, A., Stanus, E., Przedborski, S., et al. (1992) Positron emission tomography-guided stereotactic brain biopsy. *Neurosurgery* **31**, 792–7; discussion 797.

23. Levivier, M., Goldman, S., Pirotte, B., Brucher, J.M., Baleriaux, D., Luxen, A., et al. (1995) Diagnostic yield of stereotactic brain biopsy guided by positron emission tomography with

[18F]fluorodeoxyglucose. *J Neurosurg* **82**, 445–52.

24. Chandrasoma, P.T., Smith, M.M., Apuzzo, M.L. (1989) Stereotactic biopsy in the diagnosis of brain masses: comparison of results of biopsy and resected surgical specimen. *Neurosurgery* **24**, 160–5.

25. Feiden, W., Steude, U., Bise, K., Gundisch, O. (1991) Accuracy of stereotactic brain tumor biopsy: comparison of the histologic findings in biopsy cylinders and resected tumor tissue. *Neurosurg Rev* **14**, 51–6.

26. Glantz, M.J., Burger, P.C., Herndon, J.E., 2nd, Friedman, A.H., Cairncross, J.G., Vick, N.A., et al. (1991) Influence of the type of surgery on the histologic diagnosis in patients with anaplastic gliomas. *Neurology* **41**, 1741–4.

27. Pirotte, B., Goldman, S., Van Bogaert, P., David, P., Wikler, D., Rorive, S., et al. (2005) Integration of [11C]methionine-positron emission tomographic and magnetic resonance imaging for image-guided surgical resection of infiltrative low-grade brain tumors in children. *Neurosurgery* **57**, 128–39; discussion 128–39.

28. Pirotte, B., Goldman, S., Dewitte, O., Massager, N., Wikler, D., Lefranc, F., et al. (2006) Integrated positron emission tomography and magnetic resonance imaging-guided resection of brain tumors: a report of 103 consecutive procedures. *J Neurosurg* **104**, 238–53.

29. Wong, T.Z., van der Westhuizen, G.J., Coleman, R.E. (2002) Positron emission tomography imaging of brain tumors. *Neuroimaging Clin N Am* **12**, 615–26.

30. Paulus, W., Peiffer, J. (1989) Intratumoral histologic heterogeneity of gliomas. A quantitative study. *Cancer* **64**, 442–7.

31. Essig, M., Metzner, R., Bonsanto, M., Hawighorst, H., Debus, J., Tronnier, V., et al. (2001) Postoperative fluid-attenuated inversion recovery MR imaging of cerebral gliomas: initial results. *Eur Radiol* **11**, 2004–10.

32. Braun, V., Dempf, S., Tomczak, R., Wunderlich, A., Weller, R., Richter, H.P. (2000) Functional cranial neuronavigation. Direct integration of fMRI and PET data. *J Neuroradiol* **27**, 157–63.

33. Pauleit, D., Floeth, F., Hamacher, K., Riemenschneider, M.J., Reifenberger, G., Muller, H.W., et al. (2005) O-(2-[18F]fluoroethyl)-L-tyrosine PET combined with MRI improves the diagnostic assessment of cerebral gliomas. *Brain* **128**, 678–87.

34. Law, M., Yang, S., Wang, H., Babb, J.S., Johnson, G., Cha, S., et al. (2003) Glioma grading: sensitivity, specificity, and predictive values of perfusion MR imaging and proton MR spectroscopic imaging compared with conventional MR imaging. *AJNR Am J Neuroradiol* **24**, 1989–98.

35. Di Chiro, G. (1987) Positron emission tomography using [18F] fluorodeoxyglucose in brain tumors. A powerful diagnostic and prognostic tool. *Invest Radiol* **22**, 360–71.

36. Alavi, J.B., Alavi, A., Chawluk, J., Kushner, M., Powe, J., Hickey, W., et al. (1988) Positron emission tomography in patients with glioma. A predictor of prognosis. *Cancer* **62**, 1074–8.

37. Coleman, R.E., Hoffman, J.M., Hanson, M.W., Sostman, H.D., Schold, S.C. (1991) Clinical application of PET for the evaluation of brain tumors. *J Nucl Med* **32**, 616–22.

38. Goldman, S., Levivier, M., Pirotte, B., Brucher, J.M., Wikler, D., Damhaut, P., et al. (1996) Regional glucose metabolism and histopathology of gliomas. A study based on positron emission tomography-guided stereotactic biopsy. *Cancer* **78**, 1098–106.

39. Chen, W. (2007) Clinical applications of PET in brain tumors. *J Nucl Med* **48**, 1468–81.

40. Ishizu, K., Sadato, N., Yonekura, Y., Nishizawa, S., Magata, Y., Tamaki, N., et al. (1994) Enhanced detection of brain tumors by [18F]fluorodeoxyglucose PET with glucose loading. *J Comput Assist Tomogr* **18**, 12–5.

41. Spence, A.M., Muzi, M., Mankoff, D.A., O'Sullivan, S.F., Link, J.M., Lewellen, T.K., et al. (2004) 18F-FDG PET of gliomas at delayed intervals: improved distinction between tumor and normal gray matter. *J Nucl Med* **45**, 1653–9.

42. Becherer, A., Karanikas, G., Szabo, M., Zettinig, G., Asenbaum, S., Marosi, C., et al. (2003) Brain tumour imaging with PET: a comparison between [18F]fluorodopa and [11C]methionine. *Eur J Nucl Med Mol Imaging* **30**, 1561–7.

43. Weber, W.A., Wester, H.J., Grosu, A.L., Herz, M., Dzewas, B., Feldmann, H.J., et al. (2000) O-(2-[18F]fluoroethyl)-L-tyrosine and L-[methyl-11C]methionine uptake in brain tumours: initial results of a comparative study. *Eur J Nucl Med* **27**, 542–9.

44. Lahoutte, T., Caveliers, V., Camargo, S.M., Franca, R., Ramadan, T., Veljkovic, E., et al. (2004) SPECT and PET amino acid tracer influx via system L (h4F2hc-hLAT1) and its transstimulation. *J Nucl Med* **45**, 1591–6.

45. Laique, S., Egrise, D., Monclus, M., Schmitz, F., Garcia, C., Lemaire, C., et al. (2006) L-amino

acid load to enhance PET differentiation between tumor and inflammation: an in vitro study on (18)F-FET uptake. *Contrast Media Mol Imaging* **1**, 212–20.

46. Sadeghi, N., Salmon, I., Decaestecker, C., Levivier, M., Metens, T., Wikler, D., et al. (2007) Stereotactic comparison among cerebral blood volume, methionine uptake, and histopathology in brain glioma. *AJNR Am J Neuroradiol* **28**, 455–61.

47. Goldman, S., Levivier, M., Pirotte, B., Brucher, J.M., Wikler, D., Damhaut, P., et al. (1997) Regional methionine and glucose uptake in high-grade gliomas: a comparative study on PET-guided stereotactic biopsy. *J Nucl Med* **38**, 1459–62.

48. Chen, W., Delaloye, S., Silverman, D.H., Geist, C., Czernin, J., Sayre, J., et al. (2007) Predicting treatment response of malignant gliomas to bevacizumab and irinotecan by imaging proliferation with [18F] fluorothymidine positron emission tomography: a pilot study. *J Clin Oncol* **25**, 4714–21.

49. Hatakeyam, T., Kawai, N., Nishiyama, Y., Yamamoto, Y., Sasakawa, Y., Ichikawa, T., et al. (2008) (11)C-methionine (MET) and (18)F-fluorothymidine (FLT) PET in patients with newly diagnosed glioma. *Eur J Nucl Med Mol Imaging* **35**, 2009–17.

50. Saga, T., Kawashima, H., Araki, N., Takahashi, J.A., Nakashima, Y., Higashi, T., et al. (2006) Evaluation of primary brain tumors with FLT-PET: usefulness and limitations. *Clin Nucl Med* **31**, 774–80.

51. Kwee, S.A., Ko, J.P., Jiang, C.S., Watters, M.R., Coel, M.N. (2007) Solitary brain lesions enhancing at MR imaging: evaluation with fluorine 18 fluorocholine PET. *Radiology* **244**, 557–65.

52. Xiangsong, Z., Changhong, L., Weian, C., Dong, Z. (2006) PET Imaging of cerebral astrocytoma with 13N-ammonia. *J Neurooncol* **78**, 145–51.

53. Mineura, K., Sasajima, T., Kowada, M., Ogawa, T., Hatazawa, J., Shishido, F., et al. (1994) Perfusion and metabolism in predicting the survival of patients with cerebral gliomas. *Cancer* **73**, 2386–94.

54. Sadeghi, N., D'Haene, N., Decaestecker, C., Levivier, M., Metens, T., Maris, C., et al. (2008) Apparent diffusion coefficient and cerebral blood volume in brain gliomas: relation to tumor cell density and tumor microvessel density based on stereotactic biopsies. *AJNR Am J Neuroradiol* **29**, 476–82.

55. Bruehlmeier, M., Roelcke, U., Schubiger, P.A., Ametamey, S.M. (2004) Assessment of hypoxia and perfusion in human brain tumors using PET with 18F-fluoromisonidazole and 15O-H2O. *J Nucl Med* **45**, 1851–9.

56. Cher, L.M., Murone, C., Lawrentschuk, N., Ramdave, S., Papenfuss, A., Hannah, A., et al. (2006) Correlation of hypoxic cell fraction and angiogenesis with glucose metabolic rate in gliomas using 18F-fluoromisonidazole, 18F-FDG PET, and immunohistochemical studies. *J Nucl Med* **47**, 410–8.

57. Spence, A.M., Muzi, M., Swanson, K.R., O'Sullivan, F., Rockhill, J.K., Rajendran, J.G., et al. (2008) Regional hypoxia in glioblastoma multiforme quantified with 18F] fluoromisonidazole positron emission tomography before radiotherapy: correlation with time to progression and survival. *Clin Cancer Res* **14**, 2623–30.

58. Ullrich, R., Backes, H., Li, H., Kracht, L., Miletic, H., Kesper, K., et al. (2008) Glioma proliferation as assessed by 3'-fluoro-3'-deoxy-L-thymidine positron emission tomography in patients with newly diagnosed high-grade glioma. *Clin Cancer Res* **14**, 2049–55.

59. Tang, B.N., Sadeghi, N., Branle, F., De Witte, O., Wikler, D., Goldman, S. (2005) Semi-quantification of methionine uptake and flair signal for the evaluation of chemotherapy in low-grade oligodendroglioma. *J Neurooncol* **71**, 161–8.

60. Daumas-Duport, C., Scheithauer, B.W., Kelly, P.J. (1987) A histologic and cytologic method for the spatial definition of gliomas. *Mayo Clin Proc* **62**, 435–49.

61. Kelly, P.J., Daumas-Duport, C., Scheithauer, B.W., Kall, B.A., Kispert, D.B. (1987) Stereotactic histologic correlations of computed tomography- and magnetic resonance imaging-defined abnormalities in patients with glial neoplasms. *Mayo Clin Proc* **62**, 450–9.

62. Kracht, L.W., Miletic, H., Busch, S., Jacobs, A.H., Voges, J., Hoevels, M., et al. (2004) Delineation of brain tumor extent with [11C]L-methionine positron emission tomography: local comparison with stereotactic histopathology. *Clin Cancer Res* **10**, 7163–70.

63. Tang, B.N., Van Simaeys, G., Devriendt, D., Sadeghi, N., Dewitte, O., Massager, N., et al. (2008) Three-dimensional Gaussian model to define brain metastasis limits on (11) C-methionine PET. *Radiother Oncol* **89**, 270–7.

64. Delbeke, D., Meyerowitz, C., Lapidus, R.L., Maciunas, R.J., Jennings, M.T., Moots, P.L., et al. (1995) Optimal cutoff levels of F-18 fluorodeoxyglucose uptake in the differentiation

of low-grade from high-grade brain tumors with PET. *Radiology* **195**, 47–52.

65. Rosenfeld, S.S., Hoffman, J.M., Coleman, R.E., Glantz, M.J., Hanson, M.W., Schold, S.C. (1992) Studies of primary central nervous system lymphoma with fluorine-18-fluorodeoxyglucose positron emission tomography. *J Nucl Med* **33**, 532–6.

66. Kawai, N., Nishiyama, Y., Miyake, K., Tamiya, T., Nagao, S. (2005) Evaluation of tumor FDG transport and metabolism in primary central nervous system lymphoma using [18F]fluorodeoxyglucose (FDG) positron emission tomography (PET) kinetic analysis. *Ann Nucl Med* **19**, 685–90.

67. Karantanis, D., O'Eill, B.P., Subramaniam, R.M., Witte, R.J., Mullan, B.P., Nathan, M.A., et al. (2007) 18F-FDG PET-CT in primary central nervous system lymphoma in HIV-negative patients. *Nucl Med Commun* **28**, 834–41.

68. Pirotte, B., Levivier, M., Goldman, S., Brucher, J.M., Brotchi, J., Hildebrand, J. (1997) Glucocorticoid-induced long-term remission in primary cerebral lymphoma: case report and review of the literature. *J Neurooncol* **32**, 63–9.

69. Bergstrom, M., Ericson, K., Hagenfeldt, L., Mosskin, M., von Holst, H., Noren, G., et al. (1987) PET study of methionine accumulation in glioma and normal brain tissue: competition with branched chain amino acids. *J Comput Assist Tomogr* **11**, 208–13.

70. Derlon, J.M., Bourdet, C., Bustany, P., Chatel, M., Theron, J., Darcel, F., et al. (1989) [11C]L-methionine uptake in gliomas. *Neurosurgery* **25**, 720–8.

71. Mosskin, M., von Holst, H., Bergstrom, M., Collins, V.P., Eriksson, L., Johnstrom, P., et al. (1987) Positron emission tomography with 11C-methionine and computed tomography of intracranial tumours compared with histopathologic examination of multiple biopsies. *Acta Radiol* **28**, 673–81.

72. Kaplan, A.M., Bandy, D.J., Manwaring, K.H., Chen, K., Lawson, M.A., Moss, S.D., et al. (1999) Functional brain mapping using positron emission tomography scanning in preoperative neurosurgical planning for pediatric brain tumors. *J Neurosurg* **91**, 797–803.

73. Utriainen, M., Metsahonkala, L., Salmi, T.T., Utriainen, T., Kalimo, H., Pihko, H., et al. (2002) Metabolic characterization of childhood brain tumors: comparison of 18F-fluorodeoxyglucose and 11C-methionine positron emission tomography. *Cancer* **95**, 1376–86.

74. Borgwardt, L., Hojgaard, L., Carstensen, H., Laursen, H., Nowak, M., Thomsen, C., et al. (2005) Increased fluorine-18 2-fluoro-2-deoxy-D-glucose (FDG) uptake in childhood CNS tumors is correlated with malignancy grade: a study with FDG positron emission tomography/magnetic resonance imaging coregistration and image fusion. *J Clin Oncol* **23**, 3030–7.

75. Pirotte, B., Lubansu, A., Massager, N., Wikler, D., Van Bogaert, P., Levivier, M., et al. (2010) Clinical interest of integrating positron emission tomography imaging in the workup of 55 children with incidentally diagnosed brain lesions. *J Neurosurg Pediatr* **5**, 479–85.

76. Sasaki, M., Kuwabara, Y., Yoshida, T., Fukumura, T., Morioka, T., Nishio, S., et al. (1998) Carbon-11-methionine PET in focal cortical dysplasia: a comparison with fluorine-18-FDG PET and technetium-99m-ECD SPECT. *J Nucl Med* **39**, 974–7.

77. De Witte, O., Lefranc, F., Levivier, M., Salmon, I., Brotchi, J., Goldman, S. (2000) FDG-PET as a prognostic factor in high-grade astrocytoma. *J Neurooncol* **49**, 157–63.

78. Ribom, D., Eriksson, A., Hartman, M., Engler, H., Nilsson, A., Langstrom, B., et al. (2001) Positron emission tomography (11) C-methionine and survival in patients with low-grade gliomas. *Cancer* **92**, 1541–9.

79. Kim, S., Chung, J.K., Im, S.H., Jeong, J.M., Lee, D.S., Kim, D.G., et al. (2005) 11C-methionine PET as a prognostic marker in patients with glioma: comparison with 18F-FDG PET. *Eur J Nucl Med Mol Imaging* **32**, 52–9.

80. Floeth, F.W., Pauleit, D., Sabel, M., Stoffels, G., Reifenberger, G., Riemenschneider, M.J., et al. (2007) Prognostic value of O-(2-18F-fluoroethyl)-L-tyrosine PET and MRI in low-grade glioma. *J Nucl Med* **48**, 519–27.

81. Glantz, M.J., Hoffman, J.M., Coleman, R.E., Friedman, A.H., Hanson, M.W., Burger, P.C., et al. (1991) Identification of early recurrence of primary central nervous system tumors by [18F]fluorodeoxyglucose positron emission tomography. *Ann Neurol* **29**, 347–55.

82. Patronas, N.J., Di Chiro, G., Brooks, R.A., DeLaPaz, R.L., Kornblith, P.L., Smith, B.H., et al. (1982) Work in progress: [18F] fluorodeoxyglucose and positron emission tomography in the evaluation of radiation necrosis of the brain. *Radiology* **144**, 885–9.

83. Chao, S.T., Suh, J.H., Raja, S., Lee, S.Y., Barnett, G. (2001) The sensitivity and specificity of FDG PET in distinguishing recurrent brain tumor from radionecrosis in

patients treated with stereotactic radiosurgery. *Int J Cancer* **96**, 191–7.

84. Mehrkens, J.H., Popperl, G., Rachinger, W., Herms, J., Seelos, K., Tatsch, K., et al. (2008) The positive predictive value of O-(2-[18F]fluoroethyl)-L-tyrosine (FET) PET in the diagnosis of a glioma recurrence after multimodal treatment. *J Neurooncol* **88**, 27–35.

85. Terakawa, Y., Tsuyuguchi, N., Iwai, Y., Yamanaka, K., Higashiyama, S., Takami, T., et al. (2008) Diagnostic accuracy of 11C-methionine PET for differentiation of recurrent brain tumors from radiation necrosis after radiotherapy. *J Nucl Med* **49**, 694–9.

86. Chung, J.K., Kim, Y.K., Kim, S.K., Lee, Y.J., Paek, S., Yeo, J.S., et al. (2002) Usefulness of 11C-methionine PET in the evaluation of brain lesions that are hypo- or isometabolic on 18F-FDG PET. *Eur J Nucl Med Mol Imaging* **29**, 176–82.

87. Bergstrom, M., Muhr, C., Lundberg, P.O., Bergstrom, K., Lundqvist, H., Langstrom, B. (1986) Amino acid metabolism in pituitary adenomas. *Acta Radiol Suppl* **369**, 412–4.

88. Bergstrom, M., Muhr, C., Lundberg, P.O., Langstrom, B. (1991) PET as a tool in the clinical evaluation of pituitary adenomas. *J Nucl Med* **32**, 610–5.

89. Tang, B.N., Levivier, M., Heureux, M., Wikler, D., Massager, N., Devriendt, D., et al. (2006) 11C-methionine PET for the diagnosis and management of recurrent pituitary adenomas. *Eur J Nucl Med Mol Imaging* **33**, 169–78.

90. Francavilla, T.L., Miletich, R.S., Di Chiro, G., Patronas, N.J., Rizzoli, H.V., Wright, D.C. (1989) Positron emission tomography in the detection of malignant degeneration of low-grade gliomas. *Neurosurgery* **24**, 1–5.

91. Popperl, G., Gotz, C., Rachinger, W., Gildehaus, F.J., Tonn, J.C., Tatsch, K. (2004) Value of O-(2-[18F]fluoroethyl)-L-tyrosine PET for the diagnosis of recurrent glioma. *Eur J Nucl Med Mol Imaging* **31**, 1464–70.

92. Chen, W., Silverman, D.H., Delaloye, S., Czernin, J., Kamdar, N., Pope, W., et al. (2006) 18F-FDOPA PET imaging of brain tumors: comparison study with 18F-FDG PET and evaluation of diagnostic accuracy. *J Nucl Med* **47**, 904–11.

93. Hillner, B.E., Siegel, B.A., Shields, A.F., Liu, D., Gareen, I.F., Hanna, L., et al. (2008) The impact of positron emission tomography (PET) on expected management during cancer

treatment: findings of the National Oncologic PET Registry. *Cancer* **115(2)**, 410–8.

94. Popperl, G., Gotz, C., Rachinger, W., Schnell, O., Gildehaus, F.J., Tonn, J.C., et al. (2006) Serial O-(2-[(18)F]fluoroethyl)-L-tyrosine PET for monitoring the effects of intracavitary radioimmunotherapy in patients with malignant glioma. *Eur J Nucl Med Mol Imaging* **33**, 792–800.

95. Valk, P.E., Budinger, T.F., Levin, V.A., Silver, P., Gutin, P.H., Doyle, W.K. (1988) PET of malignant cerebral tumors after interstitial brachytherapy. Demonstration of metabolic activity and correlation with clinical outcome. *J Neurosurg* **69**, 830–8.

96. Popperl, G., Goldbrunner, R., Gildehaus, F.J., Kreth, F.W., Tanner, P., Holtmann-spotter, M., et al. (2005) O-(2-[18F]fluoroethyl)-L-tyrosine PET for monitoring the effects of convection-enhanced delivery of paclitaxel in patients with recurrent glioblastoma. *Eur J Nucl Med Mol Imaging* **32**, 1018–25.

97. Rozental, J.M., Levine, R.L., Nickles, R.J., Dobkin, J.A. (1989) Glucose uptake by gliomas after treatment. A positron emission tomographic study. *Arch Neurol* **46**, 1302–7.

98. De Witte, O., Hildebrand, J., Luxen, A., Goldman, S. (1994) Acute effect of carmustine on glucose metabolism in brain and glioblastoma. *Cancer* **74**, 2836–42.

99. Pirotte, B., Goldman, S., Massager, N., David, P., Wikler, D., Vandesteene, A., et al. (2004) Comparison of 18F-FDG and 11C-methionine for PET-guided stereotactic brain biopsy of gliomas. *J Nucl Med* **45**, 1293–8.

100. Pirotte, B., Goldman, S., David, P., Wikler, D., Damhaut, P., Vandesteene, A., et al. (1997) Stereotactic brain biopsy guided by positron emission tomography (PET) with [F-18]fluorodeoxyglucose and [C-11]methionine *Acta Neurochir Suppl* **68**, 133–8.

101. Massager, N., David, P., Goldman, S., Pirotte, B., Wikler, D., Salmon, I., et al. (2000) Combined magnetic resonance imaging- and positron emission tomography-guided stereotactic biopsy in brainstem mass lesions: diagnostic yield in a series of 30 patients *J Neurosurg* **93**, 951–7.

102. Levivier, M., Massager, N., Wikler, D., Devriendt, D., Goldman, S. (2007) Integration of functional imaging in radiosurgery: The Example of PET Scan *Prog Neurol Surg* **20**, 68–81.

103. Levivier, M., Massager, N., Wikler, D., Lorenzoni, J., Ruiz, S., Devriendt, D., et al. (2004) Use of stereotactic PET images in

dosimetry planning of radiosurgery for brain tumors: clinical experience and proposed classification *J Nucl Med* **45**, 1146–54.

104. Levivier, M., Wikler, D., Jr., Massager, N., David, P., Devriendt, D., Lorenzoni, J., et al. (2002) The integration of metabolic imaging in stereotactic procedures including radiosurgery: a review *J Neurosurg* **97**, 542–50.

105. Torii, K., Tsuyuguchi, N., Kawabe, J., Sunada, I., Hara, M., Shiomi, S. (2005) Correlation of amino-acid uptake using methionine PET and histological classifications in various gliomas *Ann Nucl Med* **19(8)**, 677–83.

Chapter 17

PET and PET/CT for Unknown Primary Tumors

Thomas C. Kwee, Sandip Basu, and Abass Alavi

Abstract

Carcinoma of unknown primary (CUP) is defined as histologically proven metastatic disease that, after a complete diagnostic work-up, yields no primary detectable tumor. CUP is one of the ten most frequent cancers, with overall poor outcome. Detection of the unknown primary tumor is of crucial importance in this scenario, since it might help to select and offer definitive treatment, which, in turn, may improve patient prognosis. Additional diagnostic work-up, usually consisting of a combination of several radiological and endoscopic investigations and serum tumor marker studies, can be time consuming, expensive, and pose a significant burden to the patient. The final diagnostic yield of these tests is often limited. Combined positron emission tomography/computed tomography (PET/CT), using the radiotracer ^{18}F-fluoro-2-deoxyglucose (FDG), may be of great value in the management of patients with CUP for the detection of primary tumors. This chapter gives a brief introduction to the syndrome of CUP, followed by an outline of the rationale, use, and utility of FDG-PET/CT in CUP, and concludes with a discussion on the challenges and future directions in the diagnostic management of patients with CUP.

Key words: ^{18}F-fluoro-2-deoxyglucose, Position emission tomography, Computed tomography, FDG-PET/CT, Carcinoma of unknown primary, Primary tumor detection

1. Introduction

1.1. Definition

Carcinoma of unknown primary (CUP) is defined as the presence of histologically proven metastatic disease for which the site of origin cannot be identified at the time of diagnosis (1–3). More specifically, the precise clinical definition of CUP currently refers to patients who present with histologically confirmed metastatic cancer in whom a detailed medical history, complete physical examination including pelvic and rectal examination, full blood count and biochemistry, urinalysis, stool occult blood testing, histopathological review of biopsy material with the use of immunohistochemistry, chest radiography, CT of the chest abdomen and pelvis, and, in certain cases, mammography have failed to detect the primary tumor (1–3).

Malik E. Juweid and Otto S. Hoekstra (eds.), *Positron Emission Tomography*, Methods in Molecular Biology, vol. 727, DOI 10.1007/978-1-61779-062-1_17, © Springer Science+Business Media, LLC 2011

1.2. Epidemiology

CUP is the eighth most frequent cancer in the world (accounting for 3–5% of all malignancies), and is the fourth most common cause of cancer-related death in both males and females (1–4). The annual age-adjusted incidence per 100,000 population in USA is 7–12 cases, in Australia 18–19 cases, and in the Netherlands 5.3–6.7 cases (1–4). The median age for occurrence is around 60 years and CUP is marginally more frequent in males (1–4). It should be noted that as imaging technology continues to improve, incidence of CUP will decrease, because more primary tumors will be detected in such a setting.

2. Symptomatology, Etiology, and Histopathology

Patients with CUP often have widespread metastatic disease, and are often debilitated at the time of diagnosis (1–3, 5). Constitutional symptoms such as anorexia, weight loss, and fatigue are often present, along with other clinical signs and symptoms related to the site(s) of metastatic disease (1–3, 5). Common sites of involvement at presentation include the liver, lungs, bones, and lymph nodes, but other sites may also be involved. There is considerable variation in the sites of metastases depending on the histological diagnosis (1–3, 5). Although it is widely accepted that CUP is a heterogeneous group of metastatic malignancies, it is still unclear whether CUP forms a distinct biological entity with specific genetic and phenotypic characteristics, or whether it is merely a clinical presentation of metastases in patients in whom the primary tumor cannot be detected and does not result in any visible clinical feature (1–3, 6). In addition, there are no obvious risk factors that contribute to the pathogenesis of CUP. Almost 50% of patients with CUP will be diagnosed with metastatic adenocarcinoma of well to moderate differentiation, 30% with undifferentiated or poorly differentiated carcinomas, 15% with squamous cell carcinomas, and the remaining 5% will have undifferentiated neoplasms (1–3).

3. Detection of the Primary Tumor

Detection of the primary tumor may optimize treatment planning, which, in turn, may improve patient prognosis. Furthermore, the identification of a primary tumor may reduce anxiety in both patient and physician by decreasing prognostic and therapeutic uncertainties. At present, there is no established standard protocol for additional diagnostic work-up in (subsets of) patients with CUP that has proven to be cost-effective. Patients with CUP are classified into subgroups (according to organ(s) involved and histopathological findings) in order to guide diagnostic approaches and to be able to offer optimal therapeutic management (1–3). The conventional diagnostic work-up usually consists of (a combination of several) radiological, endoscopical, and serum tumor marker studies, depending on the specific signs, symptoms, and laboratory abnormalities (1–3). However, the combination of these (often invasive) tests can be both time consuming, expensive, and pose a significant burden to the patient. Furthermore, despite extensive diagnostic work-up, a primary tumor can only be detected in a small minority of patients with CUP antemortem. In addition, autopsy studies have reported that approximately 70% of unknown primary tumors remain undetected (1–3). Of note, failure to detect the primary tumor may be due to spontaneous regression of the primary tumor (due to cellular and humoral host response) or due to its inherent small size (phenotypic and genotypic characteristics may favor metastatic spread over local tumor growth) (1–3).

4. Prognosis and Treatment

For optimal treatment planning, patients with CUP are categorized into favorable and unfavorable subgroups (1–3). Favorable subgroups include poorly differentiated carcinoma with midline distribution (extragonadal germ cell syndrome), women with papillary adenocarcinoma of the peritoneal cavity, women with adenocarcinoma involving only axillary lymph nodes, squamous cell carcinoma involving cervical lymph nodes, isolated inguinal lymphadenopathy (squamous carcinoma), poorly differentiated neuroendocrine carcinomas, men with blastic bone metastases and elevated prostate-specific antigen (adenocarcinoma), and patients with a single, small, and potentially respectable tumor (1–3). Unfavorable subgroups include adenocarcinoma metastatic to the liver and other organs, non-papillary malignant ascites (adenocarcinoma), multiple cerebral metastases (adenocarcinoma or squamous cell carcinoma), multiple lung or pleural metastases (adenocarcinoma), and multiple metastastic bone disease (adenocarcinoma) (1–3). Some favorable subgroups require specific treatment approaches and have the potential for an excellent treatment outcome (1–3). However, in general, CUP follows an aggressive biological and clinical behavior, with poor response to treatment (1–3). Improved therapy will probably await advances in the systemic therapy of non-small cell lung cancer, pancreatic cancer, and other gastrointestinal cancers, since the majority of insensitive adenocarcinomas probably arise from these primary sites (1–3, 5). Furthermore, although median survival in patients with CUP is only 6–9 months (1–3), a median survival of 23 months has been reported for patients with CUP and an identified primary tumor subsequently treated with specific therapy (7). Similarly, one study (8) reported that the 3-year survival rate for patients with cervical metastases and occult oropharyngeal primary tumors was 100% after treatment, while the patients with cervical metastases in which a primary tumor was not detected showed a survival rate of 58%. These studies (7, 8) advocate the pursuit for noninvasive imaging modalities that are able to detect a higher rate of unknown primary tumors than is currently possible.

5. FDG-PET/CT in CUP

5.1. Rationale

Since the unknown primary tumor can be located anywhere in the body in patients with CUP, a cross-sectional whole-body imaging modality is the method of choice when searching for an unknown primary tumor. In addition, whole-body cross-sectional imaging modalities potentially allow complete staging of the tumor, thereby facilitating treatment planning and possibly improving outcome. Imaging modalities that are only able to examine a limited part of the body (such as ultrasound) or planar imaging modalities (such as planar X-ray imaging) clearly have a limited role. Computed tomography (CT) and magnetic resonance imaging (MRI) are two of the main technologies that came to dominate the cross-sectional imaging of human anatomy in clinical practice. However, small lesions and pathologic changes in normal-sized structures may be missed by CT and anatomical MRI, which basically only allow for the detection of abnormal anatomy and abnormal contrast enhancement. Especially in CUP, where the primary tumor may be of small size (1–3), this is a major issue. Furthermore, image interpretation time of whole-body CT or anatomical MRI datasets may be very time consuming.

In contrast to CT and anatomical MRI, positron emission tomography (PET), using the radiotracer ^{18}F-fluoro-2-deoxyglucose (FDG), provides functional information, with excellent lesion-to-background ratio, resulting in improved sensitivity of lesion detection. This advantage of PET over CT and anatomical MRI is well reflected by the fact that, within the spectrum of macroscopic medical imaging, sensitivity ranges from the detection of millimolar to submillimolar concentrations of contrast media with CT and MRI, respectively, to picomolar concentration with PET – a 10^8 to 10^9 difference (9, 10). PET can now reach a spatial resolution of about 4–6 mm for whole-body imaging (9). Equally important is the fact that PET has an excellent lesion-to-background ratio (9, 10), which may even enable detection of lesions with a size below the spatial resolution of PET. In addition, since the vast majority of malignant cancer phenotypes exhibit an increased glucose metabolism (Warburg effect) (11), the radiotracer FDG is theoretically very useful for unknown primary tumor detection.

5.2. PET Instrumentation and Imaging Protocol

A disadvantage of FDG-PET alone is lack of anatomic information, which may impede precise localization of FDG accumulation. This may decrease diagnostic performance of FDG-PET in detecting the unknown primary tumor, and decrease tissue sampling success rate, which is necessary to establish a final histopathological diagnosis. Furthermore, unknown primary tumors with low or even no FDG uptake may be missed by FDG-PET. Complimentary anatomic information, provided by CT or MRI, may improve the diagnostic performance of FDG-PET alone, and increase tissue sampling success rate. The relatively recently introduced combined PET/CT scanner (current clinical PET/CT scanners are equipped with a 16- to 64-section multidetector-row CT unit) is rapidly replacing the stand-alone PET scanner in clinical practice. PET/CT allows obtaining both functional and anatomic images in a single examination, and is the preferred PET method of choice for the detection of primary tumors in patients with CUP. An additional advantage of PET/CT is the use of the CT images for attenuation correction of the PET emission data, which reduces whole-body scanning times from 45 to 30 min or less (12, 13); this is of great importance in patients with CUP who are generally in a poor physical condition, and may not tolerate a long examination. Furthermore, PET/CT provides low-noise attenuation correction factors, compared with those from standard PET transmission measurements using an external radiation source, and eliminates bias from emission contamination of postinjection transmission scans (13).

For the FDG-PET component of a FDG-PET/CT study, a standard protocol is used, consisting of fasting for at least 6 h before FDG administration, maximum plasma glucose levels of 150 mg/dL, avoidance of strenuous exercise prior to the examination and following injection of FDG, a standard dose of 370 MBq (or 5 MBq/kg of body weight) of FDG that is administered intravenously through an indwelling catheter inserted into an antecubital vein, data acquisition 45–60 min after FDG administration, and scanning of (at least) the head, neck, chest, abdomen, and pelvis. Care should be taken with intravenous FDG injection; aspiration of blood should be avoided, in order to minimize the chance of iatrogenic pulmonary microembolism, which may present as focal intrapulmonary FDG uptake, resembling a malignant lung lesion (14, 15). Although it is well known that in several tumors maximum FDG uptake occurs considerably later than 45–60 after FDG administration (16), there is no specific evidence yet whether it is beneficial to perform dual-time point or delayed scanning in patients with CUP. Similarly, with regard to the CT-component, there is no consensus yet whether a low-dose or an enhanced full-dose (diagnostic) CT scan should be used. A recent meta-analysis on the diagnostic performance of FDG-PET/CT for the detection of unknown primary tumors showed no significant advantage of using intravenous and oral CT contrast agents (17). Based on our experience, an enhanced full-dose CT-scan generally does not yield useful additional diagnostic information. Furthermore, CT contrast media may introduce image artifacts (18, 19). In addition, iodinated contrast agents may cause adverse reactions, including rarely occurring but life-threatening contrast-induced nephrotoxicity and anaphylactic shock (20). Therefore, the use of a low-dose CT-scan may be routinely preferred, while reserving a diagnostic CT-scan only for selected cases (e.g. in case of a high suspicion of primary lung cancer).

5.3. Image Interpretation

A careful evaluation of FDG-PET/CT findings, along with the patient's accurate history and clinical examination, is necessary to maximize diagnostic yield and minimize false-positive results. The location of the metastatic site(s) may give an indication of the location of the primary tumor. For example, in females with axillary lymph node metastasis or peritoneal carcinomatosis, primary breast or ovarian cancer may be suspected, respectively. In patients with poorly differentiated carcinoma and left supraclavicular lymph adenopathy (Virchow's node), a primary gastrointestinal tumor may be detected. Furthermore, in patients with involvement of the upper or mid-cervical lymph nodes, a primary site in the head and neck should be suspected (1–3, 5).

Regions of focally increased tracer uptake distant from the metastatic site(s) should raise the suspicion of a primary tumor. In case of equivocal findings, a maximum standardized uptake value (SUV) of >2.5 or delayed imaging may be considered to represent malignancy (17). CT images should be evaluated to accurately localize lesions with increased FDG uptake, and to detect abnormal anatomy. It is important to realize that CT-based attenuation correction may lead to misclassification of regions containing high concentrations of CT contrast medium with high-density bone (CT contrast agents have high atomic numbers relative to the atomic number of bone, and as the concentration of a contrast agent increases, its corresponding CT number will fall within the CT number range for bone), which results in overcorrection for photon attenuation, consequently leading to an overestimation of FDG uptake in the contrast-enhanced region (18, 19). Therefore, if CT contrast media are administered, it is important to evaluate both attenuation-corrected and nonattentuation-corrected images to minimize the chance of misinterpreting (FDG-PET/CT) artifacts as pathologic.

5.4. Diagnostic Performance

Autopsy studies have reported that approximately 70% of unknown primary tumors remain undetected; one plausible explanation for this phenomenon may be spontaneous regression of the primary tumor (1–3). Therefore, even a hypothetical ideal imaging modality will not be able to detect all unknown primary tumors. Nevertheless, in order to calculate estimates of diagnostic performance (i.e. primary tumor detection rate, sensitivity, and specificity), the following assumptions are often made: a true-positive result is considered when the imaging modality of interest suggested the location of the primary tumor and was subsequently confirmed. A false-positive result is considered when this location was not confirmed. Histopathological analysis of tissue obtained by biopsy or surgery is considered as the reference standard. If it is not possible to obtain histopathological proof, other imaging procedures or clinical follow-up are accepted as reference standard. A false-negative result is considered when neither the imaging modality of interest nor the reference standard could detect the primary tumor. A false-negative result is considered if the primary tumor was detected in a particular location that was negative on the imaging modality of interest (17).

A recent meta-analysis (17) showed that, overall, FDG-PET/CT is able to detect 37% of primary tumors in patients with CUP, with both sensitivity and specificity of 84%. In this meta-analysis (17), completeness of diagnostic work-up before FDG-PET/CT (i.e. complete diagnostic work-up according to the previously mentioned definition vs. incomplete diagnostic work-up), location of metastases (i.e. cervical vs. extracervical), administration of CT contrast agents (i.e. both intravenous and oral contrast vs. no intravenous or oral contrast agent, or not reported), type of FDG-PET images evaluated (i.e. both attenuation-corrected and nonattenuation-corrected images vs. attenuation-corrected images only, or not reported), and way of FDG-PET/CT review (reported blinding to reference test vs. no or unreported blinding to reference test) did not seem to influence diagnostic performance of FDG-PET/CT. However, these subgroup analyses may not have been conclusive because of the relatively small number of included studies. Furthermore, the influence of the number of CT detector rows and CT slice width on diagnostic performance could not be assessed in this meta-analysis due to incomplete reporting of studies (17).

In the same meta-analysis (17), lung (33%), oropharyngeal (16%), and pancreatic carcinoma (5%) were the most frequently detected primary tumors by FDG-PET/CT (Figs. 1–3). This is partly in line with autopsy studies in patients with CUP (21–24), which have shown that the most common locations of the primary tumor are the lung and the pancreas. The relatively high detection rate of oropharyngeal cancer by FDG-PET/CT is discrepant with the results of autopsy studies (21–24), but can be explained

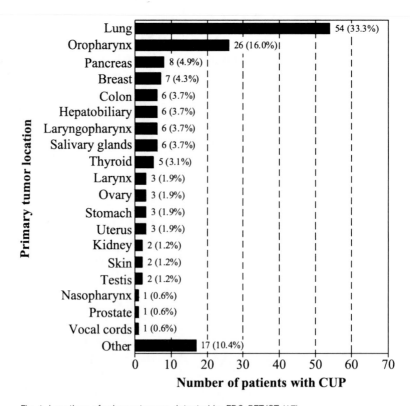

Fig. 1. Locations of primary tumors detected by FDG-PET/CT (17).

by the fact that a relatively large proportion of CUP patients in the aforementioned meta-analysis presented with cervical metastases (17), whose primary tumors are most frequently located in the oropharynx (25). Breast cancer (27%) is the most common cause of false-negative FDG-PET/CT results (Fig. 4) (17). This may be explained by the fact that small (<1 cm) and slow-growing, low-grade (breast) cancers with low or no FDG uptake (e.g. tubular carcinoma and noninvasive cancers such as ductal or lobular carcinoma in situ) may be overlooked on FDG-PET/CT (26). Therefore, in patients with CUP and a high suspicion of occult primary breast cancer, such as in case of isolated axillary lymph node metastases, an MRI-scan may be performed (which has demonstrated to be the most sensitive imaging method for detecting breast carcinoma) (27, 28), although its cost-effectiveness has not been proven yet. On the other hand, the most commonly reported locations of false-positive FDG-PET/CT results are the lung and the oropharynx (Fig. 5) (17). Interestingly, these locations are also two of the most common areas where FDG-PET/CT can detect a primary tumor (17), reflecting its imperfect specificity.

Inflammatory lesions are among the most common nononcological causes of FDG uptake in the oropharynx and lung (29). As mentioned earlier, a careful review of the patient's accurate

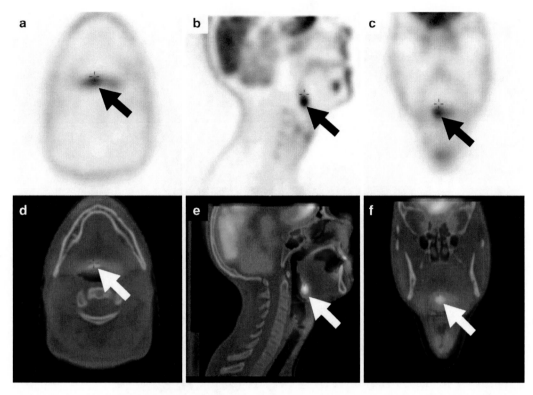

Fig. 2. FDG-PET and FDG-PET/CT in a 36-year-old man who presented with a left cervical lymph node metastasis containing squamous cell carcinoma of an unknown primary tumor. CT (not shown) could not depict a primary tumor. FDG-PET images in the axial (**a**), sagittal (**b**), and coronal plane (**c**) show the primary tumor (*black arrows*). Corresponding FDG-PET/CT images in the axial (**a**), sagittal (**b**), and coronal plane (**c**) show that the primary tumor is localized at the base of the tongue (*white arrows*). Subsequent panendoscopic examination could not depict a primary tumor. However, histopathological examination of a blind biopsy of the base of the tongue confirmed the presence of a primary tumor.

history and clinical examination is of utmost importance to increase specificity of FDG-PET/CT. In addition, the CT imaging pattern may suggest the presence of benign inflammatory disease (e.g. increased FDG uptake can be seen in lipoid pneumonia and pulmonary Langerhans cell histiocytosis, but these entities have a typical CT appearance (29)). Furthermore, accurate localization of areas with increased FDG uptake by means of CT images may decrease false-postive results (e.g. depiction of physiological muscle FDG uptake in the oropharynx (30)). Last, but not least, it has been reported that incidental pulmonary emboli are present in 4% of the general oncology population (31). Lung infarction secondary to pulmonary embolism may cause FDG uptake in the lung and mimic malignancy (29, 32). In the appropriate clinical setting, a wedge-shaped peripheral region of consolidation on CT should raise the possibility of a pulmonary infarct (29). In addition, as mentioned earlier, inappropriate intravenous FDG injection may incidentally cause iatrogenic pulmonary microembolism, with

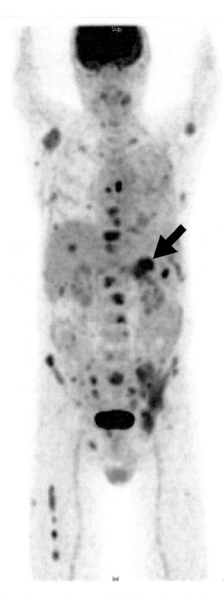

Fig. 3. FDG-PET in a 77-year-old man with a history of localized prostate carcinoma who presented with severe bone pain (back, pelvis, and legs), weight loss, and dyspnea. MRI (not shown) that was performed in an outside hospital showed pleural fluid collections, and suggested the presence of bone metastases in the lumbar vertebrae and pelvis, without clearly identifying a primary tumor. However, cytological examination of the pleural fluid revealed adenocarcinoma cells that stained positively for prostatic specific antigen, suggesting metastatic prostate cancer. FDG-PET showed widespread meta-static disease, including multiple bone lesions (mandibula, left humeral head, right glenoid, ribs, sternum, vertebrae, pelvis, and right femur), lung lesions, liver lesions, and left iliac lymph node involvement. Interestingly, FDG-PET also showed a lesion in the tail of pancreas (*black arrow*), which was histopathologically confirmed to represent a primary pancreatic adenocarcinoma.

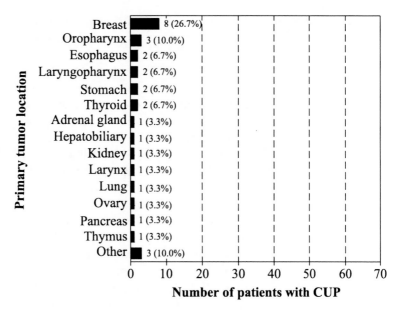

Fig. 4. Locations of false-negative FDG-PET/CT findings (17).

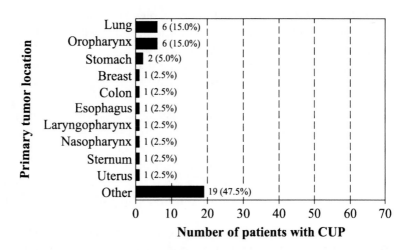

Fig. 5. Locations of false-positive FDG-PET/CT findings (17).

subsequent focal intrapulmonary FDG uptake (14, 15). In case of a focal lesion with increased FDG uptake but without corroborating anatomic evidence of the lesion on CT, the diagnosis of an iatrogenic microembolism is more likely than that of a primary lung malignancy (14, 15).

5.5. Cost-Effectiveness

Identification of the primary tumor in patients with CUP enables accurate tumor staging, which allows optimizing treatment planning; this, in turn, may improve patient prognosis. On the other hand, it should be realized that FDG-PET/CT is an expensive examination, and false-positive FDG-PET/CT findings may result in unnecessary additional invasive diagnostic procedures, which have associated morbidities and costs (33). Four studies reported the therapeutic impact of FDG-PET/CT; in these four studies, FDG-PET/CT modified therapy in 18.2–60% of patients (34–37), which is important from the viewpoint of patient management. Although one study (38) reported that the survival rate of CUP patients with at least one hypermetabolic lesion was significantly lower ($P<0.0279$) than that of the remaining CUP patients, no study has reported FDG-PET/CT-modified patient outcomes so far. Therefore, the benefit of FDG-PET/CT to patients with CUP is not clear yet. Furthermore, whole-body FDG-PET/CT is an expensive test (39), and its cost-effectiveness (i.e. a measure of how well the test fares in relation to utilization of resources (40)) is still unknown.

5.6. Utility of FDG-PET/ CT Beyond Detection of the Unknown Primary Tumor

As mentioned earlier, the utility of FDG-PET/CT for detecting a primary tumor in patients with CUP can be debated. However, it is important to realize that FDG-PET/CT is a very sensitive imaging modality for the detection of lesions throughout the entire body. Therefore, it may allow detection or exclusion of additional metastatic sites, which may have important therapeutic implications. This may particularly be of interest in patients with CUP who present with lymph node metastatic disease only (e.g. detection of initially unrecognized distant metastases can lead to a change in the treatment intent, from cure to palliation) (41). Furthermore, a baseline FDG-PET/CT may also play a valuable role for treatment monitoring following therapeutic intervention (41).

5.7. Challenges and Future Directions

The diagnostic challenge in CUP lies in maximizing the detection rate of the primary tumor while minimizing the number of false-positives. PET, using the radiotracer FDG, owes its success to clinical oncology in which whole-body scanning has a central role (9). FDG, however, is a nonspecific radiotracer that accumulates in areas of increased glycolysis that occur in both malignant and benign (mainly inflammatory) processes (29). Several new oncological radiotracers are under active investigation, including agents that are able to detect regional hypoxia, angiogenesis, or apoptosis in malignant tumors (42–44). However, these new radiotracers are probably more useful in drug development, treatment planning, and monitoring response to therapy, than for diagnostic purposes in oncology such as in CUP, since hypoxia, angiogenesis, and apoptosis also occur in inflammatory processes (45–47). Similarly, the proliferation marker ^{18}F-fluoro-3′-deoxy-3′-L-fluorothymidine is likely to be more suitable for assessing treatment response than as a diagnostic tool, because it is insensitive for detecting slow-growing tumors (48). Furthermore, CUP is a heterogeneous group of metastatic malignancies (1–3, 6), making the development of a specific radiotracer for CUP difficult. Therefore, it appears unlikely that a more specific radiotracer with at least equal sensitivity to FDG will soon become available for unknown primary tumor detection.

On the other hand, hardware improvements in PET are expected to improve the (diagnostic) management of patients with CUP. Major advances in PET technology over the past two decades include the development of whole-body PET, three-dimensional PET, new scintillator materials, improved image reconstruction methods, and the development of combined PET/CT (49). Currently, the reintroduction of time-of-flight (TOF)-PET is of great promise (50, 51). In TOF-PET, the actual time difference in the arrival of the two annihilation protons at the detectors is recorded (50). Thanks to the development of new scintillators (such as lutetium oxyorthosilicate [LSO] and lutetium-yttrium oxyorthosilicate [LYSO]), a stable timing resolution of approximately 600 ps can currently be achieved (49, 50). This can be used to constrain the reconstruction algorithm, because it localizes the annihilation site to within a few centimeters, and thus the reconstruction of that event can be weighted accordingly (49, 50). The timing information obtained by TOF-PET permits some combination of faster scanning (whole-body scanning in only 10–20 min in patients of small and average size, and whole-body scanning in 30 min in heavier patients (49, 50)), improved signal-to-noise ratio, or improved spatial resolution. Especially, the increased detectability of small lesions (49) is expected to be of great advantage in patients with CUP.

Another important issue is to reconsider the diagnostic algorithm that is used in patients who present with metastatic disease. Being a noninvasive and very sensitive tomographic whole-body imaging modality, FDG-PET/CT allows both detection of a primary tumor and, equally important, complete tumor staging. In fact, it can be argued that when a primary tumor is not detected by FDG-PET/CT, it is unlikely that it will be detected by other diagnostic tools, which are often invasive and time consuming. Thus, perhaps FDG-PET/CT should be used as a first-line imaging modality in all patients who present with metastatic disease, rather than using it after other diagnostic procedures have failed to identify a primary tumor. Future studies should investigate the utility of this shift in diagnostic paradigm.

Combined PET/CT scanners have become widely adopted in clinical practice, but are now being challenged by the promise of simultaneous (whole-body) PET/MRI (9). Regardless of the technological difficulties that have to be solved for designing a PET/MRI system (9) and its cost-effectiveness, this concept offers several advantages over PET/CT. First, the combination of

PET and MRI enables true simultaneous scanning (instead of sequential scanning with PET/CT), thereby minimizing the mismatch between PET and MRI datasets (9). Second, MRI provides superior soft-tissue contrast to CT, which may improve visualization and localization of lesions. Third, both anatomical and functional information can be obtained using MRI, which may be helpful in lesion detection and characterization. Nevertheless, several functional MRI techniques, such as perfusion-weighted MRI and MR spectroscopy are of limited use in patients with CUP, because they only offer regional tissue information, whereas the unknown primary tumor can be located anywhere in the body. However, unlike perfusion-weighted MRI and MR spectroscopy, the recently developed concept of whole-body diffusion-weighted MRI (DWI) has high potential in whole-body oncological imaging, and its application is under active investigation (51). DWI highlights areas with restricted diffusion, such as occurs in many malignancies, and may be a highly sensitive tool when searching for an unknown primary tumor (51, 52). Advantages of DWI compared to FDG-PET include a higher spatial resolution and superior evaluation of the urinary tract (where potential lesions can be obscured because of FDG accumulation) (51). Furthermore, DWI may help specifying suspicious lesions on FDG-PET. For example, the apparent diffusion coefficient (a quantitative measure of diffusion in biological tissue) has proven to be superior to the SUV in discriminating benign from malignant pulmonary nodules/masses (53). Of note, the lung is one of the most common locations of false-positive FDG-PET/CT results (Fig. 5) (51). Therefore, DWI may be a powerful adjunct to FDG-PET in a PET/MRI system when searching for an unknown primary tumor.

Last but not least, another exciting development is the use of molecular technology that allows gene expression profiling (using a quantitative reverse transcriptase polymerase chain reaction assay) in patients with CUP. Gene expression profiling has recently proven to be useful for predicting the origin of the primary tumor (54, 55). Along with further developments in the field of (functional and molecular) imaging, this may lead to an optimization of treatment planning, and, ultimately, improval of survival and quality of life of patients with CUP.

6. Conclusion

In conclusion, FDG-PET/CT is a powerful imaging modality for the detection of unknown primary tumors throughout the entire body, with an intrinsically higher sensitivity for the detection of lesions than other cross-sectional whole-body imaging modalities such as CT and anatomical MRI. Knowledge of the strengths and limitations of FDG-PET/CT, along with a careful review of clinical information, will maximize its diagnostic yield in patients with CUP. Technological advances in PET instrumentation and integration with MRI are expected to improve the detection of unknown primary tumors.

References

1. Pavlidis, N., Fizazi, K. (2009) Carcinoma of unknown primary (CUP). *Crit Rev Oncol Hematol* **69**, 271–278.

2. Pavlidis, N. (2007) Forty years experience of treating cancer of unknown primary *Acta Oncol* **46**, 592–601.

3. Pavlidis, N., Briasoulis, E., Hainsworth, J., Greco, F.A. (2003) Diagnostic and therapeutic management of cancer of an unknown primary *Eur J Cancer* **39**, 1990–2005.

4. Levi, F., Te, V.C., Erler, G., Randimbison, L., La Vecchia, C. (2002) Epidemiology of unknown primary tumours *Eur J Cancer* **38**, 1810–2.

5. Hainsworth, J.D., Greco, F.A. (1993) Treatment of patients with cancer of an unknown primary site *N Engl J Med* **329**, 257–63.

6. Van de Wouw, A.J., Jansen, R.L., Speel, E.J., Hillen, H.F. (2003) The unknown biology of the unknown primary tumour: a literature review *Ann Oncol* **14**, 191–6.

7. Raber, M.N., Faintuch, J., Abbruzzese, J.L., Sumrall, C., Frost, P. (1991) Continuous infusion 5-fluorouracil, etoposide and cis-diamminedichloroplatinum in patients with metastatic carcinoma of unknown primary origin. *Ann Oncol* **2**, 519–20.

8. Haas, I., Hoffmann, T.K., Engers, R., Ganzer, U. (2002) Diagnostic strategies in cervical carcinoma of an unknown primary (CUP). *Eur Arch Otorhinolaryngol* **259**, 325–33.

9. Zaidi, H.., Alavi, A. (2007) Current trends in PET and combined (PET/CT and PET/MR) systems design. *Pet Clin* **2**, 109–23.

10. Jones, T. (2002) Molecular imaging with PET – the future challenges. *Br J Radiol* **75**, S6–15.

11. Rohren, E.M., Turkington, T.G., Coleman, R.E. (2004) Clinical applications of PET in oncology *Radiology* **231**, 305–32.

12. Blodgett, T.M., Meltzer, C.C., Townsend, D.W. (2007) PET/CT: form and function. *Radiology* **242**, 360–85.

13. Von Schulthess, G.K., Steinert, H.C., Hany, T.F. (2006) Integrated PET/CT: current applications and future directions *Radiology* **238**, 405–22.

14. Farsad, M., Ambrosini, V., Nanni, C., Castellucci, P., Boschi, S., Rubello, D., et al. (2005) Focal lung uptake of 18F-fluorodeoxyglucose (18F-FDG) without computed tomography findings *Nucl Med Commun* **26**, 827–30.

15. Hany, T.F., Heuberger, J., von Schulthess, G.K. (2003) Iatrogenic FDG foci in the lungs: a pitfall of PET image interpretation *Eur Radiol* **13**, 2122–7.

16. Basu, S., Zaidi, H., Alavi, A. (2007) Clinical and research applications of quantitative PET imaging. *PET Clin* **2**, 161–72.

17. Kwee, T.C., Kwee, R.M. (2009) Combined FDG-PET/CT for the detection of unknown primary tumors: systematic review and meta-analysis *Eur Radiol* **19**, 731–44.

18. Ay, M.R., Zaidi, H. (2006) Assessment of errors caused by X-ray scatter and use of contrast medium when using CT-based attenuation correction in PET *Eur J Nucl Med Mol Imaging* **33**, 1301–13.

19. Antoch, G., Freudenberg, L.S., Egelhof, T., Stattaus, J., Jentzen, W., Debatin, J.F., Bockisch, A. (2002) Focal tracer uptake: a potential artifact in contrast-enhanced dual-modality PET/CT scans *J Nucl Med* **43**, 1339–42.

20. Namasivayam, S., Kalra, M.K., Torres, W.E., Small, W.C. (2006) Adverse reactions to intravenous iodinated contrast media: a primer for radiologists *Emerg Radiol* **12**, 210–5.

21. Al-Brahim, N., Ross, C., Carter, B., Chorneyko, K. (2005) The value of postmortem examination in cases of metastasis of unknown origin-20-year retrospective data from a tertiary care center. *Ann Diagn Pathol* **9**, 77–80.

22. Blaszyk, H., Hartmann, A., Bjornsson, J. (2003) Cancer of unknown primary: clinico-pathologic correlations *APMIS* **111**, 1089–94.

23. Mayordomo, J.I., Guerra, J.M., Guijarro, C., García-Prats, M.D., Gómez, A., López-Brea, M., et al. (1993) Neoplasms of unknown primary site: a clinicopathological study of autopsied patients *Tumori* **79**, 321–4.

24. Le Chevalier, T., Cvitkovic, E., Caille, P., Harvey, J., Contesso, G., Spielmann, M., et al. (1988) Early metastatic cancer of unknown

primary origin at presentation. A clinical study of 302 consecutive autopsied patients *Arch Intern Med* **148**, 2035–9.

25. Werner, J.A., Dünne, A.A., Myers, J.N. (2003) Functional anatomy of the lymphatic drainage system of the upper aerodigestive tract and its role in metastasis of squamous cell carcinoma *Head Neck* **25**, 322–32.

26. Lim, H.S., Yoon, W., Chung, T.W., Kim, J.K., Park, J.G., Kang, H.K., et al. (2007) FDG PET/CT for the detection and evaluation of breast diseases: usefulness and limitations *Radiographics* **27**, S197–213.

27. DeMartini, W., Lehman, C. (2008) A review of current evidence-based clinical applications for breast magnetic resonance imaging *Top Magn Reson Imaging* **19**, 143–50.

28. Buchanan, C.L., Morris, E.A., Dorn, P.L., Borgen, P.I., Van Zee, K.J. (2005) Utility of breast magnetic resonance imaging in patients with occult primary breast cancer *Ann Surg Oncol* **12**, 1045–53.

29. Metser, U., Even-Sapir, E. (2007) Increased (18)F-fluorodeoxyglucose uptake in benign, nonphysiologic lesions found on whole-body positron emission tomography/computed tomography (PET/CT): accumulated data from four years of experience with PET/CT. *Semin Nucl Med* **37**, 206–22.

30. Blodgett, T.M., Fukui, M.B., Snyderman, C.H., Branstetter, B.F. 4th., McCook, B.M., Townsend, D.W., et al. (2005) Combined PET-CT in the head and neck: part 1. Physiologic, altered physiologic, and artifactual FDG uptake. *Radiographics* **25**, 897–912.

31. Gladish, G.W., Choe, D.H., Marom, E.M., Sabloff, B.S., Broemeling, L.D., Munden, R.F. (2006) Incidental pulmonary emboli in oncology patients: prevalence, CT evaluation, and natural history *Radiology* **240**, 246–55.

32. Gutzeit, A., Antoch, G., Kühl, H., Egelhof, T., Fischer, M., Hauth, E., et al. (2005) Unknown primary tumors: detection with dual-modality PET/CT – initial experience. *Radiology* **234**, 227–34.

33. Schapira, D.V., Jarrett, A.R. (1995) The need to consider survival, outcome, and expense when evaluating and treating patients with unknown primary carcinoma. *Arch Intern Med* **155**, 2050–4.

34. Bruna, C., Journo, A., Netter, F., Kaminsky, M.C., Dolivet, G., Olivier, P., et al. (2007) On the interest of PET with 18F-FDG in the management of cancer of unknown primary (CUP). *Med Nucl* **31**, 242–9.

35. Wartski, M., Le Stanc, E., Gontier, E., Vilain, D., Banal, A., Tainturier, C., et al. (2007) In search of an unknown primary tumour presenting with cervical metastases: performance of hybrid FDG-PET-CT *Nucl Med Commun* **28**, 365–71.

36. Fakhry, N., Barberet, M., Lussato, D., Cammilleri, S., Mundler, O., Giovanni, A., et al. (2006) Role of [18F]-FDG PET-CT in the management of the head and neck cancers. *Bull Cancer* **93**, 1017–25.

37. Pelosi, E., Pennone, M., Deandreis, D., Douroukas, A., Mancini, M., Bisi, G. (2006) Role of whole body positron emission tomography/computed tomography scan with 18F-fluorodeoxyglucose in patients with biopsy proven tumor metastases from unknown primary site. *Q J Nucl Med Mol Imaging* **50**, 15–22.

38. Fencl, P., Belohlavek, O., Skopalova, M., Jaruskova, M., Kantorova, I., Simonova, K. (2007) Prognostic and diagnostic accuracy of [18F]FDG-PET/CT in 190 patients with carcinoma of unknown primary. *Eur J Nucl Med Mol Imaging* **34**, 1783–92.

39. Plathow, C., Walz, M., Lichy, M.P., Aschoff, P., Pfannenberg, C., Bock, H., et al. (2008) Cost considerations for whole-body MRI and PET/CT as part of oncologic staging *Radiologe* **48**, 384–96.

40. American College of Physicians (2008) Information on cost-effectiveness: an essential product of a national comparative effectiveness program. *Ann Intern Med* **148**, 956–61.

41. Basu, S., Alavi, A. (2007) FDG-PET in the clinical management of carcinoma of unknown primary with metastatic cervical lymphadenopathy: shifting gears from detecting the primary to planning therapeutic strategies *Eur J Nucl Med Mol Imaging* **34**, 427–8.

42. Lee, S.T., Scott, A.M. (2007) Hypoxia positron emission tomography imaging with 18f-fluoromisonidazole. *Semin Nucl Med* **37**, 451–61.

43. Brack, S.S., Dinkelborg, L.M., Neri, D. (2004) Molecular targeting of angiogenesis for imaging and therapy *Eur J Nucl Med Mol Imaging* **31**, 1327–41.

44. Tait, J.F. (2008) Imaging of apoptosis *J Nucl Med* **49**, 1573–6.

45. Taylor, C.T. (2008) Interdependent roles for hypoxia inducible factor and nuclear factor-kappaB in hypoxic inflammation *J Physiol* **586**, 4055–9.

46. Hopkins, N., Cadogan, E., Giles, S., McLoughlin, P. (2001) Chronic airway infection leads to angiogenesis in the pulmonary circulation *J Appl Physiol* **91**, 919–28.

47. Dockrell, D.H. (2001) Apoptotic cell death in the pathogenesis of infectious diseases *J Infect* **42**, 227–34.

48. Been, L.B., Suurmeijer, A.J., Cobben, D.C., Jager, P.L., Hoekstra, H.J., Elsinga, P.H. (2004) [18F]FLT-PET in oncology: current status and opportunities. *Eur J Nucl Med Mol Imaging* **31**, 1659–72.

49. Cherry, S.R. (2006) The 2006 Henry N. Wagner Lecture: Of mice and men (and positrons)–advances in PET imaging technology *J Nucl Med* **47**, 1735–45.

50. Surti, S., Kuhn, A., Werner, M.E., Perkins, A.E., Kolthammer, J., Karp, J.S. (2007) Performance of Philips Gemini TF PET/CT scanner with special consideration for its time-of-flight imaging capabilities *J Nucl Med* **48**, 471–80.

51. Kwee, T.C., Takahara, T., Ochiai, R., Nievelstein, R.A., Luijten, P.R. (2008) Diffusion-weighted whole-body imaging with background body signal suppression (DWIBS): features and potential applications in oncology. *Eur Radiol* **18**, 1937–52.

52. Gu, T.F., Xiao, X.L., Sun, F., Yin, J.H., Zhao, H. (2008) Diagnostic value of whole body diffusion weighted imaging for screening primary tumors of patients with metastases *Chin Med Sci J* **23**, 145–50.

53. Mori, T., Nomori, H., Ikeda, K., Kawanaka, K., Shiraishi, S., Katahira, K., et al. (2008) Diffusion-weighted magnetic resonance imaging for diagnosing malignant pulmonary nodules/masses: comparison with positron emission tomography *J Thorac Oncol* **3**, 358–64.

54. Varadhachary, G.R., Talantov, D., Raber, M.N., Meng, C., Hess, K.R., Jatkoe, T., et al. (2008) Molecular profiling of carcinoma of unknown primary and correlation with clinical evaluation *J Clin Oncol* **26**, 4442–8.

55. Horlings, H.M., van Laar, R.K., Kerst, J.M., Helgason, H.H., Wesseling, J., van der Hoeven, J.J., et al. (2008) Gene expression profiling to identify the histogenetic origin of metastatic adenocarcinomas of unknown primary *J Clin Oncol* **26**, 4435–41.

Chapter 18

Methodological Aspects of Multicenter Studies with Quantitative PET

Ronald Boellaard

Abstract

Quantification of whole-body FDG PET studies is affected by many physiological and physical factors. Much of the variability in reported standardized uptake value (SUV) data seen in the literature results from the variability in methodology applied among these studies, i.e., due to the use of different scanners, acquisition and reconstruction settings, region of interest strategies, SUV normalization, and/or corrections methods. To date, the variability in applied methodology prohibits a proper comparison and exchange of quantitative FDG PET data. Consequently, the promising role of quantitative PET has been demonstrated in several monocentric studies, but these published results cannot be used directly as a guideline for clinical (multicenter) trials performed elsewhere. In this chapter, the main causes affecting whole-body FDG PET quantification and strategies to minimize its inter-institute variability are addressed.

Key words: PET, Multicenter, Standardization, Quantification, FDG, SUV, Standardized uptake value

1. Introduction

Although visual inspection of whole-body FDG studies is and remains most important for various clinical applications, such as diagnoses and staging (1–7), the role of quantitative PET is increasingly recognized as an important tool for, e.g., response monitoring and prognoses (8–12). Various methods for quantification of FDG PET studies (13, 14), which differ in complexity regarding data collection and (mathematical) analysis, are described such as the use of tumor-to-background ratios and standardized uptake values (SUVs) on one side, and full kinetic analysis on the other, An overview of various methods for quantification of FDG PET studies can be found in, e.g., Hoekstra et al. (14).

Malik E. Juweid and Otto S. Hoekstra (eds.), *Positron Emission Tomography*, Methods in Molecular Biology, vol. 727,
DOI 10.1007/978-1-61779-062-1_18, © Springer Science+Business Media, LLC 2011

Full kinetic analysis requires dynamic PET scans and an input function, i.e., the variation of activity concentration over time in arterial blood. Occasionally, the latter can be derived directly from the dynamic scan when a large (arterial) blood pool, such as the left ventricle or aorta ascendens, is located within the field of view (FOV) of the PET scanner (15). When an image-derived input function cannot be obtained, invasive arterial sampling is required to collect this input function. Clearly, the main disadvantages of full kinetic analysis are the long (up to 60 min) dynamic scan durations covering only one bed position (generally less than 20 cm in axial direction), the need for an arterial input function, and the use of complicated kinetic analysis. Yet, full kinetic analysis can provide a quantitative measure of glucose consumption, which is corrected for differences in delivery (input function) and blood volume fraction between tumors, subjects, and scans.

The practical limitations required for full kinetic analysis prohibit its use in larger (multicenter) clinical trials and has led to the use of simplified quantitative measures, such as the SUV. SUV is the average uptake of a radiotracer at a fixed interval after tracer administration normalized by injected dose over, e.g., body weight. SUV does not require dynamic scans and can thus be used with a whole-body scanning procedure. The main advantage is that SUV provides quantitative measures from FDG PET studies in a clinically feasible setting.

Quantification based either on full kinetic analysis or on SUV, however, is affected by various acquisition, image reconstruction, and data analysis procedures (16–22). Moreover, especially in the case of SUV, patient preparation procedures and time interval between FDG administration and start of the PET study may have a large effect on SUV outcome. Various papers have investigated the impact of applied methodology on SUV outcome (16, 17, 20, 23, 24). These findings have led to the development of guidelines for both interpretation and quantification of PET studies (1, 18, 21, 25–29). In this chapter, various methodological aspects of quantification of FDG PET studies in multicenter trials are discussed. This chapter focuses on methodological aspects of PET quantification based on SUV, but some issues regarding the validation of SUV against full kinetic analysis are addressed as well.

2. Methodological Aspects of PET Quantification Using SUV

In a multicenter study, various types of PET and PET/CT scanners, which have different characteristics and performances, will be used. Sensitivities and emission scan mode (2D or 3D), image reconstruction algorithms and settings, transmission scans (based on transmission sources or CT), and attenuation and scatter correction methods may differ substantially among scanners and affect accuracy and precision of PET quantification. These differences themselves cannot be easily resolved among centers. Yet, the variability in SUV among centers can be substantially reduced by controlling the main factors affecting SUV (24). The latter can be achieved by strict standardization of patient preparation, prescription of scan acquisition parameters and FDG dosage, image reconstruction settings, and data analysis methods (1, 18, 20, 21, 26–28). Definition of specific multicenter quality control procedures and specifications is finally needed to verify scanner performance and exchangeability of SUV (21, 30).

In short, the various factors affecting SUV outcome can be classified as "biological factors," "technical factors," and "sources of errors" as was suggested by Weber et al. (20). Sources of error are, for example, calibration errors, residual unknown activities in the syringe after administration, incorrect synchronization of clocks, and paravenous administration. Thus these errors should always be avoided, not only in multicenter studies. Biological and technical factors are of more importance in a multicenter setting. Examples of biological factors are blood glucose level and FDG uptake period. Examples of technical factors are data acquisition and image reconstruction settings, applied FDG dosage, and data analysis methods. A detailed overview of factors affecting SUV is given in Weber et al. (20) and Boellaard et al. (21), and is summarized in Table 1.

Although many factors are found to affect SUV, variability of SUV in multicenter studies can be minimized by taking a number of principles into account. Standardization should focus on the following items (18, 21, 26, 28):

- Patient preparation procedures

- FDG administration procedures

- PET study statistics, image quality, and signal-to-noise ratio (SNR)

- Clinical image resolution

- Data analysis procedures and SUV normalization

- Specific multicenter quality control measures

These specific topics are briefly reviewed below. The readers of this paper are, however, encouraged to read several other papers for a more detailed overview of these topics (1, 16, 17, 19, 24, 31).

2.1. Patient Preparation Procedures

Patient preparation procedures describe all measures and procedures to be taken into account prior to FDG administration and PET study. Guidelines developed so far generally include a fasting period of at least 4 h, ample hydration prior to the study, and minimal exercise up to 24 h before FDG administration and during

Table 1
Overview of factors affecting SUV outcome

Biological factors

Blood plasma level	Lower uptake or SUV with increasing blood glucose level
Uptake period	Higher SUV at increasing time interval between injection and start of PET study
Patient motion/breathing	Image artifacts in case of mismatch in position between CT-AC and emission scan, and (possibly) lower SUV due to respiratory motion (resolution loss)
Patient comfort	Patient stress and poor waiting conditions increase uptake of FDG in muscle and/or brown fat and affects SUV quantification
Inflammation	Inflammatory processes near or at the tumor results in a false-positive increase in SUV

Technical errors

Cross-calibration between PET and dose calibrator	Systematic error in SUV equal to error in cross-calibration between PET and dose calibrator
Residual activities in administration system	Lower net administered dose resulting in incorrect lower uptake and SUV
Incorrect synchronization of clocks of PET camera and DC	Incorrect decay correction resulting in incorrect SUV
Use of injection time rather than dose calibration time	Incorrect time interval is used for decay correction of administered dose
Paravenous administration of FDG	Paravenous injection results in slow delivery of FDG to the tumor and, therefore, in incorrect SUV

Physical factors

Scan acquisition parameters	Affect signal-to-noise ratio (SNR) of PET scan
Image reconstruction settings	Insufficient convergence and lower resolution give lower SUV and increases partial volume effects. Insufficient convergence makes SUV more dependent on surrounding activity distributions
Region of interest (ROI) used to derive SUV	SUV outcome strongly depends on size and type of ROI used
Normalization factor in SUV	SUV outcomes are numerically different when using body weight, body surface area, or lean body mass as normalization factor in the SUV equation
Correction for serum glucose level in SUV calculation	Higher serum glucose levels will result in underestimation of SUV. Use of a serum glucose level correction in the SUV equation will thus result in different SUV outcomes
Use of contrast agents during CT-AC	May result in overestimation of attenuation and thus results in higher SUV (upward bias)

the uptake period. Patient height, weight, and plasma glucose concentration should be measured. A complete list of required and preferred patient preparation guidelines are given in (18, 21).

Patient preparation guidelines aim at optimizing uptake in tumors and minimizing uptake in healthy tissues such as muscle and brown fat, thereby optimizing PET study image quality for both diagnosis and quantification. Specifically for quantitative PET studies, the net administered dose, patient weight, height, and plasma glucose concentrations must be exactly known as these parameters are directly used in the SUV equation (Eqs. 1 and 2). As FDG uptake varies over time, the time interval applied between FDG administration and start of the PET study must be matched as good as possible between scans performed at various sites. Generally, an interval of 60 min with a tolerance of ±5 min is considered acceptable. When PET studies are made for response monitoring purposes, an appropriate interval between the end of therapy cycle and PET study needs to be considered as FDG uptake may vary strongly shortly after chemotherapy. In case of chemotherapy studies, a minimal interval of 14 days is generally applied (26). In case of assessing radiotherapy treatment response, intervals between treatment cycle and PET study of even 3 months may be required. The optimal interval may thus be study specific and requires further investigations (12).

2.2. FDG Administration

An accurate and reproducible FDG administration is needed to avoid paravenous injection and to minimize residual activity in the syringe or administration system. Exact knowledge of net administered dose is of utmost importance. Any inaccuracy in (real) net administered dose will result in incorrect SUV data. With this respect, care has also to be taken regarding accurate synchronization of clocks throughout the department in order to assure correct decay corrections between FDG dose calibration time and start time of the PET study.

2.3. PET Study Statistics, Image Quality, and Signal-to-Noise Ratio

The quality of a PET study depends on many technical factors. Obviously, the methodology applied for transmission and emission scanning, and (online) corrections, such as randoms and scatter corrections, affects image quality and quantification. Differences in scan statistics due to differences in scanner sensitivities, relative bed overlap in subsequent bed positions, and patient weight add to the variability in SUV as well. Poor scan statistics results in an upward bias of SUV (16).

Transmission scans are made for attenuation correction (AC) purposes and are generally performed either using transmission scan sources in case of PET systems or using a dedicated low-dose CT-AC on PET/CT systems. Obviously, when transmission scan sources are used, they need to be of sufficient strength, and transmission scan durations should be sufficient to provide an accurate and precise AC. In case of CT-AC, incorrect AC may result from patient motion (breathing), use of contrast agents during CT-AC, presence of metal implants, and truncation of the CT-AC images by the small CT FOV. Specific guidelines for PET/CT imaging are described by, e.g., Delbeke et al. (25) and in various other publications.

Emission scans can be performed in either 2D or 3D. Two-dimensional scans are performed using septa, i.e., annular shields, in the FOV, allowing the detection of lines of responses (LORs) in straight (image) planes only and thereby minimizing the contribution of scattered and random coincidences. In case of 3D scans, oblique LORs are also accepted, providing a higher sensitivity. Nowadays, almost all PET/CT scanners allow for 3D mode acquisitions only. However, 3D mode emission scans generally also suffer from higher contributions of random and scattered coincidences than 2D mode acquisitions. These "invalid" events need to be corrected, thereby potentially reducing image quality.

In a multicenter study, both PET and PET/CT scanners are likely to be used. When SUV data need to be exchanged, it is essential that all these scanners have similar performance. This can be achieved by optimizing acquisition and reconstruction settings per type of scanner and checking these settings and scanner performances using specific multicenter quality control (QC) measures (24, 32). These QC measures will be discussed in more detail later. Moreover, SUV shows an increasing upward bias with decreasing scan statistics. To minimize differences in scan statistics among centers and subjects, FDG dosage can be given as a function of patient weight, relative bed overlap of subsequent bed positions, and emission scan acquisition mode.

2.4. Clinical Image Resolution

The spatial resolution of a PET scanner is generally characterized according NEMA NU 2 2001 specifications. According to these standards, spatial resolution is measured using a point source in air, and data are reconstructed using filtered back projection while applying a voxel size of 1 mm or less. These conditions do not reflect clinical conditions, and NEMA standards thus provide a measure of (system) resolution of the PET scanner rather than the (true) spatial resolution applied in clinical practice. It should be noted, however, that the NEMA standards are important to specify the basic performance characteristics of the PET scanner and thus provide valuable information for comparison of different scanners.

The resolution seen in clinical practice is determined to a large extend by the reconstruction settings applied. Nowadays, iterative reconstruction algorithms are being almost exclusively used for reconstruction of whole-body FDG PET studies. Various parameters of these algorithms, such as number of iterations and subsets, relaxation factors, voxel size, and post-reconstruction image filter settings, determine the "clinical" spatial resolution seen in practice (22, 33). Recently, it has been observed that most PET/CT scanners provide an image resolution of approximately 7 mm FWHM when using default manufacturer-recommended settings (21). Moreover, a sufficient number of iterations (or its product with the number of subsets) are needed to ensure sufficient convergence of image reconstruction (Fig. 1a and 2).

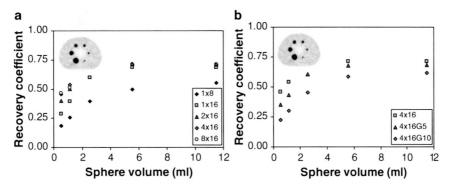

Fig. 1. Recovery coefficients as function of sphere size, measured using the NEMA NU 2 2001 image quality phantom, for a number of iterations used during image reconstruction (**a**) and for various post-reconstruction filter settings (**b**). Recovery coefficients were determined using a background corrected 50% of maximum isocount contour volume of interest. Ordered subset expectation maximization (OSEM) reconstruction settings are indicated by the product of the number of iterations and subsets. G5 represents a 5-mm FWHM Gaussian post-smoothing and G10, a 10-mm FWHM Gaussian post-smoothing.

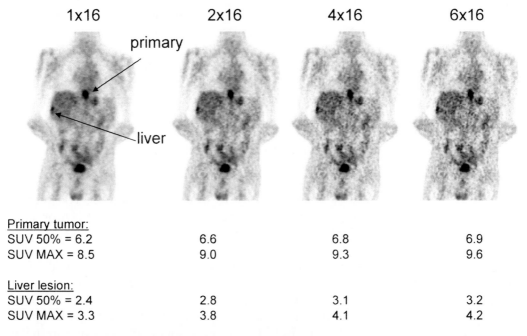

	1x16	2x16	4x16	6x16
Primary tumor:				
SUV 50% =	6.2	6.6	6.8	6.9
SUV MAX =	8.5	9.0	9.3	9.6
Liver lesion:				
SUV 50% =	2.4	2.8	3.1	3.2
SUV MAX =	3.3	3.8	4.1	4.2

Fig. 2. Clinical example on the impact of the number of iterations applied during image reconstruction on SUV outcome. Ordered subset expectation maximization (OSEM) reconstruction settings are indicated by the product of the number of iterations and subsets. Data are given for the primary tumor and a liver lesion using maximum SUV and SUV derived using a 50% (of tumor maximum) isocount contour volume of interest.

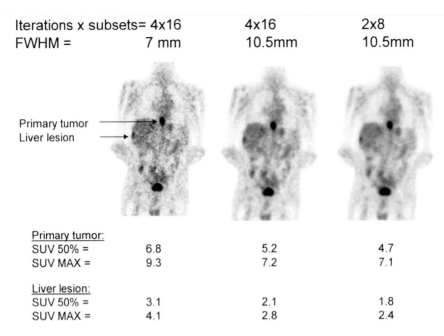

Iterations x subsets=	4x16	4x16	2x8
FWHM =	7 mm	10.5mm	10.5mm

Primary tumor:			
SUV 50% =	6.8	5.2	4.7
SUV MAX =	9.3	7.2	7.1

Liver lesion:			
SUV 50% =	3.1	2.1	1.8
SUV MAX =	4.1	2.8	2.4

Fig. 3. Clinical example of the impact of post-reconstruction filtering in combination with a number of OSEM iterations applied during image reconstruction on SUV outcome. Data are given for the primary tumor and a liver lesion using maximum SUV and SUV derived using a 50% (of tumor maximum) isocount contour volume of interest.

Insufficient convergence results in a lower resolution and an activity distribution-dependent SUV in small objects.

Difference in "clinical" resolution is probably one of the main factors contributing to variability in SUV among centers (24) (Fig. 1b and 3). Therefore, in multicenter studies, it is crucial that resolution should be matched as much as possible across centers and scanners. The latter is of utmost importance as methods to overcome the quantitative inaccuracy due to (differences in) low resolution, so-called partial volume corrections, are not yet routinely available and are not yet sufficiently accurate and precise for structures less than 3 times the "clinical" scanner resolution (for diameters of less than 20 mm). Resolution and convergence matching can be achieved by strict prescription of reconstruction settings per type of scanner and should be verified using dedicated QC phantom experiments.

2.5. Data Analysis Procedures and SUV Normalization

SUV calculations start with determining the FDG uptake from the PET study by defining a region of interest (ROI) over the tumor. Various ROI strategies have been described in the literature, such as manually defined 2D and 3D ROI, semiautomatically defined ROI based on absolute or relative thresholds, fixed-size ROI, and use of the maximum voxel within an ROI. Several other ROI methods are still under investigation. These various ROI strategies have their specific disadvantages and benefits regarding ease of use, accuracy, and precisions. Use of the maximum voxel value might be attractive as it is less dependent on the performance of manual or semiautomatic ROI procedures. However, an upward bias was reported with decreasing scan statistics (16, 31, 34) and, recently, the maximum pixel value was shown to depend on the specific software platform being used as well (35). The latter may be overcome by performing centralized data analysis for multicenter studies or by sharing dedicated multicenter ROI software programs (36). To avoid upward bias of the maximum pixel, use of small fixed-size ROI can be an alternative provided that the size of the ROI is sufficiently smaller than that of the tumors under investigation (16, 17). Clearly, the average uptake (SUV) derived from the PET study depends strongly on the ROI method being used, and the same ROI strategy should be applied across all scans and institutes in a multicenter trial.

Once the FDG uptake is derived from the PET study, the SUV can be calculated in several ways. Normalization of SUV by body weight (SUV-BW) is given in Eq. 1. Various other normalization than body weight are being used, such as lean body mass (LBM) and body surface area (BSA) (19). In case of large variations in body weight during a longitudinal study, SUV normalization with body surface area might be more accurate than with body weight, as compared to the gold standard of full kinetic analysis. Moreover, use of BSA provided a better SUV test-retest variability than SUV-BW or SUV-LBM. The most appropriate normalization factor is, however, still a matter of debate. Therefore, besides patient weight, it is recommended to measure patient height as well to allow for the application of all of the various SUV normalizations.

Finally, SUV can be corrected for plasma glucose level. Higher blood glucose levels result in lower FDG uptake in the tumor and thus lower SUV. In a monocenter setting, it was observed that the use of glucose correction provided a better correlation with full kinetic analysis outcome (14) and showed a better SUV test-retest variability, but these findings are not always replicated by other studies. Moreover, the improved test-retest variability when using plasma glucose correction was not observed in case of a multicenter study (unpublished data). Although it can be expected theoretically that the use of plasma glucose correction should improve SUV accuracy, the accuracy and precision of the plasma glucose level measurement itself should be considered as well. These measurements should therefore be performed in a clinical laboratory using validated and calibrated devices and standard procedures. Bed-side measurements do not seem to provide the required accuracy and precision for the use of SUV normalization. Even when plasma glucose levels are measured in a standardized way using validated methodology, the correction should improve accuracy without (significantly) decreasing precision.

$$SUV = \frac{ACvoi(kBq/ml)}{FDGdose(MBq)/BW(kg)} \qquad (1)$$

$$SUVglu = \frac{ACvoi(kBq/ml)}{FDGdose(MBq)/BW(kg)} \times \frac{Pglu(mmol/l)}{5.0} \qquad (2)$$

In Eqs. 1 and 2, ACvoi represents the average activity concentration within a volume of interest over the tumor, and FDG dose is the net administered dose corrected for decay between dose calibration time (not injection time) and start time of the PET study. BW represents measured body weight. In Eq. 2, the plasma glucose level (Pglu) is normalized by a population average value of 5.0 (off-rounded value).

2.6. Specific Multicenter Quality Control Measures

The quality control measures specific for multicenter PET studies should focus on three items: (a) correct functioning of PET or PET/CT camera according to specifications; (b) an accurate (within 5%) relative calibration of the PET or PET/CT scanner against the dose calibrator used for measuring patient FDG dosages; and (c) verification of activity concentration recovery coefficients as a function of sphere size to assure resolution matching among centers in a multicenter study.

Correct functioning of the PET or PET/CT scanner is generally verified on a daily basis using scanner-specific daily QC measures implemented by the manufacturer. These tests should report any hardware failures or drifts resulting in unacceptable image quality loss. Generally, methods and specifications are scanner specific and provided by the manufacturer. In case of PET/CT scanners, all daily tests should be performed for both the PET and CT components of the scanner. Clearly all tests should be passed correctly before (any) clinical use.

The relative calibration or cross-calibration of the PET or PET/CT scanner against the dose calibrator, used for measuring patient FDG dosage, provides information about potential discrepancies in calibration of PET(/CT) and that of the dose calibrator. The latter is required because separate calibration of dose calibrators, well counters, and PET/CT systems may still result in (small) discrepancies in the calibration between those devices under specific clinical conditions (30, 32). (Verification of) Cross-calibration is equally important as the calibrations of the individual devices themselves. This can be easily understood from Eq. 1. In the SUV calculation, the FDG uptake measured with PET is used in the nominator in the equation, while the injected dose measured using a dose calibrator is used in the denominator. Consequently, any discrepancy in absolute calibration results in incorrect SUV. For correct SUV data, an accurate relative (cross-) calibration is, therefore, even more important than the accuracy of the (separate) calibration of the individual devices (dose calibrator and PET scanner) themselves.

As explained earlier, differences in spatial image resolution or partial volume effects among various scanners, reconstruction methods, and settings seen within a multicenter study probably contribute the largest to inter-institute SUV variability (24). Prescriptions for acquisition and reconstruction parameters may be defined for each type of scanner to fulfill resolution and convergence criteria. However, these prescriptions will quickly become obsolete with the ongoing development of new PET/CT scanners and (reconstruction) software. Moreover, resolution is generally measured using point sources, which may provide an optimistic estimation of "clinical" resolution in case of iterative reconstruction methods. It is therefore suggested to use activity concentration recovery coefficients as a measure of resolution and convergence. The activity concentration recovery coefficient is the ratio between FDG uptake in a sphere measured by the PET or PET/CT scanner and the real FDG uptake. Recovery coefficients can be measured using, e.g., the NEMA NU 2 2001 image quality phantom containing variously sized spheres. By filling these spheres and the other compartments with known FDG solutions, the recovery coefficients can be determined as a function of sphere size (and the ROI method being used). The absolute values of these recovery coefficients and their relative change with sphere size provide a good measure of the overall partial volume effects seen under conditions that are clinically more relevant; i.e., high activity spheres in a "warm" background seem to be more representative of tumors than point sources in air. When different scanners provide similar (absolute) recovery coefficients measured in a standardized way, resolution (and partial volume effects) is sufficiently matched to allow interchangeability of SUV measures between those scanners. Acquisition and reconstruction settings should therefore be chosen per scanner such that each of these scanners meets predefined recovery coefficient specifications.

3. Discussion

3.1. Do We Need FDG PET Standardization in All Quantitative Studies?

The need for standardization of FDG PET studies may differ upon the intended clinical application. A distinction might be made regarding use of absolute SUV data for e.g. prognosis or use of relative changes in SUV in case of response monitoring. Obviously, when absolute measures of SUV are needed strict standardization amongst all scans and all centers is required to allow for exchange of SUV. Frequently it is argued that in response monitoring settings it is sufficient to apply consistency of applied methodology, i.e. acquisition, image reconstruction and data analysis methods, for all subsequent scans performed in a single subject. Various studies have, indeed, shown that the measured relative response is almost independent of applied methodology provided that the same methods and hardware are used consistently per subject (17). However, to some extend standardization of methodology in (multicenter) longitudinal studies can still be beneficial. When tumor sizes are relatively small (<5 cc) or large relative differences in tumor sizes (>50%) between subsequent scans are expected, differences in applied image resolution and ROI methods between different centers will also result in a different relative change of SUV amongst those centers. The stringency of standardization may thus also depend on the specific longitudinal study (tumor type) being conducted. However, in a study by Hoekstra et al. (37) it was shown that residual SUV, i.e. absolute SUV after or during treatment, can be used for response monitoring as well. In the latter situation absolute quantification of residual SUV is used and requires standardization in case of a multicenter trial.

3.2. Do We Need to Validate SUV and Changes in SUV Against Full Kinetic Analysis Outcome?

Various quantitative measures can be derived from FDG PET studies (13, 14, 38–40). All these quantitative measures are different regarding their complexity and underlying assumptions. Consequently, methods have different accuracies and precisions. The metabolic rate of glucose, expressed in mmol/min per ml tissue, can be derived from dynamic PET studies using compartmental kinetic analysis and represent the most accurate measure of glucose consumption, but this analysis is sensitive to noise. The Patlak method is based on linearization of the compartment model and can be applied on a voxel level allowing it to generate metabolic rate images. The Patlak method is less sensitive to noise but does not include a correction for the blood volume fraction within an ROI. Examples of more simplified methods, which can be used in combination with (static) whole-body imaging, are the simplified kinetic method by Hunter et al. (39) and SUV. The simplified kinetic method requires withdrawal of a blood sample to determine the activity concentration in (arterial) blood during the PET study. SUV is probably the most simple and clinically feasible method for quantification of FDG PET studies. However, SUV does not correct for blood volume fraction within an ROI and (changes in) shape of the input function. Consequently, the relationship between SUV, either with or without glucose correction, and metabolic rate of glucose may not be the same in all kinds of studies or between subsequent scans in a longitudinal study (38). The consequence of such a change in relationship would be that a relative change in SUV because of treatment response could either under- or overestimate actual change in metabolic rate. Therefore, in order to interpret SUV data correctly, the relation between SUV and metabolic rate should be assessed prior, during, and after treatment. The latter validation is preferably done at a single center with experience in conducting dynamic studies and full kinetic analysis prior to a larger multicenter trial (including whole-body studies only).

4. Conclusion

To date many factors affecting SUV outcome have been identified and characterized. These findings have resulted in the development of guidelines for performing PET or PET/CT studies. Most of these guidelines provide requirements to assure a minimal quality of PET or PET/CT studies. In a multicenter study, where exchange of SUV is needed, specific attention is given to minimize variability in SUV due to the use of different scanners, reconstruction and data analysis methods, and differences in their settings. Although differences in scanner hardware and reconstruction software cannot be resolved across centers, inter-institute SUV variability can be substantially reduced by standardization of FDG PET studies (21). This standardization is based on a number of principles, such as cross-scanner and institute resolution matching, which can reduce inter-institute variability in SUV measures to within 10% (21). In order to achieve this precise interchangeability, it is of utmost importance to control/standardize all factors affecting SUV outcome even when affects of individual factors seem small. Finally, a validation of the constancy of the relationship between SUV and metabolic rate should be performed prior to a multicenter study. The latter is required in order to interpret changes in SUV correctly within a larger treatment response monitoring study.

Acknowledgments

The author would like to thank Paul Kinahan, Osama Malawi, and Janet Saffer for their fruitful discussions. Adriaan Lammertsma and Otto Hoekstra are thanked for reviewing this paper and for the many helpful discussions on PET quantification. The members of the HOVON imaging workgroup are thanked for their contribution in setting up a Dutch FDG PET standardization protocol.

References

1. Fletcher, J.W., Djulbegovic, B., Soares, H.P., Siegel, B.A., Lowe, V.J., Lyman, G.H. et al. (2008) Recommendations on the use of F-18-FDG PET in oncology. *J Nucl Med* **49(3)**, 480–508.

2. Hoekstra, C.J., Stroobants, S.G., Hoekstra, O.S., Vansteenkiste, J., Biesma, B., Schramel, F.J., et al. (2003) The value of [18F]fluoro-2-deoxy-D-glucose positron emission tomography in the selection of patients with stage IIIA-N2 non-small cell lung cancer for combined modality treatment. *Lung Cancer* **39(2)**, 151–7.

3. Mijnhout, G.S., Borgstein, P.J., Hoekstra, O.S., van Diest, P.J., Pijpers, R., Meijer, S., et al. (1999) Potential value of FDG-PET for initial regional staging in melanoma. *J Invest Dermatol* **113(3)**, 514.

4. van Tinteren, H., Hoekstra, O.S., Smit, E.F., van den Bergh, J.H., Schreurs, A.J., Stallaert, R.A., et al. (2002) Effectiveness of positron emission tomography in the preoperative assessment of patients with suspected non-small-cell lung cancer: the PLUS multicentre randomised trial *Lancet* **359(9315)**, 1388–92.

5. Vansteenkiste, J.F., Stroobants, S.G. (2001) The role of positron emission tomography with 18F-fluoro-2-deoxy-D-glucose in respiratory oncology. *Eur Respir J* **17(4)**, 802–20.

6. Weber, W.A. (2006) Positron emission tomography as an imaging biomarker *J Clin Oncol* **24(20)**, 3282–92.

7. Zijlstra-Baalbergen, J.M., Hoekstra, O.S., Raaymakers, P.R., Comans, E.F., Huijgens, P.C., Hoeven, J.J., et al. (2000) FDG PET vs Ga-67 scintigraphy as a prognostic tool early during chemotherapy for non-Hodgkin's lymphoma (NHL). *J Nucl Med* **41(5)**, 278P

8. Avril, N.E., Weber, W.A. (2005) Monitoring response to treatment in patients utilizing PET *Radiol Clin North Am* **43(1)**, 189–204.

9. Borst, G., Belderbos, J., Boellaard, R., Comans, E., de Jaeger, K., Lammertsma, A., et al. (2005) Prognostic significance of the 18FDG-PET standardized uptake value for inoperable non-small cell lung cancer patients after high-dose radiotherapy. *Lung Cancer* **49**, S50.

10. Hoekstra, C.J., Paglianiti, I., Hoekstra, O.S., Smit, E.F., Postmus, P.E., Teule, G.J., et al. (2000) Monitoring response to therapy in cancer using [F-18]-2-fluouo-2-deoxy-D-glucose and positron emission tomography: an overview of different analytical methods. *Eur J Nucl Med* **27(6)**, 731–43.

11. Larson, S.M., Schwartz, L.H. (2006) 18F-FDG PET as a candidate for "qualified biomarker": functional assessment of treatment response in oncology. *J Nucl Med* **47(6)**, 901–3.

12. Weber, W.A.(2005) PET for response assessment in oncology: radiotherapy and chemotherapy *Br J Radiol* **78**, 42–9.

13. Graham, M.M., Peterson, L.M., Hayward, R.M. (2000) Comparison of simplified quantitative analyses of FDG uptake *Nucl Med Biol* **27(7)**, 647–55.

14. Hoekstra, C.J., Hoekstra, O.S., Stroobants, S.G., Vansteenkiste, J., Nuyts, J., Smit, E.F., et al. (2002) Methods to monitor response to chemotherapy in non-small cell lung cancer with F-18-FDG PET. *J Nucl Med* **43(10)**, 1304–9.

15. Hoekstra, C.J., Hoekstra, O.S., Lammertsma, A.A. (1999) On the use of image-derived input functions in oncological fluorine-18 fluorodeoxyglucose positron emission tomography studies. *Eur J Nucl Med* **26(11)**, 1489–92.

16. Boellaard, R., Krak, N.C., Hoekstra, O.S., Lammertsma, A.A. (2004) Effects of noise, image resolution, and ROI definition on the accuracy of standard uptake values: A simulation study. *J Nucl Med* **45(9)**, 1519–27.

17. Krak, N.C., Boellaard, R., Hoekstra, O.S., Twisk, J.W.R., Hoekstra, C.J., Lammertsma, A.A. (2005) Effects of ROI definition and reconstruction method on quantitative outcome and applicability in a response monitoring trial *Eur J Nucl Med Mol Imaging* **32(3)**, 294–301.

18. Shankar, L.K., Hoffman, J.M., Bacharach, S., Graham, M.M., Karp, J., Lammertsma, A.A., et al. (2006) Consensus recommendations for the use of F-18-FDG PET as an indicator of therapeutic response in patients in national cancer institute trials. *J Nucl Med* **47(6)**, 1059–66.

19. Stahl, A., Ott, K., Schwaiger, M., Weber, W.A. (2004) Comparison of different SUV-based methods for monitoring cytotoxic therapy with FDG PET *Eur J Nucl Med Mol Imaging* **31(11)**, 1471–9.

20. Weber, W.A. (2005) Use of PET for monitoring cancer therapy and for predicting outcome *J Nucl Med* **46(6)**, 983–95.

21. Boellaard, R., Oyen, W.J., Hoekstra, C.J., Hoekstra, O.S., Visser, E.P., Willemsen, A.T., et al. (2008) The Netherlands protocol for standardisation and quantification of FDG whole body PET studies in multi-centre trials

Eur J Nucl Med Mol Imaging **35(12)**, 2320–33,

22. Visvikis, D., Cheze-LeRest, C., Costa, D.C., Bomanji, J., Gacinovic, S., Ell, P.J. (2001) Influence of OSEM and segmented attenuation correction in the calculation of standardised uptake values for [18F]FDG PET. *Eur J Nucl Med* **28(9)**, 1326–35.

23. Aerts, H.J., Bosmans, G., van Baardwijk, A.A., Dekker, A.L., Oellers, M.C., Lambin, P., et al. (2008) Stability of (18)F-Deoxyglucose uptake locations within tumor during radiotherapy for NSCLC: a prospective study. *Int J Radiat Oncol Biol Phys* **71(5)**, 1402–7.

24. Westerterp, M., Pruim, J., Oyen, W., Hoekstra, O., Paans, A., Visser, E., et al. (2007) Quantification of FDG PET studies using standardised uptake values in multi-centre trials: effects of image reconstruction, resolution and ROI definition parameters. *Eur J Nucl Med Mol Imaging* **34(3)**, 392–404.

25. Delbeke, D. (2006) Procedure guideline for tumor imaging with F-18-FDG PET/CT 1.0 J Nucl Med **47(5)**, 885–95. Erratum in *J Nucl Med* **47(6)**, 903.

26. Juweid, M.E., Stroobants, S., Hoekstra, O.S., Mottaghy, F.M., Dietlein, M., Guermazi, A., et al. (2007) Use of positron emission tomography for response assessment of lymphoma: Consensus of the Imaging Subcommittee of International Harmonization Project in lymphoma *J Clin Oncol* **25(5)**, 571–8.

27. Shankar, L.K. (2006) PET standardization, NIH findings: The importance of standardization of imaging in clinical trials *J Nucl Med* **47(12)**, 57N–58N.

28. Young, H., Baum, R., Cremerius, U., Herholz, K., Hoekstra, O., Lammertsma, A.A., et al. (1999) Measurement of clinical and subclinical tumour response using [18F]-fluorodeoxyglucose and positron emission tomography: review and 1999 EORTC recommendations. European Organization for Research and Treatment of Cancer (EORTC) PET Study Group *Eur J Cancer* **35(13)**, 1773–82.

29. Schelbert, H.R., Hoh, C.K., Royal, H.D., Brown, M., Dahlbom, M.N., Dehdashti, F., et al. (1998) Procedure guideline for tumor imaging using fluorine-18-FDG. Society of Nuclear Medicine *J Nucl Med* **39(7)**, 1302–5.

30. Geworski, L., Knoop, B.O., de Wit, M., Ivancevic, V., Bares, R., Munz, D.L. (2002) Multicenter comparison of calibration and cross calibration of PET scanners *J Nucl Med* **43(5)**, 635–9.

31. Thie, J.A. (2004) Understanding the standardized uptake value, its methods, and implications for usage. *J Nucl Med* **45(9)**, 1431–4.

32. Takahashi, Y., Oriuchi, N., Otake, H., Endo, K., Murase, K. (2008) Variability of lesion detectability and standardized uptake value according to the acquisition procedure and reconstruction among five PET scanners *Ann Nucl Med* **22(6)**, 543–8.

33. Jaskowiak, C.J., Bianco, J.A., Perlman, S.B., Fine, J.P. (2005) Influence of reconstruction iterations on F-18-FDG PET/CT standardized uptake values. *J Nucl Med* **46(3)**, 424–8.

34. Lodge, M., Leal, J., Wahl, R. (2008) Quantifying metabolic tumor response to therapy: The influence of image noise on maximum and mean SUV *J Nucl Med* **49**, 108P.

35. Leal, J., Lodge, M., Wahl, R. (2008) Reproducibility of SUV max for oncologic PET: Significant differences in quantification of the SAME study between PET-only and PET-CT analysis modes *J Nucl Med* **49**, 107P.

36. Boellaard, R., Hoekstra, O.S., Lammertsma, A.A. (2008) Software tools for standardized analysis of FDG whole body studies in multicenter trials *J Nucl Med* **49**, 159P.

37. Hoekstra, C.J., Stroobants, S.G., Smit, E.F., Vansteenkiste, J., van Tinteren, H., Postmus, P.E., et al. (2005) Prognostic relevance of response evaluation using [F-18]-2-fluoro-2-deoxy-D-glucose positron emission tomography in patients with locally advanced non-small-cell lung cancer *J Clin Oncol* **23(33)**, 8362–70.

38. Lammertsma, A.A., Hoekstra, C.J., Giaccone, G., Hoekstra, O.S. (2006) How should we analyse FDG PET studies for monitoring tumour response *Eur J Nucl Med Mol Imaging* **33**, S16–S21.

39. Hunter, G.J., Hamberg, L.M., Alpert, N.M., Choi, N.C., Fischman, A.J. (1996) Simplified measurement of deoxyglucose utilization rate *J Nucl Med* **37(6)**, 950–5.

40. Sadato, N., Tsuchida, T., Nakaumra, S., Waki, A., Uematsu, H., Takahashi, N., et al. (1998) Non-invasive estimation of the net influx constant using the standardized uptake value for quantification of FDG uptake of tumours *Eur J Nucl Med* **25(6)**, 559–64.

INDEX

Malik E. Juweid and Otto S. Hoekstra (eds.), *Positron Emission Tomography*, Methods in Molecular Biology, vol. 727,
DOI 10.1007/978-1-61779-062-1, © Springer Science+Business Media, LLC 2011